Optimizing Outcomes for Liver and Pancreas Surgery

Flavio G. Rocha • Perry Shen
Editors

Optimizing Outcomes for Liver and Pancreas Surgery

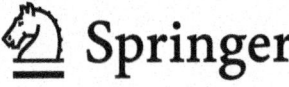 Springer

Editors
Flavio G. Rocha
Virginia Mason Medical Center
Seattle, WA, USA

Perry Shen
Wake Forest Baptist Health
Winston-Salem, NC, USA

ISBN 978-3-319-87357-2 ISBN 978-3-319-62624-6 (eBook)
DOI 10.1007/978-3-319-62624-6

Printed on acid-free paper

This Springer imprint is published by Springer Nature
The registered company is Springer International Publishing AG
The registered company address is: Gewerbestrasse 11, 6330 Cham, Switzerland

Preface

Hepatopancreatobiliary (HPB) surgery has developed as a discrete specialty within general surgery, surgical oncology, and transplantation. This is mainly due to the complexity of the diagnosis, work-up, and treatment of benign and malignant HPB disease. HPB surgeons now must master both the multidisciplinary management and the technical aspects of liver and pancreas surgery. While there are several excellent surgical textbooks and atlases in the market, a book describing a practical approach to the preoperative, intraoperative, and postoperative care of HPB patients was needed. Given the recent implementation of enhanced recovery pathways and value-added healthcare, we felt a real-world perspective on the critical aspects of HPB surgery would be of benefit to the practicing surgeon. Therefore, we assembled a panel of expert surgeons in their respective realms of liver and pancreas surgery to outline their approach to commonly encountered situations within their field. It is our sincere hope that this book will serve as a guide to residents, fellows, and even experienced HPB surgeons to improve their patient outcomes.

Seattle, WA, USA   Flavio G. Rocha
Winston-Salem, NC, USA   Perry Shen

Contents

Contributors

Peter J. Allen, MD Department of Surgery, Memorial Sloan Kettering Cancer Center, New York, NY, USA

Thomas A. Aloia, MD Department of Surgical Oncology, The University of Texas MD Anderson Cancer Center, Houston, TX, USA

Fabio Bagante, MD Department of Surgery, The Ohio State University Comprehensive Cancer Center, Columbus, OH, USA

Department of Surgery, University of Verona, Verona, Italy

William C. Chapman, MD, FACS Division of Transplant Surgery, Department of Surgery, Washington University in St. Louis, St. Louis, MO, USA

Clancy J. Clark, MD Wake Forest Baptist Health, Winston-Salem, NC, USA

Jordan M. Cloyd, MD Department of Surgery, The Ohio State University Medical Center, Columbus, OH, USA

Camilo Correa-Gallego, MD Memorial Sloan Kettering Cancer Center, New York, NY, USA

Ryan W. Day, MD Department of Surgery, Mayo Clinic Hospital in Arizona, Phoenix, AZ, USA

Mary Fischer, MD Department of Anesthesiology and Critical Care, Memorial Sloan Kettering Cancer Center, New York, NY, USA

Kathryn Fowler, MD Mallinckrodt Institute of Radiology, Washington University in St. Louis, St. Louis, MO, USA

Jan Grendar, MD Liver and Pancreas Surgery, Portland Providence Cancer Institute, Portland, OR, USA

Paul D. Hansen, MD The Oregon Clinic, Providence Portland Cancer Center, Portland, OR, USA

Justin T. Huntington, MD, MS Department of Surgery, The Ohio State University Wexner Medical Center, Columbus, OH, USA

William R. Jarnagin, MD Memorial Sloan Kettering Cancer Center, New York, NY, USA

Daniel J. Kagedan Division of General Surgery, Department of Surgery, University of Toronto, Toronto, ON, Canada

Institute of Health Policy, Management, and Evaluation, University of Toronto, Toronto, ON, Canada

Matthew H.G. Katz, MD Department of Surgical Oncology, The University of Texas MD Anderson Cancer Center, Houston, TX, USA

Adeel S. Khan, MD, FACS Division of Transplant Surgery, Department of Surgery, Washington University in St. Louis, St Louis, MO, USA

Robert C.G. Martin II, MD PhD FACS Department of Surgery, Division of Surgical Oncology, University of Louisville, Louisville, KY, USA

Division of Surgical Oncology, Upper Gastrointestinal and Hepato-Pancreatico-Biliary Clinic, University of Louisville, Louisville, KY, USA

Grant McKenzie, BS Department of Surgery, Division of Surgical Oncology, University of Louisville, Louisville, KY, USA

Timothy M. Pawlik, MD, MPH, PhD Department of Surgery, The Ohio State University Comprehensive Cancer Center, Columbus, OH, USA

Priya M. Puri, BA Department of Surgery, University of Pennsylvania Perelman School of Medicine, Philadelphia, PA, USA

Carl R. Schmidt, MD, MS Department of Surgery, The Ohio State University Wexner Medical Center, Columbus, OH, USA

Gaya Spolverato, MD Department of Surgery, The Ohio State University Comprehensive Cancer Center, Columbus, OH, USA

Department of Surgery, University of Verona, Verona, Italy

Iswanto Sucandy, MD Digestive Health Institute, Florida Hospital Tampa, Tampa, FL, USA

Allan Tsung, MD Division of Hepatobiliary and Pancreatic Surgery, University of Pittsburgh Medical Center, Pittsburgh, PA, USA

Charles M. Vollmer Jr., MD Department of Surgery, University of Pennsylvania Perelman School of Medicine, Philadelphia, PA, USA

Alice C. Wei Department of Surgery, Princess Margaret Cancer Centre, University Health Network, Toronto, ON, Canada

Department of Surgery, Toronto General Hospital, University Health Network, Toronto, ON, Canada

Division of General Surgery, Department of Surgery, University of Toronto, Toronto, ON, Canada

Institute of Health Policy, Management, and Evaluation, University of Toronto, Toronto, ON, Canada

Fitness Assessment and Optimization for Hepatopancreatobiliary Surgery

Grant McKenzie and Robert C.G. Martin II

Background

In the United States, as the large baby boomer population cohort continues to age, the number of patients presenting with hepatopancreatobiliary (HPB) malignancies has and will continue to rise into the foreseeable future. The US Census Bureau projects that the number of adults aged 65 and older is expected to increase from 46 million in 2014, to 74 million by 2030 [1]. The median age for cancer diagnosis is 66 years, making advanced age an increased risk factor for development of HPB carcinomas [2]. In agreement, cancer incidences for both liver and pancreatic cancers are expected to increase from 2010 to 2030 by 59% (liver) and 55% (pancreas), respectively [3]. Thus, in the upcoming decades, substantial healthcare resources and attention will be devoted to treating HPB malignancies.

Surgical resection continues to remain the preferred curative treatment option for HPB neoplasms. However, older patients with HPB disease are often frail and have multiple comorbidities alongside their primary malignancy, thus making aggressive surgical resections high risk for these patients. For frail and elderly patients undergoing elective procedures, perioperative care must be afforded special attention in order to decrease incidences of severe morbidity and mortality. While postoperative care is a mainstay of focus for surgical patients, preoperative assessment is often afforded less attention within the field of HPB surgery. By the use of standardized

G. McKenzie, BS
Department of Surgery, Division of Surgical Oncology, University of Louisville, Louisville, KY, USA

R.C.G. Martin II, MD, PhD, FACS (✉)
Department of Surgery, Division of Surgical Oncology, University of Louisville, Louisville, KY, USA

Division of Surgical Oncology, Upper Gastrointestinal and Hepato-Pancreatico-Biliary Clinic, University of Louisville, Louisville, KY, USA
e-mail: Robert.Martin@louisville.edu

© Springer International Publishing AG 2018
F.G. Rocha, P. Shen (eds.), *Optimizing Outcomes for Liver and Pancreas Surgery*, DOI 10.1007/978-3-319-62624-6_1

patient assessments, clinicians are able to obtain a more accurate representation of a patient's true health status, thus making it possible to identify surgical patient populations with higher risks of postoperative morbidity, mortality, increased length of hospital stay, and increased risk of being discharged to skilled nursing facilities. The aim of this chapter is to highlight current approaches to the assessment of vulnerable HPB surgical patients and elucidate ways to preoperatively optimize and treat these patients to improve surgical outcomes within the field.

Patient Assessment

Comprehensive Geriatric Assessments

The use of a patient's biological age as an indicator of their health status is not accurate in predicting postoperative complications; thus, advanced age alone should not be considered contraindicative of major HPB surgeries [4–6]. However, elderly patients have been shown to have increased 30-day morbidity and mortality when undergoing pancreatic or hepatic resections [7, 8]. As a result, more detailed and accurate measurement tools are needed to assess elderly patient health status. This may be achieved by the utilization of a comprehensive geriatric assessment (CGA). A CGA is a multidimensional diagnostic tool used to assess the medical, functional, and psychosocial status of elderly patients at risk for functional declines [9]. Such assessments give clinicians a more detailed status of a patient's health and help identify vulnerable patients at risk for poor surgical outcomes. Overall elements should include, but are not limited to, assessment of a patient's physical health, mental health, nutritional status, functional status, socioeconomic status, and environmental factors. A table of commonly used tests within a CGA is shown in Table 1.1.

While a CGA is meant to be an all-encompassing view of elderly patient health, performing a complete CGA preoperatively for all elderly patients would be an immense drain on both healthcare human and monetary resources. Depending on a CGA's components, a complete assessment can range anywhere from 30–40 min all while being performed by an experienced assessor, such as a geriatrician, physician assistant, or trained nurse [36]. In recent decades, researchers have focused on developing screening tools to help identify at-risk patients who would benefit from undergoing a CGA while filtering patients who are deemed fit. As a result, clinicians and researchers across many disciplines have been looking at which CGA components are most indicative of patient fitness levels, with hopes of identifying specific tests or metrics that best identify vulnerable individuals who may require a complete CGA. This simplistic model can be utilized in practice in a manner that is both quick and efficient, while reducing cost and resource utilization that otherwise may be wasted on screening low-risk individuals.

Functional Assessment

The functional status of patients, defined by the American College of Surgeons National Surgical Quality Improvement Program (ACS-NSQIP) as behaviors

Table 1.1 Sample of common components of geriatric assessments

Assessment condition	Assessment test used
Functional status	ADL [10]
	IADL [11]
Performance status	ECOG [12]
	SPPB [13]
Mobility	6MWT [14]
	TUG [15]
Frailty assessment	BFI [16]
	GFI [17]
	VES-13 [18]
	Fried's criteria [19]
Mental status	MMSE [20]
	BOMC [21]
	CDT [22]
	Mini-Cog [23]
	MoCA [24]
Mood/depression	GDS [25]
Nutritional assessment	MNA [26]
	SNAQ [27]
	NRS-2002 [28]
	G8 [29]
Polypharmacy	N of daily oral medications [30]
Social support	MOS-SSS [31]
Risk assessment	ASA [32]
Comorbidities	CCI [33]
	CIRS-G [34]
	Satariano's index [35]

Abbreviations: *6MWT* 6-minute walk test, *ADL* activities of daily living, *ASA* American Society of Anesthesiologists, *BFI* brief fatigue inventory, *BOMC* Blessed Orientation-Memory-Concentration, *CCI* Charlson comorbidity index, *CDT* clock-drawing test, *CIRS-G* cumulative illness rating scale-geriatrics, *ECOG* Eastern Cooperative Oncology Group, *G8* geriatric 8, *GDS* Geriatric Depression Scale, *GFI* Groningen Frailty Index, *IADL* instrumental activities of daily living, *MMSE* mini mental state examination, *MNA* mini nutritional assessment, *MoCA* Montreal Cognitive Assessment, *MOS-SSS* Medical Outcomes Study social support survey, *NRS-2002* nutritional risk screening-2002, *SPPB* short physical performance battery tests, *SNAQ* short nutritional assessment questionnaire, *TUG* timed get-up-and-go, *VES-13* Vulnerable Elders Survey-13

needed to maintain daily activities during the 30 days prior to surgery, has long been assessed by simple screening tools such as activities of daily living (ADL) and instrumental activities of daily living (IADL) to gauge the degree of a patient's independence. In patients undergoing hepatic resections and pancreaticoduodenectomy, impaired functional status was highly predictive of postoperative complications and mortality [7, 8, 37]. The timed get-up-and-go (TUG) test is another simple clinical tool used to quantify functional mobility of patients. Abnormal TUG assessment times ($\geq$20 s) have been correlated to increased postoperative morbidity in oncogeriatric surgical patients undergoing elective procedures [38]. The six-minute walk test (6MWT), which measures the distance a patient is able to walk in 6 min, is a metric of functional walking capacity. In patients undergoing colorectal resections, older age, poorer physical status, open surgery, and increased postoperative complications were associated with decreased 6MWT distances [39]. This finding supports the use of the 6MWT as an indirect measure of postoperative recovery. Cardiopulmonary exercise testing (CPET) is also used to predict postoperative outcomes in patients. In a study of patients aged 65 and older undergoing pancreatico-duodenectomy deemed as high risk, abnormal CPET results were predictive of early postoperative death and poor long-term survival for patients [40].

A patient's functional status may be affected by many different interacting domains. One clinically relevant domain, frailty, can be defined as a clinical syndrome in which three or more of the following criteria are met for a given patient: unintentional weight loss of >10 lbs within the previous year, self-reported exhaustion, weakness measured by grip strength, slow walking speed, and low levels of physical activity [19]. It is hypothesized that the mechanism through which frailty manifests is by decreasing the physiological and functional reserves of patients, thereby affecting one's ability to overcome major insults to the body, such as surgery. Surgical patients who fall into the classification of frail have been shown to have increased postoperative complications, length of hospital stay, and discharge to skilled nursing facilities [41]. For patients undergoing elective abdominal surgical procedures, patients identified as frail have recently been shown to have increased 1-year mortality and poorer surgical outcomes [42]. Several clinical screening tools for assessing frailty scores clinically have been developed, such as the Groningen Frailty Index (GFI), Vulnerable Elders Survey-13 (VES-13), and Fried's frailty criteria assessment.

Many clinicians also rely on morphometric data for assessing patient frailty status. Sarcopenia, which clinically manifests as a loss of skeletal muscle mass, strength, and decreased physical performance, is also associated with poor clinical outcomes [43]. Sarcopenia can be preoperatively assessed morphometrically by CT-based measurements for patients undergoing surgery for HPB neoplasms by use of abdominal cross-sectional muscle area, and its presence has been associated with poorer surgical outcomes [44, 45]. The use of advanced imaging technologies allows clinicians to quickly identify sarcopenia in patients that otherwise would be difficult to assess morphometrically, such as in the case of sarcopenic obese patients. In the future, radiologic imaging may become a normal part of preoperative assessment and risk stratification for patients undergoing major elective procedures [46].

Nutritional Assessment

There are a variety of nutritional status metrics that are available for predicting risk of surgical complications. Some of the more commonly used parameters include weight loss, serum protein levels, immunocompetence, and anthropometric indicators [47]. Malnutrition in patients undergoing gastrointestinal surgery has been shown to be associated with increased morbidity, and nutritional assessment scores correlate with severity of postoperative complications and length of hospital stay [48]. Several nutritional status screening assessment tools exist for clinical use, including the mini nutritional assessment examination (MNA), short nutritional assessment questionnaire (SNAQ), nutritional risk screening-2002 (NRS-2002), and geriatric 8 (G8) assessment. While no screening assessment has proven to be markedly superior above others, the NRS-2002 is favored for assessment in surgical patients and most validated in terms of predictive value [49]. In a direct comparison to the MNA assessment and serum proteins, the NRS-2002 assessment identified more elderly patients with or at risk of malnutrition [50]. The NRS-2002 screening system uses a combination of assessing patient nutrition along with quantifying the severity of disease to give a summed score of nutritional risk [28].

Mental Status

An important component of preoperative assessment for patients is mental status and cognitive assessments. One condition that cognitive assessments screen for is risk of postoperative delirium, which is an acute decline in cognitive functioning. Delirium in many cases is preventable, and its presence has been shown to be associated with many adverse surgical outcomes including increased mortality, morbidity, and discharge to rehabilitation facilities [51–53]. Leading risk factors for delirium development include dementia, cognitive impairment, functional impairment, visual impairment, history of alcohol abuse, and advanced age [54]. Patients at risk of delirium can be assessed using screening tools such as the mini mental state examination (MMSE), the Mini-Cog assessment, and the Montreal Cognitive Assessment (MoCA).

Major depression is also associated with adverse surgical outcomes. Results from the preoperative assessment of cancer in the elderly (PACE) study showed that patients with abnormal scores on the Geriatric Depression Scale (GDS) were associated with an increased risk of 30-day postoperative morbidity [55]. Identifying patients experiencing depressive symptoms may not only improve surgical outcomes but also treat an underlying disorder that often goes undiagnosed and untreated in many elderly patients.

Other Considerations

Aside from physical and cognitive assessments, there are many other domains to preoperative patient assessment that must be evaluated. With oncogeriatric patients, polypharmacy must be addressed. With advanced age and disease status comes decreased physiological capacity to metabolize and eliminate toxins; thus drug interactions can be exacerbated in patients with compromised hepatic and renal functions. It is important to evaluate and discontinue nonessential medications preoperatively to minimize the risk of any adverse drug interactions [56]. For patients undergoing intra-abdominal and HPB procedures, polypharmacy has been associated with increased length of hospital stay and risk of major postoperative complications [57, 58].

Social support is another variable that should be assessed preoperatively for patients. For geriatric patients, social support has been correlated to increased mortality risk, independent of patient age [59]. Lack of social support has also been shown to correlate to increase 30-day postoperative morbidity for elderly patients undergoing major abdominal cancer surgery [58]. Thus, preoperative assessment for elderly and frail patients should encompass a multisystem and multidisciplinary approach to maximize outcomes for these high-risk patients.

HPB Patient Assessment in Current Literature

As of yet, there is no consensus screening tool that adequately identifies vulnerable oncogeriatric surgical patients in place of a CGA nor is there consensus within the field of HPB surgery as to which components of a CGA should be used for surgical risk assessment. Several studies have shown that in patients undergoing oncogeriatric surgical procedures, CGA components can predict patients at risk for increased postoperative morbidity, mortality, complications, length of hospital stay, and risk of discharge to a skilled nursing facility [36, 38, 41, 53, 57, 58, 60–71]. However, many of these studies include a heterogeneous patient population, with only a small subset undergoing HPB surgical procedures.

Badgwell et al. (2013) attempted to prospectively record CGA variables that identified factors associated with increased perioperative risk and resource utilization in 111 elderly patients undergoing major abdominal cancer surgery. Within the study population, of 30% of patients underwent HPB surgical procedures. Variables that were found to correlate with discharge to a skilled nursing facility included weight loss ≥10% within 6 months preoperatively, American Society of Anesthesiologist (ASA) risk assessment score of ≥2, and Eastern Cooperative Oncology Group (ECOG) performance score of ≥2. Variables associated with prolonged hospital stay were weight loss ≥10%, presence of polypharmacy, and distant metastatic disease [57].

Dale et al. (2014) used CGA components to identify patients in elevated clinical risk categories undergoing pancreaticoduodenectomy. In a study population of 76 patients, researchers found that patient self-reported exhaustion was associated with major postoperative complications, surgical intensive care unit admission, and increased length of hospital stay. Scores on short physical performance battery (SPPB) tests of <10 and patient age were correlated with a discharge to a skilled nursing facility, and older age was also correlated to lower likelihood of hospital readmission [60].

Huisman et al. (2014) attempted to determine the predictive value of the timed get-up-and-go (TUG) test versus the American Society of Anesthesiologists (ASA) classification for quantifying oncogeriatric surgical patient risk assessment. Of the 263 patients undergoing elective surgery for solid abdominal tumors, 28 (10.6%) of patients underwent HPB surgical procedures. For patients with high TUG times of >20s, the risk of patients to develop major postoperative complications (Clavien-Dindo grade 3 to 5) was 50%, as opposed to 13.6% of patients with normal TUG times. For patients with abnormal ASA scores of ≥3, 24.8% of patients experienced major postoperative complications. Thus, twice as many surgical patients at risk of postoperative complications were identified using the TUG than when using the ASA classification [38].

Validating similar claims from their previous year's study and expanding the number of CGA screening assessments used, Huisman et al. (2015) investigated the accuracy of commonly used geriatric screening tools in predicting major postoperative complications in patients undergoing elective abdominal oncogeriatric surgical procedures. The study included 328 patients, of which 10.3% were HPB surgical patients, found that TUG times of >20s, ASA scores ≥3, and nutritional risk screening-2002 status were predictive of major postoperative surgical complications. The finding that once again the TUG test had good predictive value is encouraging, for this test measures basic functional mobility, coordination, and muscles strength, which can be easily and inexpensively administered by an unspecialized assessor [62].

Kaibori et al. (2016) studied how CGA components predicted postoperative complications in elderly patients undergoing elective hepatectomies for hepatocellular carcinoma treatment. In a patient population of 71, analysis showed that serum albumin levels of <4.0 g/dL, intraoperative time, intraoperative blood loss, cirrhosis, geriatric 8 (G8) scores of <14, and mini nutritional assessment (MNA) scores of <12 were all predictive of postoperative complications. Patients with G8 scores of <14 also had on average significantly higher morbidity and longer postoperative hospital stay. The G8 screening tool includes seven items from the MNA test, along with an age-related item. According to the authors, giving the test was quick, easy, and convenient that could be administered in less than 5 min by a nurse without any special geriatric training. Given the large nutritional component of the G8 test, this may indicate the importance of preoperative nutritional optimization for vulnerable patients [63].

Kenig et al. (2015) attempted to assess frailty using CGA components and measure its accuracy in predicting postoperative outcomes. In a study of 75 elderly patients undergoing elective surgery for solid abdominal tumors, of which 15% were pancreatic neoplasms, only TUG times ≥15 s and Medical Outcomes Study social support scale (MOS SSS) scores of <4 were significantly predictive of 30-day postoperative morbidity. The presence of polypharmacy (≥4 oral medications a day) was also a risk factor for major postoperative complications. This study highlights the need for frailty assessments to contain varying components of the CGA to have the best predictive outcomes for patients [58].

Lastly, Korc-Grodzicki et al. (2015) used CGA components to predict the development of postoperative delirium and other comorbidities in patients undergoing varying elective oncologic surgeries. The study population included 416 patients, of which 20% of patients underwent HPB surgeries. Charlson comorbidity index scores of ≥3, patients with a history of falls 6 months prior to surgery, instrumental activities of daily living (IADL) scores of <8, and abnormal Mini-Cog test results were all predictive of postoperative delirium. In this study, patients who developed postoperative delirium had longer median length of hospital stays and greater likelihood of discharge to a skilled nursing facility [66].

As one can see, there is a large and varied usage of CGA components to assess frailty and identify at-risk oncogeriatric surgical patients. Even between studies that use the same assessment tools, cutoff values for abnormal results may vary, making direct comparison of literature findings difficult. Additionally, almost all studies include patients with different cancer profiles, with very small percentages of study populations including HPB surgical patients. More work is needed to be done within the field of HPB surgery to identify which assessment tools are best identifying vulnerable surgical patients.

Current University of Louisville Practice

Currently, since there is no established validated screening tool, we have chosen to utilize three types of screening in our practice. Since we are a tertiary referral center and many (approx. 40%) are coming from greater than 2 h away, our initial surgical fitness screening begins prior to the first office visit, to ensure that patients do not travel long distances when they are clearly not surgical candidates based on comorbidities or frailty. Thus, the initial surgical fitness evaluation is based on whether the patient can walk a mile in 25–30 min (i.e., if on a treadmill, a mile at 2 miles an hour). This is clearly not a cardiac stress test, but a physical stamina test that we have recently validated allows us to predict postoperative recovery and accurately avoid a high incidence of permanent loss of independence in patients [72]. The ability of the patient to walk a mile in this time frame has allowed 85% of all patients to get back home and have some degree of independence.

After that initial screening, when patients are seen in the office, we then use the Groningen Frailty Indicator questionnaire, which has recently been found to be predictive in predicting morbidity and loss of independence [72, 73]. We have found that when the patient fills this questionnaire out in the office either before I have seen the patient or after I have deemed them resectable, this allows me to have an honest and accurate expectation of the risk of morbidity, which for elderly patients is critical to their decision making. The last is a simple nutritional scoring system based on greater than 3 kg weight loss and if the patient has utilized supplements in the last 3 months.

All of these tests are easily reproduced, do not require advanced training by the medical staff, and are correctable (pre-habilitation) over time either with or without neoadjuvant therapy. All of these questionnaires and evaluations are utilized multiple times in order to demonstrated and document improvement over a 2–3 months' time.

Patient Optimization and Treatment

Centralization

HPB resections are high-risk surgeries, especially when performed on elderly or frail patients. Thus, optimizing outcomes for patients undergoing such procedures is critical. Factors shown to improve outcomes at hospitals with low HPB surgical mortality are shorter operation time, low intraoperative blood loss, less blood transfusions, and quality anesthetic care [74]. It has long been established that patients undergoing complex HPB surgery at higher procedural volume institutions display better postoperative outcomes compared to medium or low volume institutions [75–78], and this finding has been more recently validated a decade later [79]. However, complex HPB surgeries can be performed at low volume institutions and achieve similar outcomes as higher volume centers; granted facilities and processes between the two institutions are the similar [80]. Elderly patients in particular seem to have significant benefit from having HPB surgeries at high volume institutions. By having procedures at a high volume centers, outcomes for elderly patients improve to levels that are comparable to younger patients [81].

In alignment with hospital volume, surgeon volume for complex HPB procedures also appears to be associated with improved patient outcomes. However, the improved outcomes only correlate to the primary procedure for which that particular surgeon has experience. High volume of expertise in one HPB area has not been shown to improve patient outcomes for other related procedures [82]. For surgeons performing pancreatoduodenectomy (PD), surgeon expertise, defined as ≥ 50 PDs performed, showed decreased patient morbidity rates as compared to procedures performed by less experienced surgeons. Conversely, in the same study, the volume of PDs a surgeon performed in a year did not correlate to any significant differences in patient morbidity or mortality [83]. Thus, it appears that once a level of expertise in performing PDs has been achieved, maintaining a high volume status does not significantly affect patient outcomes.

Many high volume institutions also double as teaching hospitals. However, even between high volume hospitals, patients undergoing complex HPB surgery have decreased mortality at teaching hospitals versus non-teaching hospitals [84]. Furthermore, Ejaz et al. has shown while resident participation in HPB surgeries may increase mean operative times and minor complication rates, there was no significant effects of resident participation in surgery and patient morbidity, mortality, or increase length of stay for patients [85]. As a result, allowing residents to participate in complex HPB surgeries does not appear to come at the expense of the patient. In summation, patients – especially elderly – should whenever possible undergo major oncologic HPB surgeries at high volume institutions at the hands of experienced surgeons to maximize patient outcomes.

Prehabilitation

Prehabilitation is an optimization process that occurs from the time of cancer diagnosis to the start of interventions for patients. The ultimate end goal of prehabilitation is to either prevent or decrease the anticipated physiological insults that result from cancer treatments [86]. For patients with HPB cancer, many will receive multimodal therapies, including combinations of chemotherapy, radiation, and surgery [87]. It is important to note that for patients receiving neoadjuvant therapies in addition to surgery, the preoperative period is also a time of recovery from the noxious effects of these systemically taxing therapeutic agents.

Current literature suggests that presurgical exercise therapy, through both aerobic and anaerobic means, can be beneficial for patients undergoing oncologic surgeries (Table 1.2) [88, 89, 92, 94, 95]. In a study of 112 patients undergoing colorectal cancer resections, Carli et al. (2014) showed that during a prehabilitation period of on average 52 days, patients who partook in 30 min of daily walking, breathing, and

Table 1.2 Summary of pre habilitation regimens

Study	Types of prehabilitation	Length of therapy	Frequency	Duration (minutes)	Intensity	Follow-up	Outcome
Carli et al. [88]	Bike/strength	Mean = 59.0 days	Daily	20–45	≥50%MHR. Volitional fatigue within 8–12 repetitions	2–4 m	Improved functional 6MWT before surgery Improved functional walking capacity in controls 4 weeks after surgery
	Walk/breathing	Mean = 45.4 days	Daily	40–45		2–4 m	Similar length of stay Similar postoperative complications Similar QOL
Kaibori et al. [63]	Aerobic exercise, diet therapy	≤1 month preop, 6 months post-op	3/week	60 min	NR	6 m	Reduced body mass, fat mass Reduced insulin resistance
	Diet therapy	≤1 month preop, 6 months post-op	NA	NA	NA	6 m	
Dronkers et al. [89]	Aerobic exercise. Resistance training, IMT	2–4 weeks	Daily	30–60 min	55–75% MHR, 11–13 on Borg scale	NR	Improved respiratory muscle endurance in preoperative period
	Home-based exercise Advice	2–4 weeks	Daily	≥30 min	NR	NR	Similar time-up-and-go, chair rise time, LASA physical activity questionnaire, physical work Capacity, and quality of life Similar postoperative complications Similar length of stay Similar QOL
Gillis et al. [90]	Aerobic/resistance training, nutritional therapy, relaxation exercises, before and after surgery	4 weeks preop, 8 weeks post-op	≥ 3/week	50 min	≥ 40% HRR, 8–12 repetitions	8 weeks	Increased walking capacity Before surgery and at 8 week post Improved recovery to baseline
	Aerobic/resistance training, nutritional therapy, relaxation exercises after surgery	8 weeks post-op	≥ 3/week	50 min	≥ 40% HRR, 8–12 repetitions	8 weeks	

Study	Intervention						Outcomes
Cho et al. [91]	Aerobic/resistance training, stretching	4 weeks	3–7/week	NR	NR	1 year	Reduced body weight, reduced postoperative complications
	Matched controls in database	None	None	None	None	None	Reduced length of stay
Kim et al. [92]	Aerobic exercise	4 weeks	Daily	20–30 mins	40–65% HRR	4 weeks	Same functional walking capacity
	Standard care	NA	NA	NA	NA	4 weeks	
Dunne et al. [93]	Aerobic exercise	4 weeks	12 sessions	30 min	Interval training alternating at less than 60% O_2 peak uptake and more than 90% O_2 at peak	4 weeks	Improved mental and overall QOL
	Standard care	NA	NA	NA	NA	4 weeks	

Length of therapy refers to therapy prior to surgery, unless otherwise noted

AT anabolic threshold, *HRR* heart rate reserve, *IMT* inspiratory muscle training, *MHR* maximal heart rate, *NACRT* neoadjuvant chemoradiotherapy, *NA* not applicable, *NR* not reported, *QOL* quality of life, *6MWT* = 6-minute walk test

statistic circulation exercises improved physical fitness levels measured by the 6-minute walk test (6MWT). Patients in the walking/breathing group also had smaller decreases in postoperative 6MWT times as compared to patients in a biking and muscle strengthening prehabilitation group [88]. Dronkers et al. (2010) showed that in a 2–4 week prehabilitation period for 42 patients undergoing colorectal cancer resections, patients who participated in two 60-min training sessions per week, consisting of inspiratory muscle training and aerobic exercise, had increased endurance and improved respiratory function during the preoperative period [89].

Kim et al. (2009) attempted to identify the most responsive measures of aerobic fitness during a 4-week prehabilitation program for 21 patients undergoing major bowel resections. Members of the prehabilitation intervention group participated in 20–30 min of daily aerobic exercise over the course of the program. Patients with initially the lowest fitness baselines showed the most improvement from the prehabilitation program in terms of aerobic fitness levels, measured by submaximal cycling economy, submaximal heart rate, and peak power output at VO_{2max} [92].

Lastly, Timmerman et al. (2011) investigated the feasibility and effectiveness of a 5-week preoperative therapeutic exercise program for 39 patients undergoing major gastrointestinal and abdominal cancer surgeries. Patients in the intervention program participated in two 120-min sessions weekly, with the program including aerobic exercise and muscle strength training. Participants in the exercise program reported higher levels of satisfaction and motivation during the prehabilitation period compared to control groups. Patient cardiorespiratory fitness, measured by the Astrand-Rhyming indirect test, and muscle strength, measured by grip strength, increased significantly during the preoperative period for patients in the prehabilitation group; however, postoperative adverse events were not reported in this study [95]. A summary of the current published prehabilitation studies is demonstrated in Table 1.3

Unfortunately, less evidence exists to support this current paradigm for HPB surgical patients. For patients with HPB malignancies, time is often of the essence, which can make delays in surgical intervention to improve patient fitness levels unwarranted. However, it may be possible in just 3 weeks to make sufficient gains in patient aerobic and strength capacities to bring about positive benefits [96].

The potential advantages of utilizing exercise programs for patient recovery extend beyond the preoperative period. It has been shown that patients who participated in self-reported exercise during cancer treatments had diminished side effects both during and after treatment, with benefits including decreased fatigue, decreased shortness of breath, and improved self-reported health [97]. Yeo et al. (2012) showed potential benefits of pancreaticoduodenectomy patients undergoing postoperative home exercise rehabilitation programs. This program included three 1-month phases, which gradually increased walking duration times each month with the goal of patients walking for 90–150 min per week in three to five sessions. Patients assigned to the home walking group demonstrated decreased fatigue, increased physical function, and increased quality of life as compared to those who did not participate in the program [98]. Thus, while specific exercise recommendations for surgical cancer patients may only be in their budding stages, current literature is pointing toward positive benefits for patients who do participate in some aspect of physical activity during their treatment plans.

Table 1.3 Current literature of surgical prehabilitation

Study	Cancer type	No. of patients	Prehabilitation intervention	Duration	Results
Carli et al. [88]	Colorectal	112	Bike/strengthening group 3–5 h per week of the following exercises: 1. Stationary cycling for 20 min 2. Weight training 3X per week for 10–15 min 3. Push-ups, sit-ups, and standing lunges until volitional fatigue	Mean of 52 days	There was no difference between two experimental programs in terms of mean functional walking capacity measured by 6-minute walk test (6MWT). Walking capacity was improved most in walk/breathing group during both the prehabilitation period and after surgery. Postoperatively, the walk/breathing group had a smaller decrease in 6MWT times
			Walk/breathing group 1. 30 min of daily walking 2. Deep breathing exercises for 5 min per day 3. Static circulation exercises		
Dronkers et al. [89]	Colorectal	42	Two 60-min training sessions weekly included: 1. Warm-up 2. Lower leg extensor muscle training 3. Inspiratory muscle training for 15 min 4. Aerobic training for 20–30 min 5. Cooldown	2–4 weeks	In the intervention group, respiratory muscle endurance increased significantly during the preoperative period. No other significant differences were measured between the groups
Kim et al. [92]	Colorectal	21	20 min of daily aerobic exercise gradually increased to 30 min over the course of the program.	4 weeks	Patients with initially low fitness levels showed improved responsive measures of aerobic fitness including increased submaximal cycling economy, submaximal heart rate, and peak power output at VO_{2max} in the prehabilitation group
Timmerman et al. [95]	Pancreatic, liver, colorectal, sarcoma, esophageal	39	Two 120-minute training sessions weekly included: 1. Aerobic exercises for 30–50 min (stationary bike, cross-trainer, treadmill) 2. Muscle strengthening with emphasis on large multijointed muscle groups	5 weeks	Program participants reported higher levels of satisfaction and motivation during the prehabilitation period. Cardiorespiratory fitness and muscle strength increased significantly during the preoperative period

Nutrition

According to the American Society for Parenteral and Enteral Nutrition (ASPEN) clinical guidelines, routine use of nutritional support therapy (NST) for patients undergoing major cancer operations is not recommended, but NST may be given perioperatively to moderate or severely malnourished patients if administered between 7 and 14 days before surgery. The benefits of the NST, however, should be weighed against the risk of the NST itself and the amount of time delaying the operation. Both of these recommendations received grading level "A," which are guidelines supported by at least two large randomized clinical trials [99]. In the large Veteran Affairs Total Parenteral Nutrition Cooperative Study published in 1991, a clinical trial of 395 patients undergoing major abdominal or thoracic surgical procedures, use of parenteral nutrition 7–15 days preoperatively and 3 days postoperatively showed no benefit in mortality or noninfectious complications for patients, and patients undergoing parenteral nutrition supplementation showed increased infectious complications as compared to control groups [100]. Currently, it appears that routine nutritional supplementation prior to surgery for patients not at nutritional risk is unwarranted.

Recently, immunonutrition has been gaining popularity in surgical spheres with its ability to enhance immune system function in immunocompromised or malnourished patients. Typical formulas contain varying components of amino acids, RNA, and omega-3 fatty acids. Most immunonutrition regimens have the amino acid arginine as a major component. Arginine is a precursor to nitric oxide, a major player in vasodilation cascades, and is implicated in cell growth and proliferation pathways involved in wound healing [101]. The use of perioperative arginine-rich supplements have been shown to reduce length of hospital stay and infectious complications in patients undergoing surgical procedures [102]. Omega-3 fatty acids EPA and DHA are involved with suppression of T-cell activation and natural killer cell activity and give rise to the anti-inflammatory agents resolvins [103, 104]. Further study of the components of immunonutritional formulas is needed to reveal the true benefits of these immune modulating supplements.

Within the field of HPB surgery, early postoperative enteral and parenteral nutritional support has been shown to decrease infectious surgical complications and length of overall hospital stay compared to total parenteral nutritional groups in patients undergoing pancreaticoduodenectomy [105]. Enteral and parenteral nutritionally supported patients also showed improved hyperglycemic control and improved gastric emptying. In general, enteral nutritional support is favored over parenteral nutrition in order to preserve gut integrity, immune function, and glycemic management [47]. In a study of patients undergoing elective abdominal procedures, patients with an NRS score of ≥ 5 who underwent parenteral nutritional support preoperatively had a significantly lower complication rate and shorter hospital stays compared to control groups [106].

ERAS

Enhanced recovery after surgery (ERAS) protocols are multidisciplinary pathways designed to maximize healthcare delivery to patients while minimizing cost [107]. ERAS protocols have been around for decades, but within recent years, they have gained increased momentum due to successes in fields outside of HPB surgery, namely, in colorectal surgery. ERAS success measures have been reported as reduced perioperative morbidity, mortality, and decreased length of hospital stay [37]. While the main goal of any surgical intervention is to return patients as close to their functional baseline status as possible, in surgical oncology, this return to baseline is possibly even more important. Many surgical patients will continue adjuvant oncologic therapies postoperatively; thus failure for patients to return to intended oncologic treatment (RIOT) due to postoperative complications has been shown to decrease disease-free and overall patient survival [108].

Within the HPB surgical field, ERAS protocols have thus far generated positive, although not resoundingly successful, outcomes for patients who a have participated in them. In a systematic review of HPB ERAS protocols by Hall et al., the general consensus across the field is the length of postoperative hospital stay can be significantly reduced by protocol implementation [109]. However, one study has shown that while using an ERAS protocol for open hepatic resection led to decreased length of hospital stay, patient readmission rates significantly increased [110]. One of the main difficulties in implementing ERAS pathways is deviation from care plans among both patients and providers. Many physicians tend to favor personal preference over evidence-based supported strategies, such as many HPB ERAS protocols calling for minimal use of intra-abdominal drains [109, 111]. Overall, both patients and physicians show positive attitudes toward ERAS components, thus supporting the continuing development of such programs [112]. More study into ERAS pathways in HPB surgery is necessitated to uncover the full potential of these clinical pathways [113].

Conclusion

There is a delicate balance within the field of HPB surgery that permits optimal and equitable treatments for vulnerable patients while avoiding unnecessary and aggressive healthcare overutilization. As healthcare within developed nations continually moves toward single-payer systems, future reimbursements will shift from fee-for-service payment models to payments based upon patient performance and clinical outcomes. Thus, early assessment and identification of patients at risk for poor clinical outcomes will become increasingly important in all fields of medicine.

With the plethora of patient assessment tools currently available to clinicians, and overall lack of standardization between healthcare institutions, it is left to surgeons to decide which screening tools best predict outcomes for vulnerable patients, as well as how to direct and manage patient optimization before surgical interventions. Opponents of more comprehensive preoperative assessments may argue that greater patient screening will lead to increased cost, administrative burden, and postponement of surgery. However, by maximizing patient fitness and nutrition on the front end of treatment, this may potentially decrease mortality, morbidity, and surgical complications, thus offsetting costs by decreasing the overall length of hospital stay and patient discharge to costly rehabilitation facilities.

Even though a patient may have recently undergone extensive assessment by primary care or geriatric physicians, due to the inaccessibility of many electronic medical record systems, these results may not be readily accessible to surgeons at outside institutions preoperatively. Hence, development of a quick, accurate, and easy to administer preoperative screening tool for vulnerable patients is necessitated. Further randomized clinical trials are also warranted in order to validate if the generalized findings of other surgical disciplines are beneficial and applicable to the unique patient population that comprises HPB surgery.

References

1. Colby SL, Ortman JM. Projections of the size and composition of the US population: 2014 to 2060. *US Census Bureau, Ed.* 2015:25–1143.
2. Horner M, Ries L, Krapcho M, et al. SEER Cancer Statistics Review, 1975–2006. Bethesda: National Cancer Institute; 2009.
3. Smith BD, Smith GL, Hurria A, Hortobagyi GN, Buchholz TA. Future of cancer incidence in the United States: burdens upon an aging, changing nation. J Clin Oncol. 2009;27(17):2758–65.
4. Melis M, Marcon F, Masi A, et al. The safety of a pancreaticoduodenectomy in patients older than 80 years: risk vs. benefits. HPB. 2012;14(9):583–8.
5. Laporte GA, Kalil AN. Liver ressection in elderly patients. Arq Bras Cir Dig: ABCD = Braz Arch Dig Surg. 2013;26(2):136–9.
6. Ramesh HS, Jain S, Audisio RA. Implications of aging in surgical oncology. Cancer J. 2005;11(6):488–94.
7. de la Fuente SG, Bennett KM, Scarborough JE. Functional status determines postoperative outcomes in elderly patients undergoing hepatic resections. J Surg Oncol. 2013;107(8):865–70.
8. de la Fuente SG, Bennett KM, Pappas TN, Scarborough JE. Pre- and intraoperative variables affecting early outcomes in elderly patients undergoing pancreaticoduodenectomy. HPB. 2011;13(12):887–92.
9. Caillet P, Canoui-Poitrine F, Vouriot J, et al. Comprehensive geriatric assessment in the decision-making process in elderly patients with cancer: ELCAPA study. J Clin Oncol. 2011;29(27):3636–42.
10. Katz S, Akpom CA. A measure of primary sociobiological functions. Int J Health Serv. 1976;6(3):493–508.
11. Lawton MP, Brody EM. Assessment of older people: self-maintaining and instrumental activities of daily living. The Gerontologist. 1969;9(3):179–86.
12. Oken MM, Creech RH, Tormey DC, et al. Toxicity and response criteria of the Eastern Cooperative Oncology Group. Am J Clin Oncol. 1982;5(6):649–56.
13. Guralnik JM, Simonsick EM, Ferrucci L, et al. A short physical performance battery assessing lower extremity function: association with self-reported disability and prediction of mortality and nursing home admission. J Gerontol. 1994;49(2):M85–94.
14. Guyatt GH, Sullivan MJ, Thompson PJ, et al. The 6-minute walk: a new measure of exercise capacity in patients with chronic heart failure. Can Med Assoc J. 1985;132(8):919–23.
15. Podsiadlo D, Richardson S. The timed "Up & Go": a test of basic functional mobility for frail elderly persons. J Am Geriatr Soc. 1991;39(2):142–8.

16. Mendoza TR, Wang XS, Cleeland CS, et al. The rapid assessment of fatigue severity in cancer patients. Cancer. 1999;85(5):1186–96.
17. Schuurmans H, Steverink N, Lindenberg S, Frieswijk N, Slaets JP. Old or frail: what tells us more? J Gerontol Ser A Biol Med Sci. 2004;59(9):M962–5.
18. Saliba D, Elliott M, Rubenstein LZ, et al. The vulnerable Elders survey: a tool for identifying vulnerable older people in the community. J Am Geriatr Soc. 2001;49(12):1691–9.
19. Fried LP, Tangen CM, Walston J, et al. Frailty in older adults evidence for a phenotype. J Gerontol Ser A Biol Med Sci. 2001;56(3):M146–57.
20. Folstein MF, Folstein SE, McHugh PR. "Mini-mental state": a practical method for grading the cognitive state of patients for the clinician. J Psychiatr Res. 1975;12(3):189–98.
21. Blessed G, Tomlinson BE, Roth M. The association between quantitative measures of dementia and of senile change in the cerebral grey matter of elderly subjects. Br J Psychiatry. 1968;114(512):797–811.
22. Watson YI, Arfken CL, Birge SJ. Clock completion: an objective screening test for dementia. J Am Geriatr Soc. 1993;41(11):1235–40.
23. Borson S, Scanlan J, Brush M, Vitaliano P, Dokmak A. The Mini-Cog: a cognitive'vital signs' measure for dementia screening in multi-lingual elderly. Int J Geriatr Psychiatry. 2000;15(11):1021–7.
24. Nasreddine ZS, Phillips NA, Bédirian V, et al. The Montreal Cognitive Assessment, MoCA: a brief screening tool for mild cognitive impairment. J Am Geriatr Soc. 2005;53(4):695–9.
25. Sheikh JI, Yesavage JA, Brooks JO, et al. Proposed factor structure of the geriatric depression scale. Int Psychogeriatr. 1991;3(01):23–8.
26. Guigoz Y, Vellas B, Garry P, Vellas B, Albarede J. Mini Nutritional Assessment: a practical assessment tool for grading the nutritional state of elderly patients. Mini Nutr Assess: MNA Nutr Elder. 1997:15–60.
27. Kruizenga H, Seidell J, De Vet H, Wierdsma N. Development and validation of a hospital screening tool for malnutrition: the short nutritional assessment questionnaire (SNAQ©). Clin Nutr. 2005;24(1):75–82.
28. Kondrup J, RASMUSSEN HH, Hamberg O, STANGA Z. Group AahEW. Nutritional risk screening (NRS 2002): a new method based on an analysis of controlled clinical trials. Clin Nutr. 2003;22(3):321–36.
29. Bellera C, Rainfray M, Mathoulin-Pelissier S, et al. Screening older cancer patients: first evaluation of the G-8 geriatric screening tool. Ann Oncol. 2012;23(8):2166–72. mdr587
30. Curtis LH, Østbye T, Sendersky V, et al. Inappropriate prescribing for elderly Americans in a large outpatient population. Arch Intern Med. 2004;164(15):1621–5.
31. Sherbourne CD, Stewart AL. The MOS social support survey. Soc Sci Med. 1991;32(6):705–14.
32. Soliani P. New classification of physical status. Anesthesiology. 1963;24:111.
33. Charlson ME, Pompei P, Ales KL, MacKenzie CR. A new method of classifying prognostic comorbidity in longitudinal studies: development and validation. J Chronic Dis. 1987;40(5):373–83.
34. Salvi F, Miller MD, Grilli A, et al. A manual of guidelines to score the modified cumulative illness rating scale and its validation in acute hospitalized elderly patients. J Am Geriatr Soc. 2008;56(10):1926–31.
35. Satariano WA, Ragland DR. The effect of comorbidity on 3-year survival of women with primary breast cancer. Ann Intern Med. 1994;120(2):104–10.
36. Chen CC, Lin MT, Liang JT, Chen CM, Yen CJ, Huang GH. Pre-surgical geriatric syndromes, frailty, and risks for postoperative delirium in older patients undergoing gastrointestinal surgery: prevalence and red flags. J Gastrointest Surg. 2015;19(5):927–34.
37. Adamina M, Kehlet H, Tomlinson GA, Senagore AJ, Delaney CP. Enhanced recovery pathways optimize health outcomes and resource utilization: a meta-analysis of randomized controlled trials in colorectal surgery. Surgery. 2011;149(6):830–40.
38. Huisman MG, van Leeuwen BL, Ugolini G, et al. "Timed Up & Go": a screening tool for predicting 30-day morbidity in onco-geriatric surgical patients? A multicenter cohort study. PLoS One. 2014;9(1):e86863.

39. Pecorelli N, Fiore JF Jr, Gillis C, et al. The six-minute walk test as a measure of postoperative recovery after colorectal resection: further examination of its measurement properties. Surg Endosc. 2016;30(6):2199–206.
40. Junejo MA, Mason JM, Sheen AJ, et al. Cardiopulmonary exercise testing for preoperative risk assessment before pancreaticoduodenectomy for cancer. Ann Surg Oncol. 2014;21(6):1929–36.
41. Makary MA, Segev DL, Pronovost PJ, et al. Frailty as a predictor of surgical outcomes in older patients. J Am Coll Surg. 2010;210(6):901–8.
42. Wagner D, Buttner S, Kim Y, et al. Clinical and morphometric parameters of frailty for prediction of mortality following hepatopancreaticobiliary surgery in the elderly. Br J Surg. 2016;103(2):e83–92.
43. Cruz-Jentoft AJ, Baeyens JP, Bauer JM, et al. Sarcopenia: European consensus on definition and diagnosis report of the European Working Group on Sarcopenia in Older People. Age Ageing. 2010;39(4):412–23. afq034
44. Peng P, Hyder O, Firoozmand A, et al. Impact of sarcopenia on outcomes following resection of pancreatic adenocarcinoma. J Gastrointest Surg. 2012;16(8):1478–86.
45. Voron T, Tselikas L, Pietrasz D, et al. Sarcopenia impacts on short- and long-term results of hepatectomy for hepatocellular carcinoma. Ann Surg. 2015;261(6):1173–83.
46. Levolger S, van Vugt J, de Bruin R, IJzermans J. Systematic review of sarcopenia in patients operated on for gastrointestinal and hepatopancreatobiliary malignancies. Br J Surg. 2015;102(12):1448–58.
47. Huhmann MB, August DA. Nutrition support in surgical oncology. Nutr Clin Pract. 2009;24(4):520–6.
48. Schiesser M, Kirchhoff P, Müller MK, Schäfer M, Clavien P-A. The correlation of nutrition risk index, nutrition risk score, and bioimpedance analysis with postoperative complications in patients undergoing gastrointestinal surgery. Surgery. 2009;145(5):519–26.
49. Rasmussen HH, Holst M, Kondrup J. Measuring nutritional risk in hospitals. Clin Epidemiol. 2010;2(1):209–16.
50. Drescher T, Singler K, Ulrich A, et al. Comparison of two malnutrition risk screening methods (MNA and NRS 2002) and their association with markers of protein malnutrition in geriatric hospitalized patients. Eur J Clin Nutr. 2010;64(8):887–93.
51. Marcantonio ER, Goldman L, Mangione CM, et al. A clinical prediction rule for delirium after elective noncardiac surgery. JAMA. 1994;271(2):134–9.
52. Korc-Grodzicki B, Root JC, Alici Y. Prevention of post-operative delirium in older patients with cancer undergoing surgery. J Geriatr Oncol. 2015;6(1):60–9.
53. Robinson TN, Wallace JI, DS W, et al. Accumulated frailty characteristics predict postoperative discharge institutionalization in the geriatric patient. J Am Coll Surg. 2011;213(1):37–42.
54. Inouye SK, Westendorp RG, Saczynski JS. Delirium in elderly people. Lancet. 2014;383(9920):911–22.
55. Audisio RA, Ramesh H, Longo WE, Zbar AP, Pope D. Preoperative assessment of surgical risk in oncogeriatric patients. Oncologist. 2005;10(4):262–8.
56. Corcoran ME. Polypharmacy in the older patient with cancer. Cancer Control. 1997;4:419–28.
57. Badgwell B, Stanley J, Chang GJ, et al. Comprehensive geriatric assessment of risk factors associated with adverse outcomes and resource utilization in cancer patients undergoing abdominal surgery. J Surg Oncol. 2013;108(3):182–6.
58. Kenig J, Olszewska U, Zychiewicz B, Barczynski M, Mituś-Kenig M. Cumulative deficit model of geriatric assessment to predict the postoperative outcomes of older patients with solid abdominal cancer. J Geriatr Oncol. 2015;6(5):370–9.
59. Seeman TE, Berkman LF, Kohout F, Lacroix A, Glynn R, Blazer D. Intercommunity variations in the association between social ties and mortality in the elderly: a comparative analysis of three communities. Ann Epidemiol. 1993;3(4):325–35.
60. Dale W, Hemmerich J, Kamm A, et al. Geriatric assessment improves prediction of surgical outcomes in older adults undergoing pancreaticoduodenectomy: a prospective cohort study. Ann Surg. 2014;259(5):960–5.

61. Hempenius L, Slaets JP, van Asselt DZ, et al. Interventions to prevent postoperative delirium in elderly cancer patients should be targeted at those undergoing nonsuperficial surgery with special attention to the cognitive impaired patients. Eur J Surg Oncol. 2015;41(1):28–33.
62. Huisman MG, Audisio RA, Ugolini G, et al. Screening for predictors of adverse outcome in onco-geriatric surgical patients: a multicenter prospective cohort study. Eur J Surg Oncol. 2015;41(7):844–51.
63. Kaibori M, Ishizaki M, Matsui K, et al. Geriatric assessment as a predictor of postoperative complications in elderly patients with hepatocellular carcinoma. Langenbeck's Arch Surg. 2016;401(2):205–14.
64. Kenig J, Richter P, Zychiewicz B, Olszewska U. Vulnerable Elderly Survey 13 as a screening method for frailty in Polish elderly surgical patient--prospective study. Pol Przegl Chir. 2014;86(3):126–31.
65. Kenig J, Zychiewicz B, Olszewska U, Richter P. Screening for frailty among older patients with cancer that qualify for abdominal surgery. J Geriatr Oncol. 2015;6(1):52–9.
66. Korc-Grodzicki B, Sun SW, Zhou Q, et al. Geriatric assessment as a predictor of delirium and other outcomes in elderly patients with cancer. Ann Surg. 2015;261(6):1085–90.
67. Kwon S, Symons R, Yukawa M, Dasher N, Legner V, Flum DR. Evaluating the association of preoperative functional status and postoperative functional decline in older patients undergoing major surgery. Am Surg. 2012;78(12):1336–44.
68. participants P, Audisio RA, Pope D, et al. Shall we operate? Preoperative assessment in elderly cancer patients (PACE) can help. A SIOG surgical task force prospective study. Crit Rev Oncol Hematol. 2008;65(2):156–63.
69. Pope D, Ramesh H, Gennari R, et al. Pre-operative assessment of cancer in the elderly (PACE): a comprehensive assessment of underlying characteristics of elderly cancer patients prior to elective surgery. Surg Oncol. 2006;15(4):189–97.
70. Revenig LM, Canter DJ, Kim S, et al. Report of a simplified frailty score predictive of short-term postoperative morbidity and mortality. J Am Coll Surg. 2015;220(5):904–11. e901.
71. Revenig LM, Canter DJ, Taylor MD, et al. Too frail for surgery? Initial results of a large multidisciplinary prospective study examining preoperative variables predictive of poor surgical outcomes. J Am Coll Surg. 2013;217(4):665–70. e661.
72. Shutt TA, Philips P, Scoggins CR, McMasters KM, Martin RC 2nd. Permanent loss of preoperative independence in elderly patients undergoing hepatectomy: key factor in the informed consent process. J Gastrointest Surg. 2016;20(5):936–44.
73. Tegels JJ, de Maat MF, Hulsewe KW, Hoofwijk AG, Stoot JH. Value of geriatric frailty and nutritional status assessment in predicting postoperative mortality in gastric cancer surgery. J. Gastrointest. Surg. 2014;18(3):439–45. discussion 445–436
74. Scally CP, Yin H, Birkmeyer JD, Wong SL. Comparing perioperative processes of care in high and low mortality centers performing pancreatic surgery. J Surg Oncol. 2015;112(8):866–71.
75. Birkmeyer JD, Siewers AE, Finlayson EV, et al. Hospital volume and surgical mortality in the United States. N Engl J Med. 2002;346(15):1128–37.
76. Gouma DJ, Van Geenen RC, van Gulik TM, et al. Rates of complications and death after pancreaticoduodenectomy: risk factors and the impact of hospital volume. Ann Surg. 2000;232(6):786–95.
77. Begg CB, Cramer LD, Hoskins WJ, Brennan MF. Impact of hospital volume on operative mortality for major cancer surgery. JAMA. 1998;280(20):1747–51.
78. Finlayson EV, Goodney PP, Birkmeyer JD. Hospital volume and operative mortality in cancer surgery: a national study. Arch Surg. 2003;138(7):721–5.
79. Colavita PD, Tsirline VB, Belyansky I, et al. Regionalization and outcomes of hepato-pancreato-biliary cancer surgery in USA. J Gastrointest Surg. 2014;18(3):532–41.
80. Kanhere H, Trochsler M, Kanhere M, Lord A, Maddern G. Pancreaticoduodenectomy: outcomes in a low-volume, specialised Hepato Pancreato biliary unit. World J Surg. 2014;38(6):1484–90.
81. van der Geest LG, Besselink MG, Busch OR, et al. Elderly patients strongly benefit from centralization of pancreatic cancer surgery: a population-based study. Ann Surg Oncol. 2016;23(6):2002–9.

82. Nathan H, Cameron JL, Choti MA, Schulick RD, Pawlik TM. The volume-outcomes effect in hepato-pancreato-biliary surgery: hospital versus surgeon contributions and specificity of the relationship. J Am Coll Surg. 2009;208(4):528–38.
83. Schmidt CM, Turrini O, Parikh P, et al. Effect of hospital volume, surgeon experience, and surgeon volume on patient outcomes after pancreaticoduodenectomy: a single-institution experience. Arch Surg. 2010;145(7):634–40.
84. Hyder O, Sachs T, Ejaz A, Spolverato G, Pawlik TM. Impact of hospital teaching status on length of stay and mortality among patients undergoing complex hepatopancreaticobiliary surgery in the USA. J Gastrointest Surg. 2013;17(12):2114–22.
85. Ejaz A, Spolverato G, Kim Y, et al. The impact of resident involvement on surgical outcomes among patients undergoing hepatic and pancreatic resections. Surgery. 2015;158(2):323–30.
86. Silver JK, Baima J. Cancer prehabilitation: an opportunity to decrease treatment-related morbidity, increase cancer treatment options, and improve physical and psychological health outcomes. Am J Phys Med Rehabil. 2013;92(8):715–27.
87. Cooper AB, Holmes HM, des Bordes JK, et al. Role of neoadjuvant therapy in the multimodality treatment of older patients with pancreatic cancer. J Am Coll Surg. 2014;219(1):111–20.
88. Carli F, Charlebois P, Stein B, et al. Randomized clinical trial of prehabilitation in colorectal surgery. Br J Surg. 2010;97(8):1187–97.
89. Dronkers JJ, Lamberts H, Reutelingsperger IM, et al. Preoperative therapeutic programme for elderly patients scheduled for elective abdominal oncological surgery: a randomized controlled pilot study. Clin Rehabil. 2010;24(7):614–22.
90. Gillis C, Li C, Lee L, et al. Prehabilitation versus rehabilitation: a randomized control trial in patients undergoing colorectal resection for cancer. Anesthesiology. 2014;121(5):937–47.
91. Cho H, Yoshikawa T, Oba MS, et al. Matched pair analysis to examine the effects of a planned preoperative exercise program in early gastric cancer patients with metabolic syndrome to reduce operative risk: the Adjuvant Exercise for General Elective Surgery (AEGES) study group. Ann Surg Oncol. 2014;21(6):2044–50.
92. Kim DJ, Mayo NE, Carli F, Montgomery DL, Zavorsky GS. Responsive measures to prehabilitation in patients undergoing bowel resection surgery. Tohoku J Exp Med. 2009;217(2):109–15.
93. Dunne DF, Jack S, Jones RP, et al. Randomized clinical trial of prehabilitation before planned liver resection. Br J Surg. 2016;103(5):504–12.
94. Singh F, Newton RU, Galvao DA, Spry N, Baker MK. A systematic review of pre-surgical exercise intervention studies with cancer patients. Surg Oncol. 2013;22(2):92–104.
95. Timmerman H, de Groot JF, Hulzebos HJ, de Knikker R, Kerkkamp HE, van Meeteren NL. Feasibility and preliminary effectiveness of preoperative therapeutic exercise in patients with cancer: a pragmatic study. Physiother Theory Pract. 2011;27(2):117–24.
96. Fearon KC, Jenkins JT, Carli F, Lassen K. Patient optimization for gastrointestinal cancer surgery. Br J Surg. 2013;100(1):15–27.
97. Mustian KM, Griggs JJ, Morrow GR, et al. Exercise and side effects among 749 patients during and after treatment for cancer: a University of Rochester Cancer Center Community Clinical Oncology Program Study. Support Care Cancer. 2006;14(7):732–41.
98. Yeo TP, Burrell SA, Sauter PK, et al. A progressive postresection walking program significantly improves fatigue and health-related quality of life in pancreas and periampullary cancer patients. J Am Coll Surg. 2012;214(4):463–75. discussion 475–467
99. August DA, Huhmann MBASPEN. Clinical guidelines: nutrition support therapy during adult anticancer treatment and in hematopoietic cell transplantation. J Parenter Enter Nutr. 2009;33(5):472–500.
100. Group VATPNCS. Perioperative total parenteral nutrition in surgical patients. N Engl J Med. 1991;325(8):525–32.
101. Evans DC, Martindale RG, Kiraly LN, Jones CM. Nutrition optimization prior to surgery. Nutr Clin Pract. 2014;29(1):10–21.
102. Drover JW, Dhaliwal R, Weitzel L, Wischmeyer PE, Ochoa JB, Heyland DK. Perioperative use of arginine-supplemented diets: a systematic review of the evidence. J Am Coll Surg. 2011;212(3):385–99. e381.

103. Hasadsri L, Wang BH, Lee JV, et al. Omega-3 fatty acids as a putative treatment for traumatic brain injury. J Neurotrauma. 2013;30(11):897–906.
104. Calder PC. Omega-3 fatty acids and inflammatory processes. Forum Nutr. 2010;2(3):355–74.
105. Zhu XH, YF W, Qiu YD, Jiang CP, Ding YT. Effect of early enteral combined with par-enteral nutrition in patients undergoing pancreaticoduodenectomy. World J Gastroenterol. 2013;19(35):5889–96.
106. Jie B, Jiang Z-M, Nolan MT, Zhu S-N, Yu K, Kondrup J. Impact of preoperative nutritional support on clinical outcome in abdominal surgical patients at nutritional risk. Nutrition. 2012;28(10):1022–7.
107. Lin D-X, Li X, Ye Q-W, Lin F, Li L-L, Zhang Q-Y. Implementation of a fast-track clinical pathway decreases postoperative length of stay and hospital charges for liver resection. Cell Biochem Biophys. 2011;61(2):413–9.
108. Aloia TA, Zimmitti G, Conrad C, Gottumukkala V, Kopetz S, Vauthey JN. Return to intended oncologic treatment (RIOT): a novel metric for evaluating the quality of oncosurgical therapy for malignancy. J Surg Oncol. 2014;110(2):107–14.
109. Hall T, Dennison A, Bilku D, Metcalfe M, Garcea G. Enhanced recovery programmes in hepato-biliary and pancreatic surgery: a systematic review. Ann R Coll Surg Engl. 2012;94(5):318–26.
110. Connor S, Cross A, Sakowska M, Linscott D, Woods J. Effects of introducing an enhanced recovery after surgery programme for patients undergoing open hepatic resection. HPB. 2013;15(4):294–301.
111. Grol R, Grimshaw J. From best evidence to best practice: effective implementation of change in patients' care. Lancet. 2003;362(9391):1225–30.
112. Hughes M, Coolsen MM, Aahlin EK, et al. Attitudes of patients and care providers to enhanced recovery after surgery programs after major abdominal surgery. J Surg Res. 2015;193(1):102–10.
113. Day RW, Cleeland CS, Wang XS, et al. Patient-reported outcomes accurately measure the value of an enhanced recovery program in liver surgery. J Am Coll Surg. 2015;221(6):1023–30. e1021–1022.

Perioperative Fluid Management for Hepatopancreatobiliary Surgery

2

Mary Fischer, Camilo Correa-Gallego, and William R. Jarnagin

Introduction

Fluid therapy is fundamental to the perioperative care of the HPB surgical patient, but the best fluid strategy remains unclear. Many questions have arisen, and much controversy has emerged regarding how much fluid should be given perioperatively, which fluids should be given, when they should be given, and whether outcomes can be influenced. In fact, one might ask whether fluid therapy can even make a difference in the ultimate oncologic outcome.

Fluid management strategies have undergone several shifts over the past 50 years. Prior to the 1960s, fluid restriction during the intraoperative period was widely practiced. In the early 1960s, it was demonstrated that major surgery was associated with fluid requirements that significantly exceeded the usual rate of fluid maintenance. As a result, fluid administration became less restrictive.

A decade later, the choice of fluid became the subject of intense debate and continued until today, as colloid versus crystalloid controversies are still raging on. In the late 1980s and early 1990s, the concept of achieving a supernormal oxygen delivery attracted much interest. More recently, there is arguably a shift toward avoiding anesthesia-related harm after surgery such as prescribing individualized goal-directed fluid therapy (GDFT).

Because preoperative fluid status and perioperative fluid shifts are difficult to measure, and "correct" therapy remains uncertain, the assessment of intravascular volume status, the maintenance of hemodynamics, and the need for transfusion for

M. Fischer, MD
Department of Anesthesiology and Critical Care, Memorial Sloan Kettering Cancer Center, New York, NY, USA

C. Correa-Gallego, MD (✉) • W.R. Jarnagin, MD
Memorial Sloan Kettering Cancer Center, New York, NY, USA
e-mail: correagj@mskcc.org

© Springer International Publishing AG 2018
F.G. Rocha, P. Shen (eds.), *Optimizing Outcomes for Liver and Pancreas Surgery*, DOI 10.1007/978-3-319-62624-6_2

patients undergoing hepatopancreatobiliary surgery remain an important clinical decision in the perioperative setting.

There are three fluid types used for fluid therapy, crystalloids, colloids, and blood. Each has its unique characteristics and part to play in fluid therapy. This chapter aims to present modern care principles and guidelines for perioperative fluid therapy; review data on outcomes as they relate to type, amount, and timing of fluid; and review fluid management specific for HPB surgery.

Conceptual Framework for Fluid Balance: Fluid Compartments

Accurate replacement of fluid deficits requires an understanding of the distribution volume of body fluids. For a person weighing 70 kg, total body water (TBW) is about 42 L (60% of weight in kg). The total body water exists within discreet but dynamic fluid compartment. Two-thirds of the TBW (28 L) is intracellular water. The remaining third (14 liters) in the extracellular compartment is divided into the intravascular (5 L, one-third) and extravascular (9 L, two-thirds) compartments. Blood is composed of around 60% plasma (extracellular compartment) and 40% red and white blood cells and platelets (intracellular compartment). Plasma consists of inorganic ions (predominantly sodium chloride), simple molecules such as urea, and larger organic molecules (predominantly albumin and the globulins) dissolved in water. Interstitial fluid bathes the cells and allows metabolic substrates and wastes to be diffused between the capillaries and cells in the tissue. Excess free interstitial fluid enters the lymphatic channels and is ultimately returned to the plasma. The majority of the interstitial water exists within a proteoglycan matrix in a gel form. The transcellular fluids are extracellular and include the cerebrospinal fluid, aqueous humor, and pleural, pericardial, and synovial fluids.

The cell wall separates the intracellular compartment from the extracellular compartment. The capillary endothelium and the walls of arteries and veins divide the extracellular compartment into the intravascular and the interstitial (tissue or extravascular) compartments. Water moves freely through cell and vessel walls and is distributed throughout all these compartments. The energy-dependent Na/K ATPase in cell walls extrudes Na and Cl and maintains a sodium gradient across the cell membrane: Na+ is an extracellular ion. The capillary endothelium is freely permeable to small ions such as Na and Cl but is relatively impermeable to larger molecules such as albumin and the semisynthetic colloids, e.g., gelatins and starches, which are therefore normally theoretically maintained in the intravascular space [1] (Fig. 2.1).

Colloid oncotic pressure (COP) is the osmotic pressure exerted by the macromolecules (the colloid molecules). Solutes that can pass freely across a semipermeable membrane do not generate any oncotic pressure – they are effectively a component of the solvent with respect to that membrane. Where membranes are selectively permeable to solutes, the water content of the fluid compartments is dictated by solute distribution as water moves down any osmotic gradient to produce isotonicity. The COP of the plasma is only one of several forces determining fluid flux at the vascular membrane. Starling in 1896 first described the forces affecting the flux of fluid across the capillary membrane [2]. These forces can be expressed in the following equation:

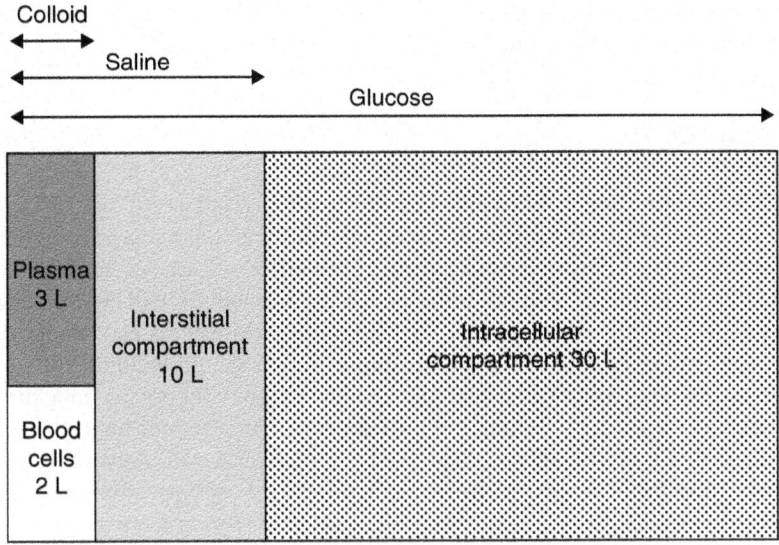

Fig. 2.1 Model for volumes of distribution of isotonic colloid, saline, and glucose solutions

$$Q_v \propto K\left[\left(P_c - P_i\right) - \sigma_c\left(\pi_c - \pi_i\right)\right]$$

in which Q_v = total flow of fluid across the capillary membrane, K = fluid filtration coefficient, P_c = capillary hydrostatic pressure, P_i = interstitial hydrostatic pressure, σ_c = reflection coefficient, π_c = capillary COP (plasma), and π_i = interstitial COP.

The filtration coefficient (K) is a function of the permeability and surface area of the capillary bed in question. The numeric value represents the net volume of fluid crossing the capillary membrane under a specific set of conditions. The reflection coefficient ($\acute{O}_c$) is a mathematical expression (from 0 to 1) of the capillary membrane's permeability to a particular substance. Thus, the reflection coefficient will vary with both the tissue bed and substance in question. If a substance is completely permeable to the capillary membrane, the reflection coefficient will be 0; if it is totally impermeable, the coefficient will be 1. For protein, the approximate reflection coefficients for liver and lung are 0.1 and 0.7, respectively [3]. The reflection coefficient for albumin, the source of 60% of the normal oncotic pressure in the pulmonary circulation, is approximately 0.7. When a pulmonary insult creates a leaky capillary state, the protein-lung reflection coefficient may decrease to approximately 0.4 [4].

The composition of administered fluids will therefore dictate their distribution. Pure water expands all body fluid compartments and therefore provides minimal expansion of the intravascular volume. Intravenous infusion of an isotonic solution of sodium chloride expands only the extracellular compartment and will increase intravascular volume by about one-fifth of the volume infused. Colloid solutions containing large molecules are maintained within the circulation, at least initially, and so provide greater intravascular volume expansion per unit infused. Lamke and Liljedahl demonstrated that 90 min following infusion of 1000 ml of 6% hetastarch, albumin, or normal saline (NS) in postoperative patients, 75% and 50% of the hetastarch and albumin, respectively, still remain in the intravascular space, whereas only less than 20% of NS remained [5].

Choice of Fluids

The choice of intravenous fluids may broadly be categorized as colloids and crystalloids. Crystalloids are effective and appropriate for the initial management of extracellular compartment losses associated with HPB surgery. Large crystalloid therapy can lead to a degree of hemodilution and a diminished COP. This reduction in plasma COP has been associated with the development of edema and transudates. It is therefore appropriate that large fluid administration should include colloid solutions in an attempt to minimize interstitial edema within vital organs. In addition to their effects on oncotic pressure, colloids are larger in size, causing the replaced volume to remain in the intravascular space for a longer duration than crystalloids. Naturally occurring protein colloids include human serum albumin, whereas hydroxyethyl starches (HES), dextrans, and gelatins comprise some of the synthetic colloids. Whether colloids may prove more beneficial over crystalloids as they are more resistant to crossing the microvascular membrane, thus requiring a lower volume for resuscitation, continues to be debated.

The Essentials of Intravenous Fluids

Crystalloids

There are at least 122 different formulations marketed in the USA for use in adult, pediatric, and veterinary clinical care. Many of these are variations of the fluids listed in Table 2.1. The crystalloid group includes aqueous dextrose, saline, and balanced salt solutions. Lactated Ringer's (LR) and Normosol solutions consist of a

Table 2.1 Electrolyte composition (mmol/l) of commonly available crystalloids

Electrolyte	Plasma	0.9% NaCl	Ringer's lactate, Hartmann's	Plasma-Lyte®	Sterofundin®
Sodium	140	154	131	140	140
Potassium	5	0	5	5	4
Chloride	100	154	111	98	127
Calcium	2.2	0	2	0	2.5
Magnesium	1	0	1	1.5	1
Bicarbonate	24	0	0	0	0
Lactate	1	0	29	0	0
Acetate	0	0	0	27	24
Gluconate	0	0	0	23	0
Maleate	0	0	0	0	5

Plasma-Lyte® from Baxter International (Deerfield, IL, USA)
Sterofundin® from B. Braun (Melsungen, Germany)

number of electrolytes that are present in the plasma, whereas 0.9% saline is made up of only sodium and chloride.

The effect of these solutions on the intravascular, extracellular, and intracellular fluid volumes varies with their electrolyte composition. The dilute solutions will expand the total body water volume because the amount of electrolytes added to the extracellular fluid is small and the cell membranes are permeable to the water.

Colloids

Hydroxyethyl Starch

The hydroxyethyl starch (HES) compounds are a group of polydisperse synthetic colloids that resembles glycogen structurally. Hetastarch is primarily excreted via the kidneys with 40–50% of the administered dose eliminated within 48 h [6].

There are four FDA-approved HES solutions on the market: 6% HES 450/0.7 in sodium chloride injection (Hespan, B. Braun Medical), 6% HES 450/0.7 in physiological solution (Hextend, BioTime), 6% HES 130/0.4 in normal saline (Voluven, Fresenius Kabi), and a generic equivalent to Hespan (Hetastarch, Teva Pharmaceuticals). The newer generation of HES solutions is the iso-oncotic plasma volume expander 6% HES 130/0.4 in 0.9% sodium chloride for injection. HES 130/0.4 has lower mean molecular weight and molar substitution, which result in no significant plasma accumulation. Increased plasma accumulation has been associated with coagulation and renal dysfunction [7].

Albumin

Albumin is a naturally occurring plasma protein which provides approximately 70% of the plasma colloid oncotic pressure in normal human subjects. Human albumin is available for infusions as either 5% or 25% solution. The 5% solution is approximately iso-oncotic with that of normal subjects, whereas the 25% solution is markedly hyper-oncotic. Human albumin is prepared from human plasma following a heating process for 10 h at 60 °C. Volume for volume, human albumin solution is more than twice as expensive as HES and significantly more expensive than crystalloid solutions, such as NS or LR, and can account for a significant portion of or addition to the total pharmacy budget in certain hospitals [8]. A human-derived product, albumin has the potential to be associated with increased risk of viral infection and prion contamination when compared with synthetic colloids [9].

Plasma protein fraction (PPF) is a 5% solution of selected proteins prepared from pooled human blood, serum, or plasma. It undergoes the same pasteurization process used for albumin and is a mixture of proteins consisting mostly of albumin in an amount equal to or greater than 83% of the total protein composition. Although albumin solution may be more purified and contains a greater percentage of albumin (>93%), the two solutions are similar in costs and used interchangeably.

Dextrans

Dextrans are high molecular weight D-glucose polymers linked by alpha 1,6 bonds into predominantly linear macromolecules. The products in current clinical use are described by their MW: dextran 40 and dextran 70 having MWs of 40,000 and 70,000 dalton, respectively.

Is There Anything New in the Choice of Fluid Solution to Administer?

Results of clinical trials comparing the effects of specific crystalloid and colloids have been conflicting but continue to raise concerns. Studies have demonstrated the predictability of acidosis following intraoperative administration of saline-based fluid [10–12]. Although the non-anion gap metabolic acidosis has historically been felt to be benign, there is now increasing evidence that it may contribute to acute renal injury [13, 14]. In a study of nearly 23,000 patients, hyperchloremic metabolic acidosis occurred in 22% of patients and was independently associated with increased morbidity and mortality [15]. Mortality at 30 days was 3% versus 1.9% in patients who did not have metabolic acidosis, and hospital lengths of stay increased by almost 1 day.

The choices of fluid administered intraoperatively can result in differences in the coagulation effects. Hespan in large volumes (>20 ml/kg) has been associated with reduced levels of coagulations factors, e.g., fibrinogen, factor VII, and von Willebrand's factor, and reduced platelet function beyond the effect of hemodilution [16, 17]. This has prompted the FDA to issue a warning against high-volume administration in its package insert.

In 2013, the FDA issued a black box warning that HES was not to be used in ICUs [18, 19]. A Cochrane review of colloid solutions and crystalloid solutions in 78 trials concluded that resuscitation with colloids did not reduce the risk of death and that HES increased mortality if the liver or kidneys were injured [20]. Another Cochrane review examined the effect on kidney function in more than 11,000 patients. HES increased the need for renal replacement therapy [21]; however, a safe volume of HES was not defined. There is no evidence that these deleterious effects of starch-based colloids occur with albumin.

Expert opinion recommends crystalloid solutions for routine surgery of short duration [22]. However, in major surgery, fluid therapy containing colloid and balanced salt solutions is recommended. In addition, although a black box warning for the use of starch solutions exists within the USA, there is limited data relative to their harm in the perioperative period. Careful consideration should occur in patients with known or acute renal injury and/or signs of coagulopathy or sepsis prior to administering starch solutions [22].

Most trials comparing different solutions have been performed among nonsurgical populations. Surgical patients are not the equivalent of the critically ill or septic patient. The trials comparing the effects of different solutions are not procedure specific. There is a lack of adequate studies in HPB surgery upon which to base a judgment whether selecting crystalloid or colloid fluid therapy influences morbidity. The ideal volume expander, whether crystalloid or colloid, for patients undergoing HPB surgery should be determined based on institution and physician preferences as there is little clinical difference between the two types when mortality is the outcome of interest. Many clinicians continue to use colloids in combination with crystalloids; however, crystalloids may be selected more often due to the high price of colloids.

Perioperative Issues Influencing Fluid Management

The assessment of intravascular volume status and optimization of hemodynamics remain an important clinical challenge [23]. This is particularly true for the intraoperative care of the patient undergoing HPB surgery, where rapid changes in hemodynamic parameters can be caused by anesthetics, blood loss, impaired cardiac contractility, and changes in systemic vascular resistance (SVR) and autonomic nervous system outflow [1].

Amount of Fluid

Traditional Practice of Intraoperative Fluid Administration

One of the most common interventions made by anesthesiologists is the administration of intravenous fluid. There are many opinions among anesthesiologists regarding fluid management in the operating room; nonetheless, as a whole, fluid administration is based on textbook guidelines for surgery-specific replacement of blood loss and maintenance fluid requirements. All anesthesiologists have some type of goal when making fluid management choices, such as maintaining adequate blood pressure, heart rate, or urine output.

Until recently, the general approach to perioperative intravascular volume management was the administration of large amounts of maintenance crystalloid fluids. This was based on the outdated premise that the preoperative patient was hypovolemic due to prolonged fasting and bowel preparation. Intraoperatively, in addition to ongoing losses from perspiration and urinary output, there was a widespread belief that surgical exposure required aggressive replacement of insensible fluid loss, often termed "third space" losses [24]. Further, hypotension during general and neuro-axial anesthesia was often treated as hypovolemia, triggering compensatory liberal intravenous (IV) fluid administration. There was the belief that the kidney would handle fluid overload but would be damaged by too little fluid [25].

Brandstrup was the first to propose an alternative to liberal intraoperative fluid management for abdominal surgery [26]. A series of trials followed that have shown patients could be managed successfully with quantities of fluids that previously would have been considered inadequate.

Are You Conservative or Liberal?

Past research to identify the perfect recipe of fluid administration during abdominal surgery suffered from standardization of regimens and the goals chosen to influence the amount of fluid prescribed. In a review of 80 prospective randomized studies comparing the effect of two different fixed fluid volumes on post-op outcome in surgery, it was concluded that there were too many differences in definitions, methodology, and results to support evidence-based guidelines for procedure-specific perioperative fixed volume regimen (yet please avoid crystalloid overload) [27]. The majority of these studies did not include a significant number of major hepatic or pancreatic resections.

Retrospective reviews of fluid management in patients undergoing pancreatectomy did not demonstrate a clinically significant association between postoperative morbidity and intraoperative fluid management [28, 29]. A prospective randomized controlled trial (RCT) of intraoperative 3% hypertonic saline (HYS) (moderately restrictive) vs 15 ml/kg/h Ringer's lactate (liberal) reported a statistically significant reduction in complications for the HYS cohort in patients undergoing pancreatectomy [30]. At our institution, a RCT of 330 patients undergoing a pancreatectomy showed no difference on perioperative complications comparing intraoperative 6 ml/kg/h (restrictive, i.e., standard) vs 12 ml/kg/h (liberal) fluid administration [31].

Studies of perioperative fluid therapy have been related to, among other things, nausea and vomiting, pain, tissue oxygenation, cardiopulmonary disorders, duration of hospital stay, and bowel recovery time. However, the relevance of each individual target depends on the examined type and extent of surgery, which in turn has an enormous influence on changes and significance of these outcome parameters. High-volume crystalloids in order to lessen postoperative nausea and vomiting and dizziness may be beneficial for a patient undergoing a laparoscopic cholecystectomy in the ambulatory setting, [32] but may not be the major goals for patients undergoing major HPB surgeries. Both Lavu and Grant showed no difference in delayed gastric emptying, pancreatic fistula, and wound infection in their recipe trials for perioperative fluid management for pancreatectomies [30, 31].

Contemporary Practice of Perioperative Fluid Administration

While liberal, standard, conservative, or restrictive has been and still remains in the eye of the beholder, contemporary fluid therapists emphasize that administering more fluid (typically crystalloid) than is needed to patients undergoing surgery has been associated with harm [25]. In order to improve patient outcome, the endpoint for fluid therapy is an adequate blood flow to all organs including traumatized tissue. Preoperative volume loading and routine replacement maintenance of highly insensible and third space losses should be abandoned in favor of rational fluid therapy [33], zero-balance fluid therapy [34], or demand-related fluid protocols [35], in order to avoid any collateral damage that may be caused by interstitial edema.

In addition, it's wrong to compare two classes of fluids, crystalloid and colloid, and instead the focus should be on when to use these fluids. Replacement of fluid should be guided by losses due to fluid shifting or acute bleeding which have to be replaced with iso-oncotic colloids, presuming the vascular barrier is intact and acknowledging that colloidal volume effects are context sensitive. While circulatory surrogates can be monitored for the replacement of plasma losses, deficits from the extracellular compartment (EC) cannot be monitored. Therefore, losses from the EC space should be replaced based on a simple protocol: use the right kind of fluid in the right amount at the right time [35].

There is evidence-based medicine to support this contemporary approach to fluid therapy. Mechanical bowel preparation and overnight fasting are becoming less common and are no longer recommended before most abdominal operations [25]. The American Society of Anesthesiologists (ASA) recommends that patients consume a clear carbohydrate beverage 2–23 h before undergoing surgery [36]. Intraoperative evaporative fluid losses during major abdominal surgery are at most 1 cc/kg/h [37]. Modern tracer studies do not support the existence of a third space [38]. Therefore, filling of this theoretical space is moot and the term should be abandoned; fluid is either intravascular or shifted into the interstitium. Conversely, the administration of excess fluid may result in tissue edema during surgery [39, 40].

Endpoints and Monitor

Focusing on intraoperative fluid management, the challenge is to find the optimal balance while achieving two primary rational goals: establish and maintain central euvolemia, and avoid administering inadequate or excessive fluid with a high salt content. Hypovolemia may lead to hypoperfusion, bowel ischemia, organ dysfunction, and increased adverse outcomes. Conversely, if we allow patients to become overloaded with fluid, edema, organ dysfunction, postoperative ileus, and increased adverse outcomes may result [41] (Fig. 2.2).

The standard approach used to achieve these goals uses maintenance background fluid therapy that replenishes fluid lost by urinary output as well as perspiration. Blood loss and fluid shifts during major surgery may require additional fluid usually as fluid boluses. It is accepted practice to adjust the dose of fluid in response to some form of endpoint. Conventional endpoints include urine output, blood pressure, and heart rate. For the higher-risk patient or higher-risk surgery, basic invasive monitoring such as arterial pressure and central venous pressure may be added.

Despite these clear physiologic goals and rational thinking, traditional perioperative fluid management strategy is unreliable. Excess fluid may be administered under conditions that are incorrectly interpreted as fluid deficit. Empiric fluid management strategy has the potential of leading to overload, thus prolonging mechanical ventilation and hospital length of stay (LOS), and causing worse overall outcomes [42]. If there are complications from fluid management, then the protocol, monitoring, or the parameters guiding our choices are flawed.

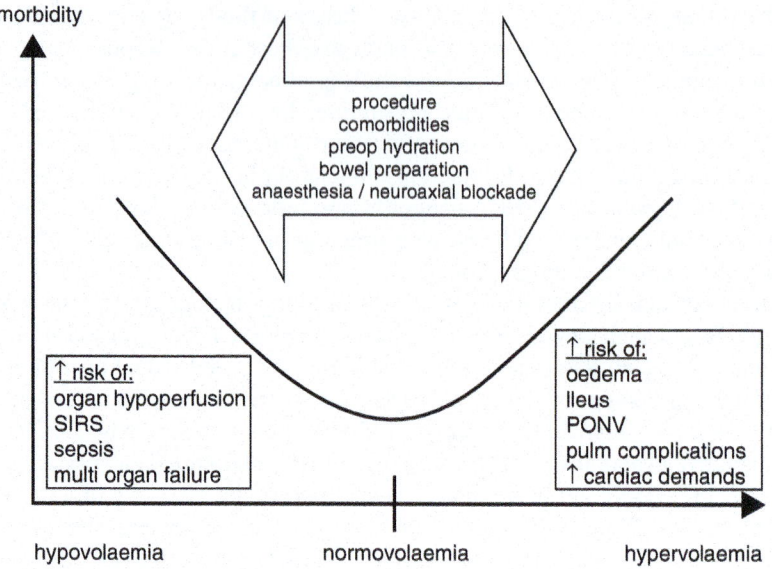

Fig. 2.2 Fluid load vs outcomes

Monitoring Fluid Volume and Determining Fluid Needs

Traditional Static Parameters

The key question to ensure tissue perfusion and circulatory optimization is whether administration of fluids would result in a clinically relevant increase in cardiac output (CO), thereby enhancing tissue perfusion and oxygen delivery [1, 23]. Furthermore, a strategy that does not require an empiric fluid challenge in order to determine whether fluid administration would increase cardiac output has the obvious benefit of preventing fluid administration and volume overload-induced complications in patients who are "fluid nonresponsive" [43]. Unfortunately, methods that have been used over the past decades to assess volume status and volume responsiveness are unreliable [1, 42–46]. The most rudimentary measure used, the mean arterial pressure (MAP), provides little useful information regarding actual blood flow or oxygen delivery [1]. Similarly, measurement of central venous pressure (CVP) via placement of a central catheter in combination with urine output is loose and highly indirect measures with a large degree of temporal lag that correlate very poorly with CO [1].

Blood Pressure and Heart Rate

Despite well-known limitations in assessing changes in heart rate and blood pressure during blood loss, the clinical diagnosis of hypovolemia is still often based on these two parameters and their response to a fluid challenge [47]. Because blood pressure is a regulated variable, a normal blood pressure does not necessarily reflect hemodynamic stability. Today we know that blood pressure is not the same as blood volume. A healthy patient may lose up to 25% of blood volume before there is a decrease in arterial pressure or an increase in heart rate [48]. Volume expansion-induced changes in arterial pressure-derived parameters are inconclusive for the detection of an increase in cardiac output and thus should not be used for fluid responsiveness evaluation in routine clinical care of patients undergoing high-risk surgery [49]. Similarly, these conventional measurements do not predict the development of complications [50, 51].

Urine Output (UOP)
The common assumption is that urine output has to be maintained above a certain level to prevent acute kidney injury (AKI), and therefore, low urine output should be treated with crystalloid boluses [52, 53]. Yet, in the perioperative period, oliguria defined as UOP < 0.5 ml/kg/h is extremely common and often occurs as a neurohormonal response to surgical stress, rendering it an unreliable marker of volume status. Kheterpal et al. in a large retrospective analysis showed that 85% of postoperative patients not developing AKI had a UOP less than 0.5 ml/kg/h, surprisingly significantly more patients than those who developed AKI (75%) [54]. The incidence of AKI and its impact on 30-day mortality differs among different types of abdominal surgeries [55]. While permissive oliguria during low CVP (LCVP)-assisted hepatectomy is associated with a transient biochemical alteration in estimated glomerular filtration rate, clinically relevant renal dysfunction is a very uncommon event [56].

Central Venous Pressure (CVP)
Although central venous pressure (CVP) is used almost universally to guide fluid therapy in hospitalized patients, there is very little evidence that supports the use of CVP to guide perioperative fluid therapy. CVP and pulmonary artery occlusion pressure (PAOP) or "wedge" pressure were designed to estimate volume status of the right and left ventricles. Unfortunately, CVP or PAOP has not shown adequate correlation with volume or flow status [57].

Dramatic changes in systemic hemodynamics may not be associated with any significant changes in CVP. The venous system contains approximately 70% of the total blood volume and is 30 times more compliant than arterial system; therefore, changes in blood volume within the veins are associated with relatively small changes in venous pressure.

Marik et al. [58], in an excellent meta-analysis, recommended that CVP not be used in the perioperative course because of its lack of accuracy. As demonstrated by his study, only about a half of patients administered with a fluid bolus will demonstrate a positive hemodynamic response to the intervention [58]. With a ROC of 0.56, the play of coin toss will be as helpful as CVP in predicting which patients will respond to a fluid challenge. If fluid resuscitation is guided by CVP, it is likely that patients will have volume overload and pulmonary edema. Insufficient data exists demonstrating any benefit of using CVP as a target for achieving goal-directed hemodynamic management or for improving patient outcomes. It is this imbalance of risk versus benefit that has influenced hepatobiliary anesthesiologists at our institution to abandon routine central venous line placement even while routinely practicing fluid-restricted liver resection.

Goal-Directed Therapy in the Perioperative Phase

Historical Perspective

Major surgery exposes patients to periods of cardiovascular insufficiency, either because of anesthesia-induced loss of vasomotor tone and baroreceptor responsiveness or because of blood loss and mechanical obstruction to blood flow. In all cases cardiac output (CO) will fall, and if the heart rate remains constant, stroke volume will fall as well as global oxygen delivery (DO_2), and then end-organ dysfunction may occur.

Until about 20 years ago, it was felt that these concerns about microcirculation were primarily academic and did not affect patient outcome. However, in the 1980s, Shoemaker observed that in postoperative surgical patients, once routine parameters like blood pressure and heart rate were stabilized, survivors had a consistently higher CO and DO_2 than those who subsequently died [59]. There is a surgery-associated reduction of global DO_2 that affects patient outcome. The initial trial to target what they referred to as survivor levels of DO_2 was successful [60]; subsequent trials resulted in worse outcomes [61–66]. It was assumed at the time that the risks associated with aggressive resuscitation and vasoactive drug therapies needed to achieve these levels of DO_2 could be detrimental. The trial by Gutierrez et al. [67] demonstrated that targeted threshold values of DO_2 were only effective at reducing long-term mortality if applied before the development of end-organ failure. Thus, presurgical intraoperative resuscitation to target goal-directed therapy has been termed preoptimization to connote that treatment begins before the stress is created.

Boyd's landmark study and numerous others showed that targeting DO_2 values above 600 ml/min/m^2 before the stress of surgery could decrease morbidity and mortality in high-risk surgical patients [68]. While initial results were encouraging, the acceptance of preoptimization strategies for surgical patients did not catch on. Preoptimization requires additional monitoring to measure DO_2 requiring one to treat those targets. In the 1980s, such monitoring always meant the insertion of a pulmonary artery catheter (PAC) . PAC itself caused increased major morbidity and mortality, which undermined interest in the concept of using physiological targets to optimize cardiovascular performance and improve outcomes. Over the intervening years, less invasive monitors (esophageal Doppler and pulse waveform contour analysis) capable of capturing flow-based hemodynamic variables have renewed interest in individualized goal-directed fluid therapy (GDFT) [43, 58, 69].

Frank-Starling Respiratory Variations: Dynamic Flow-Related Parameters

Positive pressure ventilation induces cyclic changes in intrathoracic pressures that transiently affect venous return, resulting in cyclic changes in stroke volume. During mechanical ventilation, respiratory variations in the arterial pressure are related to volume status. The degree of respiratory variations in systolic pressure, pulse pressure, stroke volume, and aortic flow accurately reflects volume (preload) responsiveness. These dynamic predictors of volume responsiveness are often referred to as systolic pressure variation (SPV), pulse pressure variation (PPV), and stroke volume variation (SVV). These dynamic flow-related parameters are more accurate than the static traditional parameters to identify fluid responsiveness [70]. Today most cardiac monitors analyze the arterial waveform automatically calculating the degree of these respiratory variations and providing a continuous numeric representation of the patient's volume status and volume responsiveness [71].

Perioperative goal-directed fluid therapy (PGDT) is a clinician-directed protocol that uses measurements of advanced hemodynamic parameters during surgery to guide fluid management [71]. The accurate assessment of hemodynamic parameters – SV, SVV, and CO – allows for individualized volume management and decreases variability among clinicians because fluids are given only when there is demonstrable fluid responsiveness. PGDT is based on the physiological principles outlined in the Frank-Starling curve describing the relationship between stroke volume and preload. These principles are based on the fact that SV is 1 of the 2 determinants of CO and that SV is the first parameter to change when a patient has volume loss. The natural phenomenon of SVV, which occurs due to normal changes in SV resulting from respiratory cycle – induced changes in venous return – acts as a small endogenous physiologic fluid challenge and can be used as an assessment of the Frank-Starling state (i.e., fluid responsiveness) of the left ventricle without the need for an empirical fluid challenge with exogenous fluids [70–73]. Because arterial pulse pressure is directly proportional to SV, SVV or PPV can be used to predict increases in CO in response to fluid administration with numbers roughly <8% corresponding to fluid nonresponsiveness and >14% corresponding to responsiveness [74, 75]. This strategy has the advantage of easy and relatively noninvasive monitoring through placement of a peripheral arterial catheter.

The Protocol

Fundamentally the only reason to give a patient a fluid challenge is to increase the stroke volume. This assumes that the patient is on the ascending portion of the Frank-Starling curve and has "recruitable" cardiac output. Once the left ventricle is functioning near the plateau on the Frank-Starling curve, fluid loading has little effect on cardiac output and only serves to increase tissue edema and to promote tissue dysoxia [43].

Two concepts drive GDFT: cardiac output optimization or preload dependence optimization. It has been suggested that giving fluid until the patient has reached the plateau of the Frank-Starling curve may be the way of preventing both hypovolemia and fluid overload. In clinical practice, this approach consists of giving fluid until flow parameters reach a plateau value (to prevent hypovolemia) and then to stop giving any additional fluid volume (to prevent fluid overload). Patients who respond to a fluid challenge with an increase in SV of more than 10% are considered fluid responsive and may benefit from more fluid challenges. Euvolemic patients will

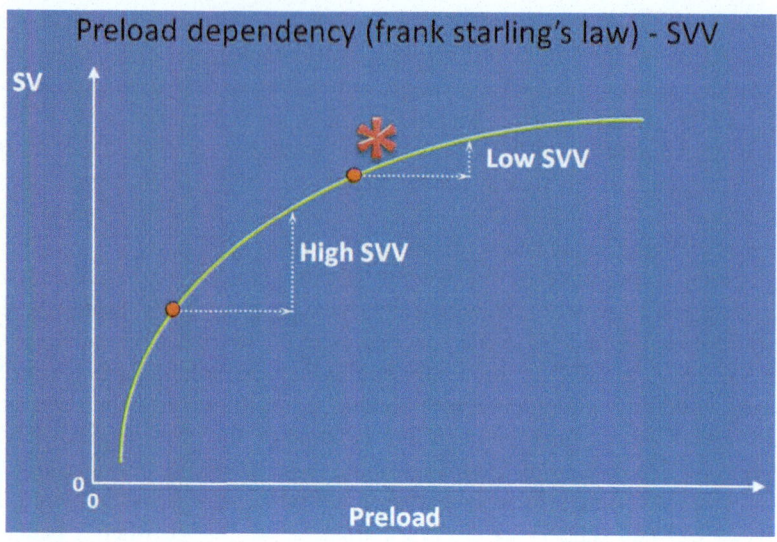

Fig. 2.3 Preload dependency

exhibit a change in SV < 10%. These patients are considered replete and fluid administration should stop [43].

Dynamic predictors of fluid responsiveness are not markers of blood volume, nor markers of cardiac preload, but markers of the position on the Frank-Starling curve during mechanical ventilation. In this regard, they have been proposed to identify when the plateau of the Frank-Starling relationship is reached without the need to give fluid or measure flow. High respiratory variations reflect that the heart is working on the steep part of the relationship (indicating preload dependence), whereas low respiratory variations reflect that the heart is working on the plateau of the relationship (indicating a preload independence) [43] (Fig. 2.3).

Preload dependence optimization (SVV or PPV minimization) dictates the fluid boluses aiming at keeping the value below a threshold number. There is a wide range of protocols available for the perioperative setting. They take into account patient risk and type of surgery, vascular access, and the hemodynamic monitor chosen [76] (Fig. 2.4).

Benefit of Perioperative Goal-Directed Therapy (PGDT)

Recent research has demonstrated the clinical benefit of PGDT on patient recovery, including postsurgical complications and reduced hospital length of stay (LOS) [77]. A stratified meta-analysis of 5021 patients from 34 randomized controlled trials compared a restrictive fluid therapy approach with either a liberal fluid therapy without hemodynamic goals (11 studies, 1160 patients) or PGDT (23 studies, 3861 patients) [77]. The outcomes for patients receiving liberal use of fluid without

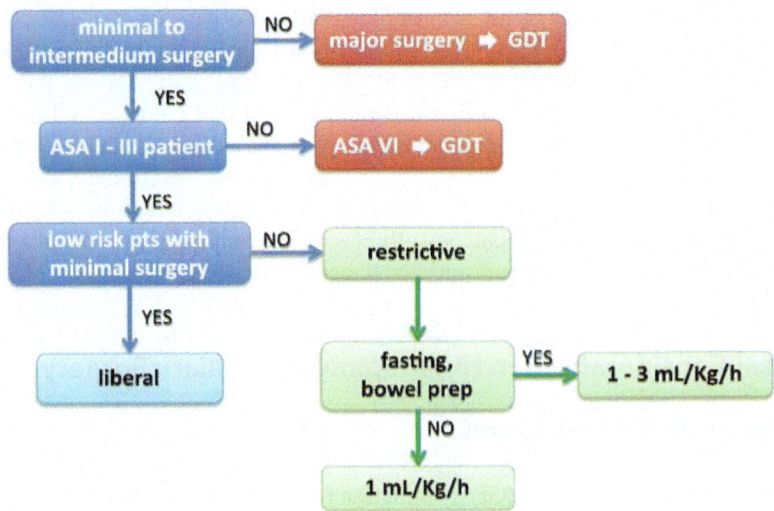

Fig. 2.4 Fluid flow chart

hemodynamic goals were not equivalent to those for patients receiving PGDT, although patients in the PGDT and liberal therapy groups received more fluid than patients in the restrictive groups, but with very different effects. Patients in the liberal fluid group had a higher risk for pneumonia and an increased time to first bowel movement [77]. Patients in the PGDT group had a lower risk for pneumonia, fewer renal complications, and shorter LOS. Liberal use of fluids during surgery produced inferior patient outcomes relative to PGDT [77]. Other studies of PGDT demonstrated reduced gastrointestinal complications and reduced infections relative to control conditions [78, 79].

The recently completed OPTIMISE trial evaluated 734 high-risk patients who underwent major gastrointestinal surgery with or without PGDT [41]. After adjusting for risk factors, compliance with the protocol, and excluding the ten patients per center who discontinued the trial, the decrease in postsurgical complications was significant [41]. The primary outcome, a composite measure of complications at 30 days postsurgery, trended toward lower values in the PGDT group relative to usual care (36.6% vs 43.4%; $p = 0.07$). Similarly, 180-day mortality was reduced in patients in the PGDT group relative to usual care (7.7% vs 11.6%, respectively; $p = 0.08$) [41]. These results suggest that PGDT could positively affect recovery and long-term survival after surgery. Other studies also have indicated PGDT benefits long-term outcomes [80].

Based on the growing evidence supporting PGDT and the need for professional guidance and education, clinical societies have published guidelines for operative fluid management in Europe. In 2015, the International Fluid Optimization Group published a consensus statement focusing on perioperative fluid therapy that recommended that all anesthesiologists should have a perioperative fluid plan using an algorithm guided by the most appropriate and accurate monitor [22]. While acknowledging that the benefits of perioperative goal-directed fluid therapy have yet to be proven, these experts believe the bulk of clinical research supports the implementation of a two-step GDT plan containing colloid and balanced solutions for major surgery. All anesthesiologists should implement a two-step GDT plan which is to begin immediately after induction of anesthesia. First, determine if the patient requires hemodynamic support or augmentation of cardiovascular function. Second, if the need is apparent and the patient is fluid responsive, fluid bolus therapy should be considered and guided by appropriate changes in stroke volume.

Special Considerations in Hepatopancreatobiliary Surgery

Pancreatic Anastomotic Leak

Postoperative gastrointestinal (GI) dysfunction is a frequent complication in surgical patients. Although the pathogenesis of GI complications is multifactorial [81], gut hypoperfusion, secondary to hypovolemia or cardiac dysfunction, plays a key role. While healthy patients may tolerate a 25–30% decrease in blood volume without changes in systemic arterial pressure or heart rate, splanchnic perfusion is compromised after 10–15% reduction in intravascular volume [82]. Selective vasoconstriction of mesenteric arterioles, mediated primarily by the renin-angiotensin system, contributes to the maintenance of systemic arterial pressure and the perfusion of non-mesenteric organs [83].This response occurs at the expense of splanchnic hypoperfusion that often outlasts the period of the hypovolemic insult or low-flow state, promoting abdominal organ damage. GI dysfunction presents with clinical signs and symptoms ranging from impaired motility [81] and inability to tolerate enteral diet to ischemic injury [84]. The type of surgery is important. For example, in abdominal surgery, poor oxygen delivery is significantly associated with anastomotic leak [82], especially in GI segments highly dependent on oxidative phosphorylation [85].

One of the postoperative GI complications of particular interest for pancreatic surgery, anastomotic leak, would seem to be the one most affected by excessive fluid administration. Hypervolemia (typically too much crystalloid) can damage the glycocalyx, a layer of membrane-bound proteoglycans and glycoproteins that coats healthy vascular endothelium and plays an important role in managing vascular permeability by acting as a second barrier to extravasation [86]. The most common manifestation of hypervolemia is edema of the gut wall and prolonged ileus. A study in rats undergoing a bowel resection and anastomosis showed that excessive crystalloid results in submucosal intestinal edema, lower anastomotic bursting pressure, and a decrease in the structural stability of intestinal anastomosis in the early postoperative period [87]. PGDT has been advocated as the strategy to best maintain oxygen delivery and minimize splanchnic hypoperfusion, and a meta-analysis of major surgeries has shown it decreases major and minor GI complications in the perioperative period [79].

At our institution, a hemodilution (HD) RCT for patients undergoing pancreatectomy in which the HD group received more fluid than the liberal arm of our RCT of liberal vs restrictive fluid therapy, there was an increased incidence of pancreaticoduodenectomy anastomotic leak (ANH 21% vs STD 7.7%) [88]. The strength in these studies may be bringing us closer to identifying a safe range of intraoperative fluids that do not effect this significant morbidity for patients undergoing pancreatectomy at high-volume centers. Both trials used traditional empiric endpoints. The authors know of no trials that have looked at PGDT and its effect on anastomotic leak for pancreatectomy.

Hepatectomy

A relationship between intraoperative blood loss, transfusion, and morbidity has been consistently shown for hepatic resection [89, 90]. In order to minimize blood loss, it is common anesthesia practice to perform liver resections with the central venous pressure less than 5 mmHg. Fluid management is an important aspect of LCVP anesthesia. The liver anesthesiologist that practices LCVP must be familiar with the physiology of the venous system in order to maintain hemodynamic stability. Unstressed blood volume is a sequestered volume that does not directly participate in venous return. Splanchnic veins and the liver with their high density of alpha adrenergic receptors play the role in maintaining a ratio between stressed and unstressed blood volume [91]. CVP can only be decreased by decreasing stressed volume which can only be done either from hypovolemia or venodilation. In order to maintain hemodynamics, decreased stressed volume and venous return can be restored by fluid infusion to fill up the increased venous capacity or venoconstriction. The clinical advantage of using a vasopressor is that it maintains tissue blood flow but avoids fluid infusion and liver congestion. Some extent of tolerance of permissive hypovolemia, and oliguria, as well as permissive relative hypotension is often needed. One cannot confuse the temporary improvement of blood pressure with liberal fluid or transfusion with an outcome benefit. However, a clinician that practices LCVP should realize that this restrictive fluid approach decreases the margin of safety. Up to 1000 cc of blood may be lost without change in standard hemodynamic parameters. However, beyond this point, even minor reduced venous return (preload) caused by the Pringle maneuver, vena cava compression or blood loss, or lifting the liver, can lead to sudden hemodynamic deterioration.

Using central venous catheters in order to practice LCVP, anesthetic technic has been very popular. Prior to liver transection, the CVP would be lowered to <5 mmHg by fluid restriction and/or pharmacologic manipulation and then raised at completion of transection in order to reach euvolemia. The numeric measurement of CVP itself is not reliable to determine volume status or responsiveness, and we have abandoned its routine use [46].

Early proactive GDT may compromise the effectiveness of LCVP on blood loss. The only GI complication that was not influenced by GDFT in Giglio's meta-analysis (which included no liver surgery) was liver injury [79]. The author hypothesized that this may be because the liver has flow protection already: the hepatic artery buffer. When the Pringle maneuver to minimize intraoperative blood loss is combined with LCVP, some degree of hypoperfusion may lead to liver tissue injury. Whether PGDT for liver surgery can rescue patients from this insult is unknown.

PGDT has been studied for liver resections as an approach to return to euvolemia after transection of the liver, and it was shown to be beneficial as part of an ERAS program [92, 93]. The authors recently completed a RCT using SVV minimization in the operating room to resuscitate patients undergoing LCVP-assisted hepatectomy. It allowed less fluid to be given intraoperatively without harm; however, there was no effect on 30-day morbidity among randomized groups, despite the fact that total intraoperative fluid was found to be independently associated with postoperative morbidity [94].

Perioperative Blood Manangement

Current Transfusion Management

It is becoming apparent that the risks associated with blood transfusion are not outweighed by the potential benefits in many surgical patients who are routinely transfused. Studies have shown that clinical outcomes in patients who are treated without (or with less) allogeneic blood transfusion are often comparable or better than the outcomes of similar patients who are transfused or receive more blood. As such, restrictive transfusion strategies are being increasingly recommended by practice guidelines [95]. Nonetheless, there has been a need for a more systematic approach with emphasis on improving patient outcomes (as opposed to mere focusing on usage of blood components) . Patient blood management (PBM) has recently been recognized by the World Health Organization (WHO) as a means to promote the availability of transfusion alternatives. However, the scope of PBM goes beyond transfusions as reflected by its definition: the timely application of evidence-based medicine designed to maintain hemoglobin concentration, optimize hemostasis, and minimize blood loss in an effort to improve patient outcome. This definition is derived from the observation that the vast majority of transfusion in the perioperative period can be attributed to low preoperative hemoglobin levels, excessive surgical blood loss, and inappropriate transfusion practices [96].

Accordingly PBM is built on four principles, anemia management, optimization of coagulation, adoption of blood conservation strategies, and patient-centered decision, with the single goal of measurable improved patient outcome [97]. In 2011, the Department of Health and Human Services stressed the importance of strengthening blood management systems to promote rational use of blood, cut down on the number of unnecessary transfusions, reduce transfusion risks, improve patient care, and save hospital resources. The American Board of Internal Medicine foundation, dedicated to advancing medical professionalism to improve health care, is endorsed by both the American Board of Anesthesiology and Surgery and has launched the Choosing Wisely campaign regarding optimal blood use [98].

Red cell transfusion is independently associated with adverse short-term outcomes for major HPB surgery [89, 90, 99, 100]. While the correlation of transfusion with complications should not be interpreted as causation, every effort should be made to reduce avoidable transfusions in these patients. A RCT from our institution looking at the effect of acute normovolemic hemodilution during liver surgery showed an effect on transfusion rate however did not reduce short-term or long-term morbidity [101, 102]. A restrictive approach to blood transfusion with a threshold of 7 g/dl has been shown to reduce blood use and not cause harm in liver resection patients [103].

Conclusion

While there is limited data to drive fluid management in this patient population, a rational approach that uses reliable monitoring devices and individualized physiologic endpoints should be advocated. To this end, it is imperative to consider different types of IV fluids as medications with specific indications, dosages, and adverse effects. There is no universal formula that applies to all hepatopancreatobiliary patients; rather, as discussed, the clinical situation should drive the type and amount of fluid administered.

During the operative and immediate postoperative period, it is essential to have a dedicated anesthesia team that specializes in these kinds of procedures and understands the physiology involved. The induced hemodynamic lability that inevitably accompanies LCVP-assisted liver resection leaves no room for error and requires quick, efficient, and safe management of potential complications. In the postoperative period, the approach to fluid management should similarly be guided by a rational approach that takes into consideration the consequences of both intravascular depletion and fluid overload.

References

1. Grocott MP, Mythen MG, Gan TJ. Perioperative fluid management and clinical outcomes in adults. Anesth Analg. 2005;100(4):1093–106.
2. Starling EH. On the absorption of fluids from the connective tissue spaces. J Physiol. 1896;19(4):312–26.
3. Wittmers LE Jr, Bartlett M, Johnson JA. Estimation of the capillary permeability coefficients of inulin in various tissues of the rabbit. Microvasc Res. 1976;11(1):67–78.
4. Brigham KL. Mechanisms of lung injury. Clin Chest Med. 1982;3(1):9–24.
5. Lamke LO, Liljedahl SO. Plasma volume changes after infusion of various plasma expanders. Resuscitation. 1976;5(2):93–102.
6. Yacobi A, Stoll RG, Sum CY, Lai CM, Gupta SD, Hulse JD. Pharmacokinetics of hydroxyethyl starch in normal subjects. J Clin Pharmacol. 1982;22(4):206–12.
7. Jungheinrich C, Scharpf R, Wargenau M, Bepperling F, Baron JF. The pharmacokinetics and tolerability of an intravenous infusion of the new hydroxyethyl starch 130/0.4 (6%, 500 mL) in mild-to-severe renal impairment. Anesth Analg. 2002;95(3):544–51. table of contents

8. Tarin Remohi MJ, Sanchez Arcos A, Santos Ramos B, Bautista Paloma J, Guerrero Aznar MD. Costs related to inappropriate use of albumin in Spain. Ann Pharmacother. 2000;34(10):1198–205.

9. Mishler JM. Synthetic plasma volume expanders--their pharmacology, safety and clinical efficacy. Clin Haematol. 1984;13(1):75–92.

10. Prough DS, White RT. Acidosis associated with perioperative saline administration: dilution or delusion? Anesthesiology. 2000;93(5):1167–9.

11. Rehm M, Orth V, Scheingraber S, Kreimeier U, Brechtelsbauer H, Finsterer U. Acid-base changes caused by 5% albumin versus 6% hydroxyethyl starch solution in patients undergoing acute normovolemic hemodilution: a randomized prospective study. Anesthesiology. 2000;93(5):1174–83.

12. Waters JH, Bernstein CA. Dilutional acidosis following hetastarch or albumin in healthy volunteers. Anesthesiology. 2000;93(5):1184–7.

13. Chowdhury AH, Cox EF, Francis ST, Lobo DN. A randomized, controlled, double-blind crossover study on the effects of 2-L infusions of 0.9% saline and plasma-lyte(R) 148 on renal blood flow velocity and renal cortical tissue perfusion in healthy volunteers. Ann Surg. 2012;256(1):18–24.

14. Yunos NM, Bellomo R, Hegarty C, Story D, Ho L, Bailey M. Association between a chloride-liberal vs chloride-restrictive intravenous fluid administration strategy and kidney injury in critically ill adults. JAMA. 2012;308(15):1566–72.

15. McCluskey SA, Karkouti K, Wijeysundera D, Minkovich L, Tait G, Beattie WS. Hyperchloremia after noncardiac surgery is independently associated with increased morbidity and mortality: a propensity-matched cohort study. Anesth Analg. 2013;117(2):412–21.

16. Martin G, Bennett-Guerrero E, Wakeling H, Mythen MG, el-Moalem H, Robertson K, et al. A prospective, randomized comparison of thromboelastographic coagulation profile in patients receiving lactated Ringer's solution, 6% hetastarch in a balanced-saline vehicle, or 6% hetastarch in saline during major surgery. J Cardiothorac Vasc Anesth. 2002;16(4):441–6.

17. Treib J, Haass A, Pindur G, Grauer MT, Seyfert UT, Treib W, et al. Influence of low molecular weight hydroxyethyl starch (HES 40/0.5-0.55) on hemostasis and hemorheology. Haemostasis. 1996;26(5):258–65.

18. Estrada CA, Murugan R. Hydroxyethyl starch in severe sepsis: end of starch era? Crit Care. 2013;17(2):310.

19. Zarychanski R, Abou-Setta AM, Turgeon AF, Houston BL, McIntyre L, Marshall JC, et al. Association of hydroxyethyl starch administration with mortality and acute kidney injury in critically ill patients requiring volume resuscitation: a systematic review and meta-analysis. JAMA. 2013;309(7):678–88.

20. Perel P, Roberts I, Ker K. Colloids versus crystalloids for fluid resuscitation in critically ill patients. Cochrane Database Syst Rev. 2013;2 doi:10.1002/14651858.CD000567.pub6.

21. Mutter TC, Ruth CA, Dart AB. Hydroxyethyl starch (HES) versus other fluid therapies: effects on kidney function. Cochrane Database Syst Rev. 2013;7 doi:10.1002/14651858.CD007594.pub3.

22. Navarro LH, Bloomstone JA, Auler JO Jr, Cannesson M, Rocca GD, Gan TJ, et al. Perioperative fluid therapy: a statement from the international fluid optimization group. Perioper Med. 2015;4:3.

23. Hamilton MA. Perioperative fluid management: progress despite lingering controversies. Cleve Clin J Med. 2009;76(Suppl 4):S28–31.

24. Shires T, Williams J, Brown F. Acute change in extracellular fluids associated with major surgical procedures. Ann Surg. 1961;154:803–10.

25. Miller TE, Roche AM, Mythen M. Fluid management and goal-directed therapy as an adjunct to enhanced recovery after surgery (ERAS). Can J Anaesth. 2015;62(2):158–68.

26. Brandstrup B, Tonnesen H, Beier-Holgersen R, Hjortso E, Ording H, Lindorff-Larsen K, et al. Effects of intravenous fluid restriction on postoperative complications: comparison of two perioperative fluid regimens: a randomized assessor-blinded multicenter trial. Ann Surg. 2003;238(5):641–8.

27. Holte K, Kehlet H. Fluid therapy and surgical outcomes in elective surgery: a need for reassessment in fast-track surgery. J Am Coll Surg. 2006;202(6):971–89.

28. Grant FM, Protic M, Gonen M, Allen P, Brennan MF. Intraoperative fluid management and complications following pancreatectomy. J Surg Oncol. 2013;107(5):529–35.
29. Melis M, Marcon F, Masi A, Sarpel U, Miller G, Moore H, et al. Effect of intra-operative fluid volume on peri-operative outcomes after pancreaticoduodenectomy for pancreatic adenocarcinoma. J Surg Oncol. 2012;105(1):81–4.
30. Lavu H, Sell NM, Carter TI, Winter JM, Maguire DP, Gratch DM, et al. The HYSLAR trial: a prospective randomized controlled trial of the use of a restrictive fluid regimen with 3% hypertonic saline versus lactated Ringers in patients undergoing pancreaticoduodenectomy. Ann Surg. 2014;260(3):445–53; discussion 53–5
31. Grant F, Brennan MF, Allen PJ, DeMatteo RP, Kingham TP, D'Angelica M, et al. Prospective randomized controlled trial of liberal vs restricted perioperative fluid management in patients undergoing pancreatectomy. Ann Surg. 2016;264(4):591–8.
32. Holte K, Klarskov B, Christensen DS, Lund C, Nielsen KG, Bie P, et al. Liberal versus restrictive fluid administration to improve recovery after laparoscopic cholecystectomy: a randomized, double-blind study. Ann Surg. 2004;240(5):892–9.
33. Chappell D, Jacob M, Hofmann-Kiefer K, Conzen P, Rehm M. A rational approach to perioperative fluid management. Anesthesiology. 2008;109(4):723–40.
34. Brandstrup B, Svendsen PE, Rasmussen M, Belhage B, Rodt SA, Hansen B, et al. Which goal for fluid therapy during colorectal surgery is followed by the best outcome: near-maximal stroke volume or zero fluid balance? Br J Anaesth. 2012;109(2):191–9.
35. Miller TE, Roche AM, Gan TJ. Poor adoption of hemodynamic optimization during major surgery: are we practicing substandard care? Anesth Analg. 2011;112(6):1274–6.
36. American Society of Anesthesiologists C. Practice guidelines for preoperative fasting and the use of pharmacologic agents to reduce the risk of pulmonary aspiration: application to healthy patients undergoing elective procedures: an updated report by the American Society of Anesthesiologists Committee on Standards and Practice Parameters. Anesthesiology. 2011;114(3):495–511.
37. Lamke LO, Nilsson GE, Reithner HL. Water loss by evaporation from the abdominal cavity during surgery. Acta Chir Scand. 1977;143(5):279–84.
38. Jacob M, Chappell D, Rehm M. The 'third space' – fact or fiction? Best Pract Res Clin Anaesthesiol. 2009;23(2):145–57.
39. Bellamy MC. Wet, dry or something else? Br J Anaesth. 2006;97(6):755–7.
40. Edwards MR, Mythen MG. Fluid therapy in critical illness. Extreme Physiol Med. 2014;3:16.
41. Pearse RM, Harrison DA, MacDonald N, Gillies MA, Blunt M, Ackland G, et al. Effect of a perioperative, cardiac output-guided hemodynamic therapy algorithm on outcomes following major gastrointestinal surgery: a randomized clinical trial and systematic review. JAMA. 2014;311(21):2181–90.
42. Hamilton MA, Cecconi M, Rhodes A. A systematic review and meta-analysis on the use of preemptive hemodynamic intervention to improve postoperative outcomes in moderate and high-risk surgical patients. Anesth Analg. 2011;112(6):1392–402.
43. Cannesson M. Arterial pressure variation and goal-directed fluid therapy. J Cardiothorac Vasc Anesth. 2010;24(3):487–97.
44. Connors AF Jr, Dawson NV, Shaw PK, Montenegro HD, Nara AR, Martin L. Hemodynamic status in critically ill patients with and without acute heart disease. Chest. 1990;98(5):1200–6.
45. Hoeft A, Schorn B, Weyland A, Scholz M, Buhre W, Stepanek E, et al. Bedside assessment of intravascular volume status in patients undergoing coronary bypass surgery. Anesthesiology. 1994;81(1):76–86.
46. Marik PE, Baram M, Vahid B. Does central venous pressure predict fluid responsiveness? A systematic review of the literature and the tale of seven mares. Chest. 2008;134(1):172–8.
47. McGee S, Abernethy WB 3rd, Simel DL. The rational clinical examination. Is this patient hypovolemic? JAMA. 1999;281(11):1022–9.
48. Pizov R, Eden A, Bystritski D, Kalina E, Tamir A, Gelman S. Arterial and plethysmographic waveform analysis in anesthetized patients with hypovolemia. Anesthesiology. 2010;113(1):83–91.

49. Le Manach Y, Hofer CK, Lehot JJ, Vallet B, Goarin JP, Tavernier B, et al. Can changes in arterial pressure be used to detect changes in cardiac output during volume expansion in the perioperative period? Anesthesiology. 2012;117(6):1165–74.
50. Pearse R, Dawson D, Fawcett J, Rhodes A, Grounds RM, Bennett ED. Early goal-directed therapy after major surgery reduces complications and duration of hospital stay. A randomised, controlled trial [ISRCTN38797445]. Crit Care. 2005;9(6):R687–93.
51. Shoemaker WC, Appel PL, Kram HB, Waxman K, Lee TS. Prospective trial of supranormal values of survivors as therapeutic goals in high-risk surgical patients. Chest. 1988;94(6):1176–86.
52. Nisanevich V, Felsenstein I, Almogy G, Weissman C, Einav S, Matot I. Effect of intraoperative fluid management on outcome after intraabdominal surgery. Anesthesiology. 2005;103(1):25–32.
53. Sear JW. Kidney dysfunction in the postoperative period. Br J Anaesth. 2005;95(1):20–32.
54. Kheterpal S, Tremper KK, Englesbe MJ, O'Reilly M, Shanks AM, Fetterman DM, et al. Predictors of postoperative acute renal failure after noncardiac surgery in patients with previously normal renal function. Anesthesiology. 2007;107(6):892–902.
55. Kim M, Brady JE, Li G. Variations in the risk of acute kidney injury across intraabdominal surgery procedures. Anesth Analg. 2014;119(5):1121–32.
56. Correa-Gallego C, Berman A, Denis SC, Langdon-Embry L, O'Connor D, Arslan-Carlon V, et al. Renal function after low central venous pressure-assisted liver resection: assessment of 2116 cases. HPB. 2015;17(3):258–64.
57. Kumar A, Anel R, Bunnell E, Habet K, Zanotti S, Marshall S, et al. Pulmonary artery occlusion pressure and central venous pressure fail to predict ventricular filling volume, cardiac performance, or the response to volume infusion in normal subjects. Crit Care Med. 2004;32(3):691–9.
58. Marik PE, Cavallazzi R, Vasu T, Hirani A. Dynamic changes in arterial waveform derived variables and fluid responsiveness in mechanically ventilated patients: a systematic review of the literature. Crit Care Med. 2009;37(9):2642–7.
59. Bland RD, Shoemaker WC, Abraham E, Cobo JC. Hemodynamic and oxygen transport patterns in surviving and nonsurviving postoperative patients. Crit Care Med. 1985;13(2):85–90.
60. Shoemaker WC, Appel PL, Kram HB. Tissue oxygen debt as a determinant of lethal and nonlethal postoperative organ failure. Crit Care Med. 1988;16(11):1117–20.
61. Gattinoni L, Brazzi L, Pelosi P, Latini R, Tognoni G, Pesenti A, et al. A trial of goal-oriented hemodynamic therapy in critically ill patients. SvO2 Collaborative Group. N Engl J Med. 1995;333(16):1025–32.
62. Hayes MA, Timmins AC, Yau EH, Palazzo M, Hinds CJ, Watson D. Elevation of systemic oxygen delivery in the treatment of critically ill patients. N Engl J Med. 1994;330(24):1717–22.
63. Heyland DK, Cook DJ, King D, Kernerman P, Brun-Buisson C. Maximizing oxygen delivery in critically ill patients: a methodologic appraisal of the evidence. Crit Care Med. 1996;24(3):517–24.
64. McKinley BA, Kozar RA, Cocanour CS, Valdivia A, Sailors RM, Ware DN, et al. Normal versus supranormal oxygen delivery goals in shock resuscitation: the response is the same. J Trauma. 2002;53(5):825–32.
65. Tuchschmidt J, Fried J, Astiz M, Rackow E. Elevation of cardiac output and oxygen delivery improves outcome in septic shock. Chest. 1992;102(1):216–20.
66. Velmahos GC, Demetriades D, Shoemaker WC, Chan LS, Tatevossian R, Wo CC, et al. Endpoints of resuscitation of critically injured patients: normal or supranormal? A prospective randomized trial. Ann Surg. 2000;232(3):409–18.
67. Gutierrez G, Palizas F, Doglio G, Wainsztein N, Gallesio A, Pacin J, et al. Gastric intramucosal pH as a therapeutic index of tissue oxygenation in critically ill patients. Lancet. 1992;339(8787):195–9.
68. Boyd O, Grounds RM, Bennett ED. A randomized clinical trial of the effect of deliberate perioperative increase of oxygen delivery on mortality in high-risk surgical patients. JAMA. 1993;270(22):2699–707.
69. Garcia X, Pinsky MR. Clinical applicability of functional hemodynamic monitoring. Ann Intensive Care. 2011;1:35.
70. Cannesson M, Aboy M, Hofer CK, Rehman M. Pulse pressure variation: where are we today? J Clin Monit Comput. 2011;25(1):45–56.

71. McGee WT. A simple physiologic algorithm for managing hemodynamics using stroke volume and stroke volume variation: physiologic optimization program. J Intensive Care Med. 2009;24(6):352–60.
72. Michard F, Boussat S, Chemla D, Anguel N, Mercat A, Lecarpentier Y, et al. Relation between respiratory changes in arterial pulse pressure and fluid responsiveness in septic patients with acute circulatory failure. Am J Respir Crit Care Med. 2000;162(1):134–8.
73. Tavernier B, Makhotine O, Lebuffe G, Dupont J, Scherpereel P. Systolic pressure variation as a guide to fluid therapy in patients with sepsis-induced hypotension. Anesthesiology. 1998;89(6):1313–21.
74. Cannesson M, Musard H, Desebbe O, Boucau C, Simon R, Henaine R, et al. The ability of stroke volume variations obtained with Vigileo/FloTrac system to monitor fluid responsiveness in mechanically ventilated patients. Anesth Analg. 2009;108(2):513–7.
75. Derichard A, Robin E, Tavernier B, Costecalde M, Fleyfel M, Onimus J, et al. Automated pulse pressure and stroke volume variations from radial artery: evaluation during major abdominal surgery. Br J Anaesth. 2009;103(5):678–84.
76. Della Rocca G, Vetrugno L, Tripi G, Deana C, Barbariol F, Pompei L. Liberal or restricted fluid administration: are we ready for a proposal of a restricted intraoperative approach? BMC Anesthesiol. 2014;14:62.
77. Corcoran T, Rhodes JE, Clarke S, Myles PS, Ho KM. Perioperative fluid management strategies in major surgery: a stratified meta-analysis. Anesth Analg. 2012;114(3):640–51.
78. Dalfino L, Giglio MT, Puntillo F, Marucci M, Brienza N. Haemodynamic goal-directed therapy and postoperative infections: earlier is better. A systematic review and meta-analysis. Crit Care. 2011;15(3):R154.
79. Giglio MT, Marucci M, Testini M, Brienza N. Goal-directed haemodynamic therapy and gastrointestinal complications in major surgery: a meta-analysis of randomized controlled trials. Br J Anaesth. 2009;103(5):637–46.
80. Rhodes A, Cecconi M, Hamilton M, Poloniecki J, Woods J, Boyd O, et al. Goal-directed therapy in high-risk surgical patients: a 15-year follow-up study. Intensive Care Med. 2010;36(8):1327–32.
81. Mythen MG. Postoperative gastrointestinal tract dysfunction. Anesth Analg. 2005;100(1):196–204.
82. Hamilton-Davies C, Mythen MG, Salmon JB, Jacobson D, Shukla A, Webb AR. Comparison of commonly used clinical indicators of hypovolaemia with gastrointestinal tonometry. Intensive Care Med. 1997;23(3):276–81.
83. Takala J. Determinants of splanchnic blood flow. Br J Anaesth. 1996;77(1):50–8.
84. Kusano C, Baba M, Takao S, Sane S, Shimada M, Shirao K, et al. Oxygen delivery as a factor in the development of fatal postoperative complications after oesophagectomy. Br J Surg. 1997;84(2):252–7.
85. Testini M, Scacco S, Loiotila L, Papa F, Vergari R, Regina G, et al. Comparison of oxidative phosphorylation in the anastomosis of the small and large bowel. An experimental study in the rabbit. Euro Surg Res. Europaische chirurgische Forschung Recherches chirurgicales europeennes. 1998;30(1):1–7.
86. Becker BF, Chappell D, Jacob M. Endothelial glycocalyx and coronary vascular permeability: the fringe benefit. Basic Res Cardiol. 2010;105(6):687–701.
87. Marjanovic G, Villain C, Juettner E, zur Hausen A, Hoeppner J, Hopt UT, et al. Impact of different crystalloid volume regimes on intestinal anastomotic stability. Ann Surg. 2009;249(2):181–5.
88. Fischer M, Matsuo K, Gonen M, Grant F, Dematteo RP, D'Angelica MI, et al. Relationship between intraoperative fluid administration and perioperative outcome after pancreaticoduodenectomy: results of a prospective randomized trial of acute normovolemic hemodilution compared with standard intraoperative management. Ann Surg. 2010;252(6):952–8.
89. Jarnagin WR, Gonen M, Fong Y, DeMatteo RP, Ben-Porat L, Little S, et al. Improvement in perioperative outcome after hepatic resection: analysis of 1,803 consecutive cases over the past decade. Ann Surg. 2002;236(4):397–406; discussion –7.
90. Kooby DA, Stockman J, Ben-Porat L, Gonen M, Jarnagin WR, Dematteo RP, et al. Influence of transfusions on perioperative and long-term outcome in patients following hepatic resection for colorectal metastases. Ann Surg. 2003;237(6):860–9; discussion 9–70.

91. Gelman S. Venous function and central venous pressure: a physiologic story. Anesthesiology. 2008;108(4):735–48.
92. Hughes MJ, McNally S, Wigmore SJ. Enhanced recovery following liver surgery: a systematic review and meta-analysis. HPB. 2014;16(8):699–706.
93. Jones C, Kelliher L, Dickinson M, Riga A, Worthington T, Scott MJ, et al. Randomized clinical trial on enhanced recovery versus standard care following open liver resection. Br J Surg. 2013;100(8):1015–24.
94. Correa-Gallego C, Tan KS, Arslan-Carlon V, Gonen M, Denis SC, Langdon-Embry L, et al. Goal-directed fluid therapy using stroke volume variation for resuscitation after low central venous pressure-assisted liver resection: a randomized clinical trial. J Am Coll Surg. 2015;221(2):591–601.
95. Perkins HA, Busch MP. Transfusion-associated infections: 50 years of relentless challenges and remarkable progress. Transfusion. 2010;50(10):2080–99.
96. Shander A, Javidroozi M, Perelman S, Puzio T, Lobel G. From bloodless surgery to patient blood management. Mt Sinai J Med. 2012;79(1):56–65.
97. Shander A, Javidroozi M. Blood conservation strategies and the management of perioperative anaemia. Curr Opin Anaesthesiol. 2015;28(3):356–63.
98. Callum JL, Waters JH, Shaz BH, Sloan SR, Murphy MF. The AABB recommendations for the Choosing Wisely campaign of the American Board of Internal Medicine. Transfusion. 2014;54(9):2344–52.
99. Cannon RM, Brown RE, St Hill CR, Dunki-Jacobs E, Martin RC 2nd, McMasters KM, et al. Negative effects of transfused blood components after hepatectomy for metastatic colorectal cancer. Am Surg. 2013;79(1):35–9.
100. Kingham TP, Correa-Gallego C, D'Angelica MI, Gonen M, DeMatteo RP, Fong Y, et al. Hepatic parenchymal preservation surgery: decreasing morbidity and mortality rates in 4,152 resections for malignancy. J Am Coll Surg. 2015;220(4):471–9.
101. Correa-Gallego C, Gonen M, Fischer M, Grant F, Kemeny NE, Arslan-Carlon V, et al. Perioperative complications influence recurrence and survival after resection of hepatic colorectal metastases. Ann Surg Oncol. 2013;20(8):2477–84.
102. Jarnagin WR, Gonen M, Maithel SK, Fong Y, D'Angelica MI, Dematteo RP, et al. A prospective randomized trial of acute normovolemic hemodilution compared to standard intraoperative management in patients undergoing major hepatic resection. Ann Surg. 2008;248(3):360–9.
103. Wehry J, Cannon R, Scoggins CR, Puffer L, McMasters KM, Martin RC. Restrictive blood transfusion protocol in liver resection patients reduces blood transfusions with no increase in patient morbidity. Am J Surg. 2015;209(2):280–8.

Perioperative Pain Management for Hepatopancreaticobiliary Surgery

3

Clancy J. Clark

Introduction

Postoperative pain is a major barrier to rapid recovery and source of serious postoperative morbidity and mortality after liver and pancreas surgery. Pain is also a barrier to reaching recovery milestones. Reports indicate that inadequate pain management occurs up to 50% of patients [1]. Postoperative pain varies widely from procedure to procedure, as well as among patients who undergo the same procedure. Pain associated with surgical procedures is a recognized risk factor for chronic neuropathic pain.

Optimal outcomes after hepatopancreaticobiliary surgery require a well-developed postoperative pain management program in addition to excellent surgical technique and standardized care pathways. As HPB surgeons we strive to not only decrease postoperative morbidity and mortality but facilitate a patient's return to normality and a state of independency in activities of daily living [2]. While prior pain management programs have focused on the interests of institutions and providers (i.e., length of stay, readmission, and cost), patient-centered outcomes are critically important. Numerous pain management options are now available during the perioperative period (Table 3.1). The following chapter will review the most common perioperative pain management strategies and recommendations for providing optimal care.

Medications

Meta-analyses demonstrate that combination regimens, such as acetaminophen and NSAIDs, have better pain control than single agents [4]. While multidrug regimens (polypharmacy) may improve outcomes on face value, it is inaccurate to assume

C.J. Clark, MD (✉)
Wake Forest Baptist Health, Winston-Salem, NC, USA
e-mail: cjclark@wakehealth.edu

© Springer International Publishing AG 2018
F.G. Rocha, P. Shen (eds.), *Optimizing Outcomes for Liver and Pancreas Surgery*, DOI 10.1007/978-3-319-62624-6_3

Table 3.1 Perioperative pain
management options

Medications
Nonsteroidal anti-inflammatory drugs (NSAIDs)
Acetaminophen
Gabapentin
Opioids
Regional anesthesia
Epidural
Intrathecal
Transverse abdominis plane block
Wound catheters

additive effects for each additional medication particularly with cross-reactivity and individual drug-associated adverse effects. Similarly, the objective evaluation of heterogeneous multidrug trials poses significant challenge. Many of these studies are difficult to interpret, and current meta-analysis techniques are unable to evaluate multiple outcomes in setting of various drug iterations.

Nonsteroidal Anti-inflammatory Drugs

Nonsteroidal anti-inflammatory drugs (NSAIDs) are a drug class including ibuprofen and ketorolac that have both analgesic and antipyretic effects. NSAIDs inhibit the activity of cyclooxygenase-1 (COX-1) and cyclooxygenase-2 (COX-2). Several NSAIDs are selective COX-2 inhibitors, such as celecoxib. Through this inhibition, prostaglandins and thromboxanes are not synthesized leading to beneficial effects in the postoperative patient. Meta-analyses demonstrate that selective (celecoxib) and nonselective (ibuprofen) NSAIDs decrease opioid use and decrease opioid-associated postoperative adverse events [5, 6].

Unfortunately, NSAIDs with COX-1 inhibition can lead to severe gastrointestinal bleeding and increased risk of anastomotic leak after gastrointestinal surgery. Three observation retrospective cohort studies have demonstrated increased risk of anastomotic leak with NSAID from less than 5% to over 20% [7]. Perioperative ketorolac can improve short-term (less than 24 h) pain but has been associated with an increased risk of postoperative bleeding [8]. Dyspepsia is also common among NSAID users. Therefore, NSAIDs are generally avoided if other non-opioid alternatives are available. If necessary, NSAIDs are limited to short intervals less than 2 weeks or COX-2 inhibitors are used.

Acetaminophen (Paracetamol)

Acetaminophen is an effective opioid-sparing analgesic with antipyretic properties. Acetaminophen is metabolized by the cytochrome p450 pathway in the liver producing N-acetyl-p-benzoquinone imine (NAPQI) which is further conjugated by glutathione. Given well-recognized liver toxicity, acetaminophen dosing is limited to 4 g per 24-h period. Intravenous acetaminophen has earlier plasma and cerebral spinal fluid peaks compared with oral formulations and has gained popularity among gastrointestinal surgery patients [9]. Due to high cost, intravenous acetaminophen use is often restricted by many hospital pharmacies. With increasing need for opioid alternatives, the use of intravenous acetaminophen will continue to rise and can play an important role in multimodal pain management strategies for the NPO patient.

Patients and primary care providers frequently avoid postoperative acetaminophen in liver resection patients; however, this is not founded. Acetaminophen metabolism is altered with larger liver resections, but no deficiency in glutathione is observed [10]. With preserved liver function, acetaminophen is safe during the postoperative period for hepatobiliary patients. Clearly in the setting of acute hepatitis, impaired liver function, or liver failure, acetaminophen should be avoided.

Gabapentin

Gabapentin is an oral non-opioid analgesic used in the treatment of chronic neuropathic conditions, such as diabetic neuropathy and epilepsy. In the 1970s, a German chemist, Gerhardt Satzinger, designed a series of compounds to mimic gamma-aminobutyric acid (GABA) [11]. Gabapentin, (1-aminomethyl-cyclohexyl)-acetic acid, emerged as a potent antiseizure compound (Fig. 3.1). It was further developed and ultimately marketed by Parke-Davis (now Pfizer) in 1994 for the treatment of epilepsy. Following reports of improved pain control for postherpetic neuralgia and diabetic neuropathy, gabapentin was approved by the FDA in the United States for management of neuropathic pain in 2002 [13, 14].

Although the exact mechanism of action of gabapentin is not clear, it appears to bind alpha$_2$-delta subunit of voltage-gated calcium ion channels resulting in altered neurotransmitter signaling [15]. Gabapentin does not appear to bind GABA$_A$ or

Fig. 3.1 Gabapentin 2D structure [12]

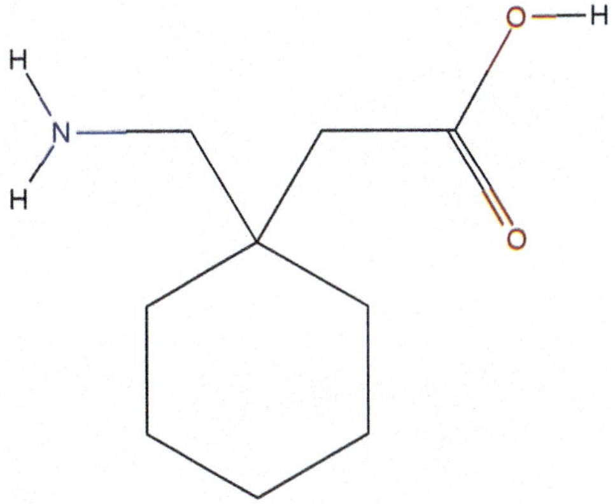

GABA$_B$ receptors or alter GABA uptake or metabolism. Gabapentin bioavailability is inversely proportional to its dose and not dependent on food. Interestingly, humans do not metabolize gabapentin, and it is excreted in the urine following first-order kinetic elimination. The half-life of gabapentin is between 5 and 9 h [15]. Gabapentin metabolism is not altered by liver dysfunction.

Over 130 studies have evaluated the benefit of gabapentin for postoperative analgesia. In general, gabapentin use within 24 h of operation will decrease opioid use [16]. Timing and dosage of gabapentin varies from study to study, but most convenient is administration in preoperative holding just before surgery. In addition to analgesic effects, gabapentin appears to improve postoperative nausea, anxiety, and patient satisfaction.

Gabapentin is well tolerated with few serious adverse effects. Side effects include sedation and dizziness and are dose and time related. Importantly, rapid discontinuation of high-dose gabapentin can result in significant withdrawal similar to alcohol or benzodiazepines including irritability, agitation, diaphoresis, and palpitations [15].

Opioids

Opioid-related adverse drug events contribute to poor surgical outcomes after liver and pancreas surgery [17]. Table 3.2 outlines the most commonly recognized adverse events following opioid administration. Opioids directly suppress the central respiratory drive resulting in elevation of carbon dioxide leading to apnea and even death. This ventilatory impairment is exacerbated by numerous factors including

Table 3.2 Opioid-related adverse drug effects [18]

Arrhythmias
Constipation
Cough
Dry mouth
Endocrinopathy
Histamine release
Ileus
Immunomodulation
Increased intracranial pressure
Myoclonus
Nausea and vomiting
Neurotoxicity
Pruritus
Respiratory depression
Rigidity
Serotonin syndrome
Urinary retention
Withdrawal symptoms

disease-related fatigue, sleep apnea, chronic lung disease, and benzodiazepines. Route of narcotic administration will result in variable extent of respiratory depression with intramuscular delivery having a lower rate of depression compared with intravenous administration including patient-controlled analgesia (PCA).

While the etiology of postoperative ileus is multifactorial (inflammatory, hormonal, metabolic), acute and chronic opioid exposure directly impacts bowel function. Postoperative ileus results in prolonged hospitalization and increased cost and resource utilization. Hospitalization costs nearly double with postoperative ileus, $8,316 vs. $15,914 [19]. Narcotics interact with mu- and kappa-opioid receptors resulting in decreased gut transit, increased sphincter tone (e.g., sphincter of Oddi), and increased non-pulsatile bowel tone. These effects are dose dependent where length of stay and proportion with postoperative ileus increase with increasing doses of narcotic [20]. Barletta et al. demonstrated that, despite surgical technique (laparoscopic vs. open), patients receiving more than 2 mg/day of hydromorphone had significantly longer length of stay [21]. Most medications including metoclopramide, erythromycin, naloxone, and methylnaltrexone have not decreased the postoperative ileus or length of stay [20]. Alvimopan, a peripherally acting mu-receptor antagonist, may be able to mitigate the adverse effects of opioids on the gastrointestinal tract. However, results are mixed with alvimopan and may only reduce length of stay by several hours [17].

In the management of pancreaticobiliary disease, classic teaching of pain management recommended meperidine over morphine to minimize opioid-induced sphincter of Oddi contraction. Early indirect measures of sphincter of Oddi function using radionuclide scintigraphy (hepato-iminodiacetic acid (HIDA) scan) or bile duct pressures via T-tube following cholecystectomy demonstrated increased bile duct pressures and delayed emptying with administration of opioids. In the 1980s, ERCP enabled direct measurement of the sphincter of Oddi. These follow-up manometry studies demonstrated no significant difference in sphincter of Oddi between meperidine and morphine; however, direct manometry may not reflect the dynamic peristalsis of the sphincter [22]. Goff, who performed these early experiments, suggested that the sphincter may act more like a pump than a valve [23].

Despite significant intrigue with the impact of opioids on the sphincter of Oddi and potential benefits of meperidine, meperidine is not used in clinical practice due to serious seizure side effects. General opioid-sparing strategies are likely more beneficial in reducing sphincter of Oddi dysfunction.

Regional Anesthesia

Given the direct association between higher systemic opioid exposure and worse postoperative outcomes and adverse drug events, alternative modalities of analgesia have been employed including regional anesthetics, such as local infusion catheters and patient-controlled epidural anesthesia. Regional neurologic blockade provides potential for opioid sparing while improving pain relief, anti-inflammatory effects, attenuation of catabolism, improved mobilization, decreased postoperative ileus, and fewer pulmonary complications [2]. Given the diverse anesthetic modalities in regional anesthesia, a team-based approach is required to determine the appropriate regional anesthetic technique for each specific liver or pancreas operation in any given hospital. Several of the regional anesthetic modalities commonly using in HPB surgery are reviewed here.

Three categories of regional analgesia should be considered: first, central neuraxial techniques including epidural and intrathecal anesthesia; second, regional analgesia, such as transverse abdominis plane blocks and celiac plexus block; and, lastly, local analgesia including local injection and wound catheters.

Epidural

Epidural analgesia is widely used in abdominal surgery. The catheter is typically placed by a regional anesthesiologist in a specialized regional anesthesia holding area or the operating room before induction of general anesthesia. Reports of epidural analgesia and sedation only for hepatobiliary surgery have been described but not widely accepted [24]. Epidural analgesia is more commonly combined with general anesthetic and continued for 3–5 days postoperatively. Following discharge from the postoperative care unit, patients then receive a continuous epidural infusion but also are able to self-administer anesthesia using a pump device with fixed dosing and lockout mechanism. The infusion may contain anesthetic only (bupivacaine) or combined with opioid. Type of infusion and dosing of analgesia varies greatly from institution to institution resulting in variable rates of "functional" epidural and incidence of adverse events. Epidural analgesia causes a sympathetic blockage that may lower central venous pressure. Given continuous infusions and potential for hypotension, epidural analgesia can be resource intensive.

Numerous single institution studies demonstrate improved outcomes with functional epidurals. Large national studies using hospital administrative data, however, do not paint such an optimistic picture of epidurals with longer length of stay and increased hospital costs [20]. Functioning epidurals with appropriate level analgesia can decrease pulmonary complications, deep vein thrombosis, pulmonary embolism, cardiac morbidity, blood loss, acute renal failure, and ileus [25]. Benefits of epidural analgesia are thwarted by dislodgement, partial blocks, and early discontinuation secondary to hypotension. With conflicting results routine use of epidural analgesia for hepatobiliary and pancreatic surgery is not widely accepted.

The sympathetic blockage of epidural analgesic results in relative hypotension. Numerous studies have demonstrated an increased administration of intravenous fluids in patients with epidurals compared to controls. This predictable response to epidural analgesia is challenging for a junior resident and programs new to epidural infusions. Asymptomatic hypotension in a patient with an epidural does not require aggressive fluid resuscitation. Clear communication with the regional anesthesia team is required. High-performing programs have an on-call regional anesthesia team that rounds on the wards daily (preferably in the morning). The regional/acute pain anesthesia team can work closely with the surgeon to evaluate epidural function, volume status, and potential complications.

Generally, epidural use is safe in liver surgery; however, elevations in INR during postoperative recovery after major hepatectomy can delay epidural removal in up to 50% of patient and result in administration of fresh frozen plasma [26]. Epidural hematoma may occur with INR more than 1.5 during intentional and accidental catheter removal. With transition to laparoscopic-assisted and totally laparoscopic approaches to liver resection, patient-controlled epidural analgesia is less applicable given increasingly shorter lengths of stay.

In contrast to liver surgery, epidural analgesia is frequently used in pancreatic surgery. In the DISPACT trial, 20 of 23 European centers routinely used thoracic epidurals for postoperative pain management following distal pancreatectomy [27]. Multiple studies demonstrate improved outcomes with patient-controlled epidural analgesia; and it is commonly integrated into ERAS pathways for pancreatectomy. In a meta-analysis of 125 trials, epidural analgesia decreased postoperative mortality (OR 0.6 CI 0.39–93) [28]. Epidural analgesia is also associated with decreased risk of cardiac dysrhythmias, deep venous thrombosis, pneumonia, and postoperative ileus. However, epidural dysfunction, as described by Traverso and colleagues, occurs in 49% of pancreatectomy patients and can lead to increased complications [29]. Epidural hypofunction (poor pain control, need for opioid infusion) results in increased pancreas-related complications (pancreatic leak). Epidural hyperfunction (hypotension, oliguria) results in increased non-pancreas-related complications. Therefore, objective assessment of epidural function during the postoperative period is vital and should be considered a specific outcome measure in evaluating the success of an acute pain management program.

Intrathecal

Given practical challenges of patient-controlled epidural analgesia in an era of shorter hospitalization and ERAS, intrathecal single-shot analgesia has been proposed as an alternative. Intrathecal anesthesia is administered immediately preoperatively by lumbar puncture and combined with patient-controlled analgesia during the postoperative period. Analgesic can include a combination of opioid and bupivacaine. This approach can decrease staffing for an after-hours acute pain service and potentially avoid complications associated with coagulopathy and liver surgery. For liver surgery, preoperative intrathecal morphine injection is safe with no increased complications [30, 31]. In a prospective observational study by Kasivisvanathan et al., intrathecal analgesia compared with epidural analgesia decreased length of stay and time to mobilization for patient undergoing hepatic resection [32]. While these early results are promising, no randomized controlled trials have yet evaluated postoperative outcomes or length of stay for patients undergoing hepatobiliary and pancreatic surgery.

Transverse Abdominis Plane Block

Transverse abdominis plane (TAP) block has gained substantial popularity and common practice at our institution for minimally invasive hepatobiliary surgery. Anatomically, thoracic nerves T7 to T11 travel through a neurovascular plane between the internal oblique and transversus abdominis muscles to innervate the skin, muscle, and parietal peritoneum of the abdomen. For example, T10 supplies sensation to the umbilicus. Regional anesthetic to the abdominal wall historically relied on anatomic landmarks and fascial "pops" to identify the correct location. In an era of obesity, traditional techniques can be challenging. Ultrasound-guided delivery of anesthetic has improved outcomes and function of TAP blocks.

The TAP block achieves anesthesia by disrupting nerve signaling before the sensory nerves enter the musculature of the anterior abdominal wall. Original landmarks for catheter insertion for TAP blocks were the lumbar triangle of Petit with boundaries being external oblique, latissimus dorsi, and iliac crest. Using ultrasound guidance, a needle can be inserted into the plane between the internal oblique and transversus abdominis (Fig. 3.2). In real time, this potential plane is separated

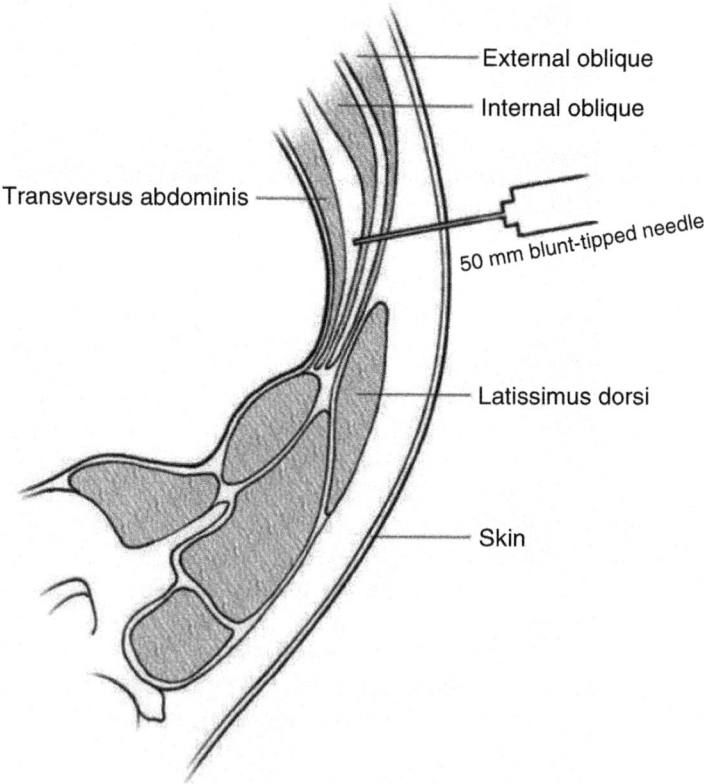

Fig. 3.2 Transverse abdominal plane block [33]

with local anesthetic. Bilateral anesthetic is required for abdominal operations and takes approximately 60 min for maximal effect [33].

Recent meta-analyses and a 2010 Cochrane Review indicate that TAP blocks lower the total opioid requirement in the first 24 h after surgery [34, 35]. In a meta-analysis of 12 randomized controlled trials, TAP blocks reduced postoperative morphine consumption by 9.1 mg (95% CI −16.83, −1.45, $p = 0.02$) and lowered pain scores at 24, 36, and 48 h [35]. Decreased opioid use should result in lower opioid-associated adverse events including nausea and vomiting; however, these benefits are not seen with the short duration of action with TAP blocks. Importantly, TAP blocks will not improve visceral pain. Outcomes with TAP blocks are comparable to single-shot intrathecal morphine or locally infiltrated anesthetic [34, 36]. TAP blocks may benefit from decreased chronic pain given administration as preemptive anesthetic [35].

Celiac Plexus Block

Epigastric pain radiating to the back is a common presentation for patients with pancreatic cancer and typically suggests unresectable disease. For patients with severe pain that has failed opioid and non-opioid analgesia, celiac plexus block can provide sustained relief. Pancreatic cancer may directly invade adjacent nerve sheaths and neural ganglia resulting in pain. Pancreatic duct obstruction or intestinal obstruction can also result in severe pain. Celiac plexus neurolysis can ablate visceral associated pain. Percutaneous, endoscopic, or surgical approaches have been described [37]. Most commonly, celiac plexus block is performed using endoscopic ultrasound guidance. For surgeons, chemical splanchnicectomy can be easily performed if unresectable disease is identified. A needle is inserted into the periaortic celiac ganglia of the retroperitoneum, and 20 mL of 50% alcohol is injected on either side of the aorta. For awake patients, local anesthetic should be injected first given pain associated with alcohol injection.

Celiac plexus block can provide improved pain and decreased opioid consumption [37]. Potential short-term risks of celiac block include incomplete block, hematoma, and infection. Long-term risk of diarrhea can occur but uncommon [37].

Wound Incision and Intramuscular Pain Catheters

Catheter-based intramuscular infusion of anesthetic (bupivacaine) has been used in hepatobiliary and pancreatic surgery, but exact benefit is not clear. The catheters are inserted at time of closure into the subcutaneous space or deep in the intramuscular plane of either the rectus, internal oblique, or transverse abdominis. Experience with such catheters is limited for hepatobiliary and pancreatic surgery [26]. In a meta-analysis of four studies, epidural analgesia has superior pain control on postoperative day 1 but similar pain control on postoperative days 2 and 3 following liver surgery [38]. Wound catheters, however, had lower overall complications.

Long-Term Risks

Opioid addiction is a serious concern and now recognized by governmental agencies and patients alike. Opioid exposure during the perioperative period is a recognized risk factor for developing opioid dependence [39]. Chronic pain after surgery varies from operation to operation and well recognized following procedures such as inguinal hernia repair. Chronic postoperative pain is defined by the following criteria: (1) pain developed after surgical procedure, (2) at least 2 months duration, and (3) other causes of pain excluded, such as malignancy or infection [39]. Chronic pain is directly linked with chronic opioid use and dependence.

Chronic pain develops through normal processes of healing. Surgery can lead to prolonged changes in both the peripheral and the central nervous system [1]. Inflammatory mediators released into the wound alter the function of afferent nerve endings resulting in lower threshold for activation. This can result in a hyperactive nociceptor response. The risk factors for a maladaptive pain response include pain prior to surgery, genetic variation, psychologic vulnerability, younger age, and female [39].

Strategies to decrease maladaptive chronic pain include preemptive analgesia and centrally acting anesthetics. Administration of analgesia before surgical incision conceptually blocks the initial nociceptive signaling. Randomized controlled trials of local and regional anesthetics combined with general anesthesia have demonstrated long-term analgesic benefits [39].

Gabapentin has developed improved postoperative pain control and also reduction in narcotic use following surgery. In fact, gabapentin has been shown to reduce chronic pain at 3 months postoperatively [16].

Special Considerations

In the setting of hepatic dysfunction including acute liver failure, end-stage liver disease, and orthotopic liver transplantation, pharmacokinetics and pharmacodynamics are altered. Plasma concentrations of opioids vary greatly, and perioperative analgesic requirements will be decreased. Hepatic clearance of a medication is dependent on hepatic extraction (hepatic enzyme activity) and hepatic blood flow [40]. Cirrhosis not only can impact hepatocyte function but also alter hepatic blood flow due to cellular regeneration and intrahepatic vasculature distortion. Therefore, dosing of opioids and benzodiazepines need to be carefully monitored in the compromised liver.

The Multidisciplinary Team

Implementation of an evidence-based strategy for optimal postoperative pain management requires critical assessment of the evidence with careful consideration of existing institutional resources. This will require a multidisciplinary team with key stakeholders including anesthesiologists (in and out of the operating room), nurses, discharging planning coordinators, pharmacist, and surgical team. Additional team members may include nutrition, respiratory therapy, and clinical informatics. Omission of key players will result in poor compliance with recommendations and protocols leading to significant dissatisfaction among team members and patients. The multidisciplinary team will need to be flexible and have a foundation knowledge in cycles of process improvement. Members will also need to abandon biases and focus on the evidence including economic impact, feasibility, and resource utilization. Barriers to successful implementation of a comprehensive pain management plan for hepatopancreaticobiliary surgery patients will need to factor preoperative (e.g., high opioid exposure), intraoperative (e.g., volume manage with the pharmacologic sympathectomy of an epidural), and postoperative (liver insufficiency) barriers (Table 3.3).

Table 3.3 Summary of postoperative pain management options for hepatopancreaticobiliary patients

Modality	Recommendation	Grade of recommendation[a]
Medications		
Nonsteroidal anti-inflammatory drugs (NSAIDS)	Avoid NSAIDs if possible given increased risk of anastomotic leak	B
Acetaminophen	Recommended in patients with normal liver function. Safe non-opioid for postoperative pain management	B
Gabapentin	Recommended perioperative analgesic. Safe, well-tolerated non-opioid that decreases postoperative short- and long-term pain	A
Opioids	Minimize utilization. High-risk postoperative analgesic associated with increased worse outcomes and increased postoperative costs	A
Regional anesthesia		
Epidural – liver resection	Provides improved postoperative pain control but may increase length of stay and costs	B
Epidural – pancreatic resection	Preferred anesthetic for open pancreas surgery. Provides improved postoperative pain control and may decrease postoperative complications	B
Intrathecal	Good alternative to epidural anesthetic. Provides postoperative pain control comparable to epidural without associated complications in liver surgery	B
Transverse abdominis plane (TAP) block	Preferred for minimally invasive procedures. Decreases postoperative opioid use and opioid-associated adverse events and is a good option for minimally invasive liver surgery	A
Wound pain catheters	Not preferred postoperative regional anesthetic. Provides improved pain control for first day after surgery but no improvement in long-term pain management	A

[a]OCEBM Levels of Evidence Working Group. "The Oxford 2011 Levels of Evidence." Oxford Centre for Evidence-Based Medicine. http://www.cebm.net/index.aspx?o=5653

Successful postoperative pain management programs frequently include an acute pain management team that rounds on patients daily and early in the morning. Close coordinated care with an acute pain management team enables rapid assessment of incomplete and nonfunctional epidurals, modification of dosage based on unanticipated complications including respiratory compromise, and discharge planning for patients with existing high-dose narcotic requirements.

In addition, assessment of clinical outcomes and program implementation should be embedded in the pain management plan. Documentation of opioid-related adverse drug events, respiratory complications, narcotic utilization, and protocol compliance is invaluable and enables future program assessment. While capturing outcome data can help guide process improvement, members of the multidisciplinary team must agree on clinical outcome definitions a priori. For example, failed epidural can be defined as (1) epidural removal for any reason or (2) epidural removal for incomplete block based on objective sensory assessment. Scheduled review and evaluation of clinical outcomes data can thus enable an optimal patient experience.

Enhanced Recovery After Surgery

Enhanced recovery after surgery (ERAS) is a multidisciplinary, multimodality treatment pathway that has been implemented broadly in the case of surgical patients. Successfully programs in pancreatic and liver surgery have decreased length of stay and improved clinical outcomes [41].

Recent 2016 guidelines by the ERAS Society specifically outline current evidence and recommendations for optimal postoperative pain management in liver surgery that support use of intrathecal (spinal) or wound infusion catheters [42]. Despite recognized improved pain control, ERAS Society recommendations are less enthusiastic regarding patient-controlled epidural anesthetic given potential delay in removal with elevated INR/prothrombin time and reported increased risk of kidney failure secondary to hypotension.

For pancreatic surgery, ERAS programs have recognized the importance of preoperative education and setting of expectations. Preoperative analgesia and coordinated management of regional anesthesia can improve outcomes. Opioid-sparing strategies decreased sphincter of Oddi dysfunction, decrease ileus, and minimize respiratory complications. Importantly, a well-developed perioperative pain management program is only one component in a successful pancreatic ERAS pathway.

Future

Pharmacologic Interventions

In recent years, intravenous lidocaine has demonstrated some promise in decreased postoperative length of stay and ileus [43]. In addition to being a local anesthetic and anti-arrhythmic, lidocaine has analgesic and anti-hyperalgesic effects. Typically, patients receive an intraoperative bolus followed by an infusion for up to 24 h. Meta-analysis of randomized controlled trials of intravenous lidocaine infusion demonstrated decreased postoperative pain and decreased postoperative opioid consumption [9]. Lidocaine infusions have yet to be evaluated specifically in liver and pancreatic surgery.

Non-pharmacologic Interventions

Novel approaches to postoperative pain management that look beyond conventional pharmacologic interventions have been proposed. Acupuncture, hypnosis, and music therapy have been used as adjunctive therapy for management of postoperative pain and may reduce total opioid consumption and associated adverse events [9]. Efficiency of acupuncture therapy is highly debated given unclear mechanism of action of postoperative patients. Music therapy and hypnosis can reduce the physiologic response to pain and anxiety associated with surgery; however, the optimal timing and duration of such interventions remain unknown. While current evidence is weak and outcomes debated, non-pharmacological adjunctive pain management techniques are generally low cost and low risk with significant potential for future patients.

Conclusions

Optimal perioperative pain management for patients undergoing hepatobiliary and pancreatic surgery requires a team-based approach using multimodal therapy and regional analgesia. Epidural analgesic remains an important aspect of evidence-based ERAS programs for pancreatectomy but is being replaced by TAP blocks and intrathecal injections for both open and laparoscopic liver resection. Opioid-sparing regimens that include acetaminophen and gabapentin can improve outcomes and decrease adverse events associated with narcotics. Importantly, the specific pain management program at any given institution must be guided by institution resources, case mix, patient population, and provider expertise.

Bibliography

1. Weinbroum AA. Non-opioid IV adjuvants in the perioperative period: pharmacological and clinical aspects of ketamine and gabapentinoids. Pharmacol Res [Internet]. 2012;65(4):411–29. Available from: http://dx.doi.org/10.1016/j.phrs.2012.01.002
2. Aarts M, Okrainec A, Wood T. Enhanced recovery after surgery guideline. Minerva Anestesiol. 2014;80(11):1228–33.
3. Kehlet H, Dahl JB. The value of "multimodal" or "balanced analgesia" in postoperative pain treatment. Anesth Analg. 1993;77:1048–56.
4. Ong CKS, Seymour RA, Lirk P, Merry AF. Combining paracetamol (acetaminophen) with nonsteroidal antiinflammatory drugs: a qualitative systematic review of analgesic efficacy for acute postoperative pain. Anesth Analg. 2010;110(4):1170–9.
5. DAHL JB, Nielsen RV, Wetterslev J, Nikolajsen L, Hamunen K, Kontinen VK, et al. Postoperative analgesic effects of paracetamol, NSAIDs, glucocorticoids, gabapentinoids and their

combinations: a topical review. Acta Anaesthesiol Scand [Internet]. 2014;58(10):1165–81. Available from: http://doi.wiley.com/10.1111/aas.12382

6. Khan JS, Margarido C, Devereaux PJ, Clarke H, McLellan A, Choi S. Preoperative celecoxib in noncardiac surgery. Eur J Anaesthesiol [Internet]. 2016;33(3):204–14. Available from: http://www.embase.com/search/results?subaction=viewrecord&from=export&id=L6081617 36%255Cn. http://dx.doi.org/10.1097/EJA.0000000000000346%255Cn. http://findit.library. jhu.edu/resolve?sid=EMBASE&issn=13652346&id=doi:10.1097%252FEJA.000000000000 0346&atitle=Preo

7. Rushfeldt CF, Sveinbjørnsson B, Søreide K, Vonen B. Risk of anastomotic leakage with use of NSAIDs after gastrointestinal surgery. Int J Color Dis. 2011;26(12):1501–9.

8. Kagedan DJ, Ahmed M, Devitt KS, Wei AC. Enhanced recovery after pancreatic surgery: a systematic review of the evidence. HPB. 2015;17(1):11–6.

9. Tan M, Law LS-C, Gan TJ. Optimizing pain management to facilitate Enhanced recovery after surgery pathways. Can J Anaesth [Internet]. 2014;62(2):203–18. Available from: http://link. springer.com/10.1007/s12630-014-0275-x

10. Hughes MJ, Harrison EM, Jin Y, Homer N, Wigmore SJ. Acetaminophen metabolism after liver resection: a prospective case-control study. Dig Liver Dis [Internet]. 2015;47(12):1039– 46. Available from: http://www.ncbi.nlm.nih.gov/pubmed/26362614

11. Thorpe A, Taylor C. Calcium channel a2–d ligands: gabapentin and pregabalin. In: Taylor J, Triggle D, editors. Comprehensive medical chemistry II. 1st ed. Oxford: Elsevier; 2007. p. 227–46.

12. NIH. Gabapentin [Internet]. PubChem. Open Chemistry Database. 2016 [cited 2016 Jan 1]. Available from: https://pubchem.ncbi.nlm.nih.gov/compound/gabapentin#section=Top.

13. Rowbotham M, Harden N, Stacey B, Bernstein P, Magnus-Miller L. Gabapentin for the treatment of postherpetic neuralgia: a randomized controlled trial. JAMA [Internet]. 1998;280(21):1837–42. Available from: http://www.ncbi.nlm.nih.gov/pubmed/9846778

14. Backonja M, Beydoun A, Edwards KR, Schwartz SL, Fonseca V, Hes M, et al. Gabapentin for the symptomatic treatment of painful neuropathy in patients with diabetes mellitus: a randomized controlled trial. JAMA [Internet]. 1998;280(21):1831–6. Available from: http://www. ncbi.nlm.nih.gov/pubmed/9846777

15. Chang CY, Challa CK, Shah J, Eloy JD. Gabapentin in acute postoperative pain management. Biomed Res Int. 2014;2014(2):1–7.

16. Doleman B, Heinink TP, Read DJ, Faleiro RJ, Lund JN, Williams JP. A systematic review and meta-regression analysis of prophylactic gabapentin for postoperative pain. Anaesthesia. 2015;70(10):1186–204.

17. Barletta JF. Clinical and economic burden of opioid use for postsurgical pain: focus on ventilatory impairment and ileus. Pharmacotherapy. 2012;32(9):3–9.

18. Erstad BL, Puntillo K, Gilbert HC, Grap MJ, Li D, Medina J, et al. Pain management principles in the critically ill. Chest [Internet]. 2009;135(4):1075–86. Available from: http://www. ncbi.nlm.nih.gov/pubmed/19349403

19. Asgeirsson T, El-badawi KI, Mahmood A, Barletta J, Luchtefeld M, Senagore AJ. Postoperative ileus: it costs more than you expect. J Am Coll Surg [Internet]. 2010;210(2):228–31. Available from: http://dx.doi.org/10.1016/j.jamcollsurg.2009.09.028

20. Barletta JF, Senagore AJ. Reducing the burden of postoperative ileus: evaluating and implementing an evidence-based strategy. World J Surg. 2014;38(8):1966–77.

21. Barletta JF, Asgeirsson T, Senagore AJ. Influence of intravenous opioid dose on postoperative ileus. Ann Pharmacother. 2011;45(7–8):916–23.

22. Thompson DR. Narcotic analgesic effects on the sphincter of Oddi: a review of the data and therapeutic implications in treating pancreatitis. Am J Gastroenterol. 2001;96(4):1266–72.

23. Goff JS. The human sphincter of Oddi. Physiology and pathophysiology. Arch Intern Med [Internet]. 1988;148(12):2673–7. Available from: http://www.ncbi.nlm.nih.gov/ pubmed/3058076

24. Yu G, Wen Q, Qiu L, Bo L, Yu J. Laparoscopic cholecystectomy under spinal anaesthesia vs. general anaesthesia: a meta-analysis of randomized controlled trials. BMC Anesthesiol [Internet]. 2015;15(1):176. Available from: http://www.biomedcentral.com/1471-2253/15/176

25. Moraca RJ, Sheldon DG, Thirlby RC. The role of epidural anesthesia and analgesia in surgical practice. Ann Surg. 2003;238(5):663–73.
26. Tzimas P, Prout J, Papadopoulos G, Mallett SV. Epidural anaesthesia and analgesia for liver resection. Anaesthesia. 2013;68(6):628–35.
27. Bruns H, Rahbari NN, Löffler T, Diener MK, Seiler CM, Glanemann M, et al. Perioperative management in distal pancreatectomy: results of a survey in 23 European participating centres of the DISPACT trial and a review of literature. Trials. 2009;10:58.
28. Popping DM, Elia N, Van Aken HK, Marret E, Schug SA, Kranke P, et al. Impact of epidural analgesia on mortality and morbidity after surgery: systematic review and meta-analysis of randomized controlled trials. Ann Surg [Internet]. 2014;259(6):1056–67. Available from: http://shibboleth.ovid.com/secure/?T=JS&CSC=Y&NEWS=N&PAGE=fulltext&D=medl&AN=24096762 http://sfx.kcl.ac.uk/kings?sid=OVID:medline&id=pmid:&id=doi:10.1097%252FSLA.0000000000000237&genre=article&atitle=Impact+of+epidural+analgesia+on+mortality+and+morbidity
29. Sugimoto M, Nesbit L, Barton JG, William TL. Epidural anesthesia dysfunction is associated with postoperative complications after pancreatectomy. J Hepatobiliary Pancreat Sci. 2016;23(2):102–9.
30. Clark CJ, Ali SM, Zaydfudim V, Jacob AK, Nagorney DM. Safety of an enhanced recovery pathway for patients undergoing open hepatic resection. PLoS One [Internet]. 2016;11(3):e0150782. Available from: http://www.ncbi.nlm.nih.gov/pubmed/26950852
31. De Pietri L, Siniscalchi A, Reggiani A, Masetti M, Begliomini B, Gazzi M, et al. The use of intrathecal morphine for postoperative pain relief after liver resection: a comparison with epidural analgesia. Anesth Analg. 2006;102(4):1157–63.
32. Kasivisvanathan R, Abbassi-Ghadi N, Prout J, Clevenger B, Fusai GK, Mallett SV. A prospective cohort study of intrathecal versus epidural analgesia for patients undergoing hepatic resection. HPB. 2014;16(8):768–75.
33. Yarwood J, Berrill A. Nerve blocks of the anterior abdominal wall. Contin Educ Anaesth Crit Care Pain. 2010;10(6):182–6.
34. Jakobsson J, Wickerts L, Forsberg S, Ledin G. Transversus abdominal plane (TAP) block for postoperative pain management: a review. F1000Res [Internet]. 2015;4(F1000 Faculty Rev):1359. Available from: http://f1000research.com/articles/4-1359/v1
35. Abdallah FW, Laffey JG, Halpern SH, Brull R. Duration of analgesic effectiveness after the posterior and lateral transversus abdominis plane block techniques for transverse lower abdominal incisions: a meta-analysis. Br J Anaesth. 2013;111(5):721–35.
36. Keir A, Rhodes L, Kayal A, Khan OA. Does a transversus abdominis plane (TAP) local anaesthetic block improve pain control in patients undergoing laparoscopic cholecystectomy? A best evidence topic. Int J Surg [Internet]. 2013;11(9):792–4. Available from: http://dx.doi.org/10.1016/j.ijsu.2013.05.039
37. Arcidiacono PG, Calori G, Carrara S, McNicol ED, Testoni PA. Celiac plexus block for pancreatic cancer pain in adults. Cochrane Database Syst Rev. 2011;3:CD007519. doi: 10.1002/14651858.CD007519.pub2. Review. PubMed PMID: 21412903.
38. Bell R, Pandanaboyana S, Prasad KR. Epidural versus local anaesthetic infiltration via wound catheters in open liver resection: a meta-analysis. ANZ J Surg. 2015;85(1–2):16–21.
39. Reddi D. Preventing chronic postoperative pain. Anaesthesia. 2016;71:64–71.
40. Pai S-L, Aniskevich S, Rodrigues ES, Shine TS. Analgesic considerations for liver transplantation patients. Curr Clin Pharmacol [Internet]. 2015;10(1):54–65. Available from: http://www.ncbi.nlm.nih.gov/pubmed/24521192
41. Hughes MJ, McNally S, Wigmore SJ. Enhanced recovery following liver surgery: a systematic review and meta-analysis. HPB (Oxford) [Internet]. 2014;16(8):699–706. Available from: http://www.ncbi.nlm.nih.gov/pubmed/24661306
42. Melloul E, Hübner M, Scott M, et al. Guidelines for perioperative care for liver surgery: Enhanced Recovery After Surgery (ERAS) society recommendations. World J Surg. 2016;40(10):2425–40. doi:10.1007/s00268-016-3700-1.
43. Marret E, Rolin M, Beaussier M, Bonnet F. Meta-analysis of intravenous lidocaine and postoperative recovery after abdominal surgery. Br J Surg. 2008;95(11):1331–8.

Determination and Optimization of Liver Function and Volume for Extended Hepatectomy

4

Adeel S. Khan, Kathryn Fowler, and William C. Chapman

Introduction

Considerable advances have been made in hepatic surgery in the last two decades [1]. More and more patients are now undergoing resections for primary and secondary hepatic malignancies with increasing safety. Advances in diagnostic imaging modalities, patient selection, and anesthetic and surgical techniques have led to improved outcomes after liver resection with significant reduction in perioperative mortality, which now ranges between 1% and 5% in most major centers [1, 2]. However, despite all these improvements, hepatic surgery still carries a certain risk of post-hepatectomy liver failure (PHLF), which remains the major cause of morbidity and mortality after major liver resection [3–6]. The risk of PHLF is higher in patients with underlying parenchymal disease and in those undergoing extended resections (at least five hepatic segments) and appears to be related primarily to quality and volume of the liver remnant after resection (future liver remnant [FLR]) [5–8]. The significance of hepatic insufficiency is even more pronounced when complex biliary or vascular reconstructions are required as part of the hepatectomy [6, 7, 9].

A.S. Khan, MD, FACS • W.C. Chapman, MD, FACS (✉)
Division of Transplant Surgery, Department of Surgery, Washington University in St. Louis, St. Louis, MO, USA
e-mail: AKhan24@wustl.edu; chapmanw@wustl.ed

K. Fowler, MD
Mallinckrodt Institute of Radiology, Washington University in St. Louis, St. Louis, MO, USA
e-mail: fowlerk@wustl.edu

© Springer International Publishing AG 2018
F.G. Rocha, P. Shen (eds.), *Optimizing Outcomes for Liver and Pancreas Surgery*, DOI 10.1007/978-3-319-62624-6_4

Post-Hepatectomy Liver Failure (PHLF)

There is no consensus on the exact definition of PHLF. In general PHLF is characterized as failure of one or more of the synthetic and excretory functions of the liver that include hypoalbuminemia, prolonged prothrombin time, elevated serum lactate, and/or hepatic encephalopathy [1–4].

The incidence of PHLF ranges anywhere between 0 and 32% in different case series in literature and is determined by a number of factors [2, 3, 5, 9]. Jarnagin reported PHLF of 5% in patients without chronic liver disease [10], whereas the incidence PHLF can reach upward of 20% in patients with chronic liver disease or cirrhosis [5]. PHLF is an important predictor of postoperative mortality and is the cause of post-resection mortality up to 75% of the time [4]. Balzan et al. in 2005 established the 50–50 criteria, which utilize prothrombin (PT) index <50% (international standardized ration [INR] > 1.7) and serum bilirubin >50 umol/L (2.9 mg/dl) on postoperative day 5 after liver resection to give an estimate of PHLF-related mortality risk. The authors observed a 59% risk of mortality when the 50–50 criteria were fulfilled compared to 1.2% when they were not met (sensitivity 69.6% and specificity 98/5%) [11]. These results have been validated in other studies since then, and the 50–50 criteria remains a fairly accurate predictor of mortality from PLF after major liver resection [1, 3, 4]. Mullen et al. reviewed post-hepatectomy outcomes in 1509 patients and showed that a peak serum bilirubin concentration of >7 mg/dl after resection was associated with a more than 30% chance of dying from liver failure (sensitivity 93.3% and specificity 94.3%) [12].

In 2011, the International Study Group of Liver Surgery (ISGLS) defined PHLF as increased INR and hyperbilirubinemia on or after the fifth postoperative day and provided a severity grade depending on the impact on patient's clinical course and management. PHLF grade A reflects a postoperative deterioration that does not require a change in the patient's clinical management and is not associated with any increase in perioperative mortality. Patients with PHLF grade B show a deviation from the regular postoperative clinical pathway, but invasive treatment is not required, while patients who develop PHLF and require invasive procedure are classified as grade C. The risks of perioperative mortality with grades B and C are 12% and 54%, respectively [13].

Pathogenesis of PHLF

Liver resection results in loss of functional liver mass, and varying amounts of regeneration and death are seen in remaining hepatocytes. In most instances, regeneration outweighs cell death, and both liver mass and function are restored rapidly [14]. Nadalin et al. reported restoration of liver mass up to 74% of initial volume after right hepatectomy for living donor liver transplantation [15]. The ability of a liver to regenerate after resection is dependent on its ability to limit cell death, to preserve or recover an adequate synthetic function, and to enhance its regenerative power [14]. Factors like hepatic parenchymal congestion, hepatic ischemia-reperfusion injury, and reduced phagocytic ability negatively impact the ability of hepatocytes to regenerate after major hepatectomy [4, 6, 11, 15, 16].

Risk Factors for PHLF

Table 4.1 summarizes the major risk factors for development of PHLF.

Patient-Related Factors

Male sex has been shown to double the risk for development of PHLF likely due to circulating levels of sex hormones. Testosterone is also thought to have an immune-depressive effect, which predisposes to septic complications [4, 10]. Relationship between age and risk of development of PHLF is a little controversial, but data suggests that *advanced age* (≥ 65 years) increases risk for PHLF and post-resection mortality [11]. This increased risk can partly be attributed to increased comorbidities and limited regenerative capacity of hepatocytes in the elderly [3]. Little et al. showed increased postoperative mortality in *diabetics* after liver resection with 80% of deaths attributable to PHLF [17]. Similarly *obesity* (BMI ≥ 30) has shown to be a significant predictor of PHLF [18], while malnutrition can be associated with an altered immune response and a reduction in hepatocyte regenerative capacity after resection [1].

Liver-Related Factors

Patients with *steatosis* have been shown to have a higher risk of developing PHLF compared to those without (14% vs 4%) [19]. This increased risk is thought to be due to impaired hepatic microcirculation and decreased resistance to ischemia-reperfusion injury [4]. Similarly cholestasis, due to either biliary obstruction or parenchymal liver disease, can significantly increase morbidity (50% vs 15%),

Table 4.1 Risk factors for post-hepatectomy liver failure (PHLF)

Patient-related factors	Male gender
	Age (>65 years)
	Diabetes mellitus
	Obesity (BMI > 30)
	Malnutrition
Liver-related factors	Cholestasis
	Steatosis
	Cirrhosis
	Chemotherapy-associated hepatotoxicity
Surgery-related factors	Intraoperative blood loss (>1000 ml)
	Prolonged operating time
	Prolonged intraoperative hypotension
	Prolonged inflow occlusion
	Vascular reconstruction
	Ex vivo resection
	Small remnant liver volume
	Postoperative sepsis

mortality (5–13% vs 0–6%), and PHLF (5–17% vs 0–3%) when compared to patients without cholestasis [9, 20]. Patients with *cirrhosis* of the liver also demonstrate decreased levels of hepatocyte regeneration and growth after major liver resection. This, in combination with a wide range of comorbid conditions that exist in cirrhotic patients, like portal hypertension, jaundice, malnutrition, and coagulopathy, results in high mortality rate (5–6.5%) and PHLF (5–10%) after major liver resection [4, 7]. Several clinical studies have shown increased morbidity and PHLF-related death following liver resection in patients who received *neoadjuvant chemotherapy* prior to hepatectomy [4]. The hepatotoxic effects of oxaliplatin (sinusoidal obstruction syndrome) and irinotecan (steatohepatitis) are well documented [4, 21]. However, the benefits of neoadjuvant therapy on tumor burden may counterbalance the increased morbidity. Additionally, though controversial, the toxic effects on the liver related to chemotherapy may be reversible with cessation of therapy.

Surgery-Related Factors

Increased intraoperative bleeding (>1000 ml), need for *blood transfusion* during surgery, *prolonged operative time,* and prolonged *ischemia* (from hypotension or hepatic inflow occlusion) have all been shown to predispose to PHLF and increase morbidity and mortality after major liver resection [3, 10, 16]. Vascular reconstructions as part of liver resection or ex vivo liver resection are also associated with increased rates of PHLF and mortality [1]. *Sepsis* in the postoperative period can similarly predispose to PHLF and increased mortality by prolonging ischemia and directly inhibiting hepatocyte regeneration [1, 4]. Removal of too much liver can result in a *small-for-size syndrome (SFSS)* where remaining mass of liver is insufficient to maintain normal liver function. Many mechanisms have been proposed to explain this phenomenon with the "hyperperfusion theory" being the most widely accepted explanation [22]. According to this theory, the surge in sinusoidal blood flow following reduction in parenchymal volume results in a cycle of sinusoidal dilation, sheer stress, centrilobular necrosis, prolonged cholestasis, impaired synthetic function, and inhibition of cell proliferation, all of which can negatively impact hepatic function [22].

The safe limits for liver resection are still a debated issue; the minimal volume of remnant liver (functional liver remnant [FLR]) varies from patient to patient and is dependent on liver function and underlying liver disease [2–6, 23].

The Functional (Future) Liver Remnant (FLR)

Although many variables influence the risk of PHLF, the preoperative evaluation of the FLR volume is considered by many to be the most important modifiable predictor of PHLF [2–6, 15, 23]. FLR is defined as a percentage of remaining functional liver volume compared with preoperative functional liver volume (total liver volume with tumor volume subtracted) [2, 23]. Several studies indicate that the FLR volume serves as a predictor of remnant liver function, and consequently FLR volume is widely used as a surrogate for the risk of developing PHLF [2–6, 23]. The extent of resection has shown to correlate closely with rates of PHLF and death, with 80% deaths from PHLF occurring after resection of more than 50% of liver volume [18, 24, 25]. Schnidl et al. in 2005 described a proportional increase in incidence of PHLF with increasing numbers of segments resected. The authors reported PHLF rates of less than 1% in patients with no underlying parenchymal disease who underwent resection of 1–2 segments, 10% when 4 segments were resected, and an increase to 30% with removal of 5 or more segments [26].

Though the exact volume of FLR required to preserve sufficient liver function is unknown, in general, FLR of ≥20% in otherwise healthy liver is associated with good post-resection outcomes. Abdalla et al. showed a 50% incidence of PHLF in patients who underwent extended right hepatectomy with FLR volumes ≤20% versus only 13% for patients with FLR ≥ 20% [27]. This cutoff for safe hepatic resection was confirmed by Kishi et al., who described a significant increase in PHLF and death in patients with FLR volumes ≤20% (34% and 11%) compared to patients with FLR of 20–30% (10% and 3%), respectively [28]. These results were reflected in the 2006 expert consensus statement and a minimum safe limit of FLR of 20% was recommended for liver resection with normal liver [29].

The recommendations for safe FLR are less clear in patients with chronic liver disease and cirrhosis. Safe limits of resection are not only dependent on the nature of the underlying disease but also on its severity and impact on overall liver function. Current data suggests that safe limits for FLR for patients with mild steatosis, cholestasis, and early cirrhosis (Child's-Pugh A) are in the range of 30–35%, and 40% for severe steatosis and cholestasis [3, 21, 30, 31]. Schroeder et al. reported the superiority of the Child-Pugh scoring system to the MELD score in predicting short-term morbidity and mortality after liver resection [32]; however, others have shown preoperative MELD score of greater than 11 to be a highly reliable and accurate predictor of PHLF [33]. In patients with cirrhosis but no functional impairment or portal hypertension resection of up to 50%, liver volume can be safe [34]. However, in patients with more advanced cirrhosis (Child's-Pugh B or C), even small resections can result in PHLF [1]. A percutaneous liver biopsy of the FLR prior to hepatectomy can give valuable information on the extent of parenchymal disease and can impact extent of resection. In patients requiring resections beyond the safe limit of volume criteria, strategies like portal vein embolization (PVE) must be considered prior to surgery [1, 23, 31, 34].

Assessment of FLR: Liver Volumetry

Given the high variability between individuals in the ratio and size of liver segments, a thorough preoperative volumetric evaluation of the FLR is essential to avoid PHLF. In the western population, the right liver typically accounts for approximately two thirds (65%) of the total liver volume and the left liver accounting for about one third (35%). However, a great deal of heterogeneity can exist in liver volumes with the right liver contributing anywhere from 49% to 82% and the left liver contributing between 17% and 49% [6, 35].

Multiple imaging modalities are available to assess the FLR volume including scintigraphy, ultrasound, computed tomography (CT) scan, and magnetic resonance imaging (MRI). These studies can also aid in identification of underlying liver disease and vascular anatomy, which may influence extent of resection. CT-guided three-dimensional reconstructions allow visualization of vasculature including hepatic venous outflow, tumor localization, and size and facilitate operative planning [36]. Three-dimensional CT volumetric estimation is performed by manually outlining the liver margin from which the area can be derived and then multiplied by the slice thickness [1, 4, 36]. Several vendors provide 3-D packages that allow volumetric analysis (Fig. 4.1). The sensitivity of volumetric assessment can be additionally enhanced by combination of body surface area (BSA) and body weight (BW) calculations [37]. Volumes of interest are total liver volume (TLV), FLR, and tumor volume (TV). TV is usually subtracted from TLV to provide the functional liver volume (FLV), which is a more accurate measurement for calculating FLR and determining need for volume optimization [37–39]. It should be noted that while volume has been closely studied and is a strong predictor of postoperative outcome, it is basically a surrogate measure for function.

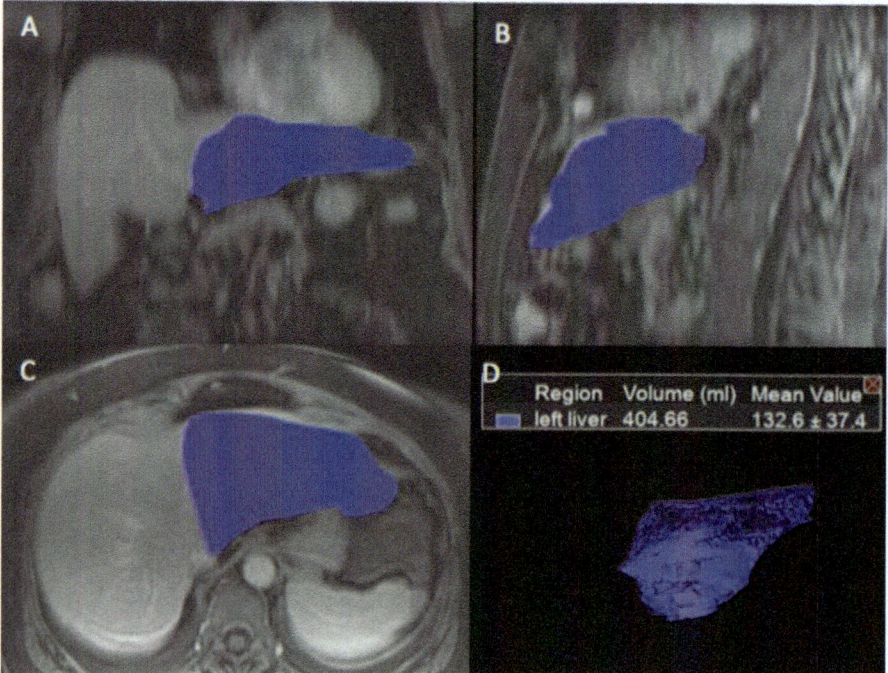

Fig. 4.1 Images (**a**–**c**) demonstrate a tint overlay of the region contoured on a post-contrast MR image to provide volumetric assessment for preoperative planning. The final volume will reflect the remnant liver volume (**d**), which can be used to calculate functional liver reserve. These images were generated on Vitrea Core advanced viewer (Vital Images, Minnetonka, Minnesota, USA)

Assessment of Liver Function Prior to Resection

Liver function may be considered the ground truth for predicting reserve following a major hepatectomy. It is reduced in patients with underlying liver disease, and therefore, determining the synthetic function of the liver is considered by many to be as important as volumetry especially in patients with parenchymal disease [40]. Many quantitative tests have been described to assess function of the liver; however, they are rarely applied in clinical practice due to limited availability, complexity, and cost.

The *indocyanine green (ICG) clearance* is considered to be one of the most powerful predictive tests of operative mortality after hepatectomy in some parts of the world but is not widely used in western countries. ICG retention in 15 min (ICGR15) depends on hepatic perfusion rate and is one of the most frequently used parameters in decision-making protocol before liver resection [3]. ICGR above 15–20% is generally indicative of impaired hepatic functional reserve, and these patients might benefit from leaving a larger FLR [41].

Galactose elimination test, lidocaine-monoethylglycinexylidide (MEGX) test, and the C-aminopyrine breath test are some of the other tests that have been described for assessment of liver function in operative planning [42].

Strategies for Optimization of FLR

Figure 4.2 gives an overview of the algorithm for assessment of a patient for volume optimization strategies prior to planned hepatectomy.

Portal Vein Embolization (PVE)

PVE is commonly used in the patients requiring extensive liver resection but have insufficient FLR volume on preoperative testing. The procedure involves occluding portal venous flow to the side of the liver with the lesion thereby redirecting portal flow to the contralateral side, in an attempt to cause hypertrophy and increase the volume of the FLR prior to hepatectomy [43] (Fig. 4.3). PVE was first described by Kinoshita and later reported by Makuuchi as a technique to facilitate hepatic resection of hilar cholangiocarcinoma [44, 45]. The technique is now widely used by surgeons all over the world to optimize FLR volume before major liver resections.

PVE works because the extrahepatic factors that induce liver hypertrophy are carried primarily by the portal vein and not the hepatic artery [43]. The increase in FLR size seen after PVE is due to both clonal expansion and cellular hypertrophy, and the extent of post-embolization liver growth is generally proportional to the degree of portal flow diversion [46]. The mechanism of liver regeneration after PVE is a complex phenomenon and is not fully understood. Although the exact trigger of liver regeneration remains unknown, several studies have identified periportal inflammation in the embolized liver as an important predictor of liver regeneration [47].

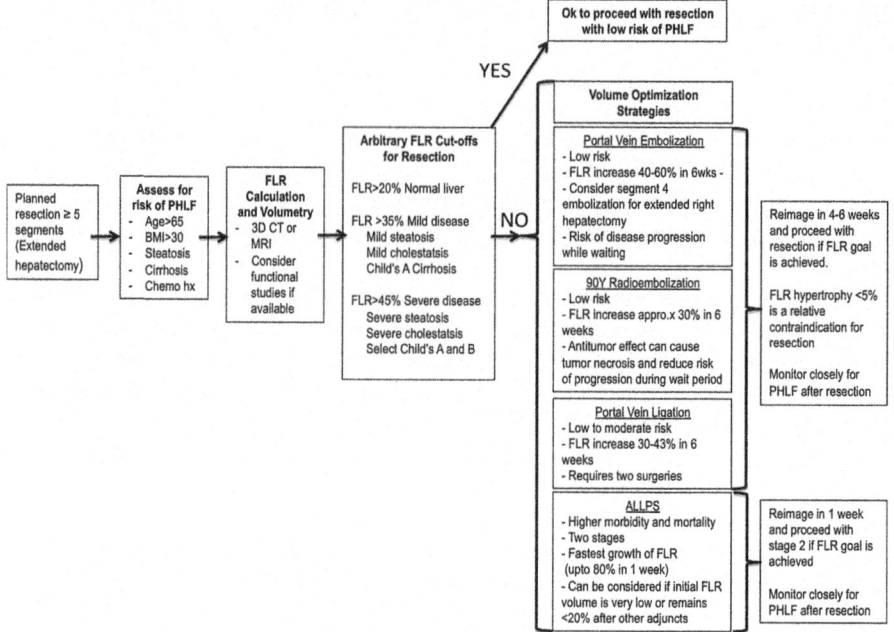

Fig. 4.2 Algorithm for assessment of a patient for consideration for volume optimization strategies

PVE is technically feasible in 99% of the patients with low risk of complications [48]. Studies have shown the FLR to increase by a median of 40–62% after a median of 34–37 days after PVE, and 72.2–80% of the patients are able to undergo resection as planned [49, 50]. It is generally indicated for patients being considered for right or extended right hepatectomy in the setting of a relatively small FLR. It is rarely required before extended left hepatectomy or left trisectionectomy, since the right posterior section (segments 6 and 7) comprises about 30% of total liver volume [51]. PVE is usually performed through percutaneous transhepatic access to the portal venous system, but there is considerable variability in technique between centers. The access route can be ipsilateral (portal access at the same side being resected) with retrograde embolization or contralateral (portal access through FLR) with antegrade embolization. The type of approach selected depends on a number of factors including operator preference, anatomic variability, type of resection planned, extent of embolization, and type of embolic agent used. Many authors prefer ipsilateral approach especially for right-sided tumors as this technique allows easy catheterization of segment 4 branches when they must be embolized and also minimizes the theoretic risk of injuring the FLR vasculature or bile ducts through a contralateral approach and potentially making a patient ineligible for surgery [43, 46, 47, 52]. However, majority of the studies on contralateral PVE show it to be a safe technique with low complication rate [53–55]. Di Stefano et al. reported a large series of contralateral PVE in188 patients and described 12 complications (6.4%),

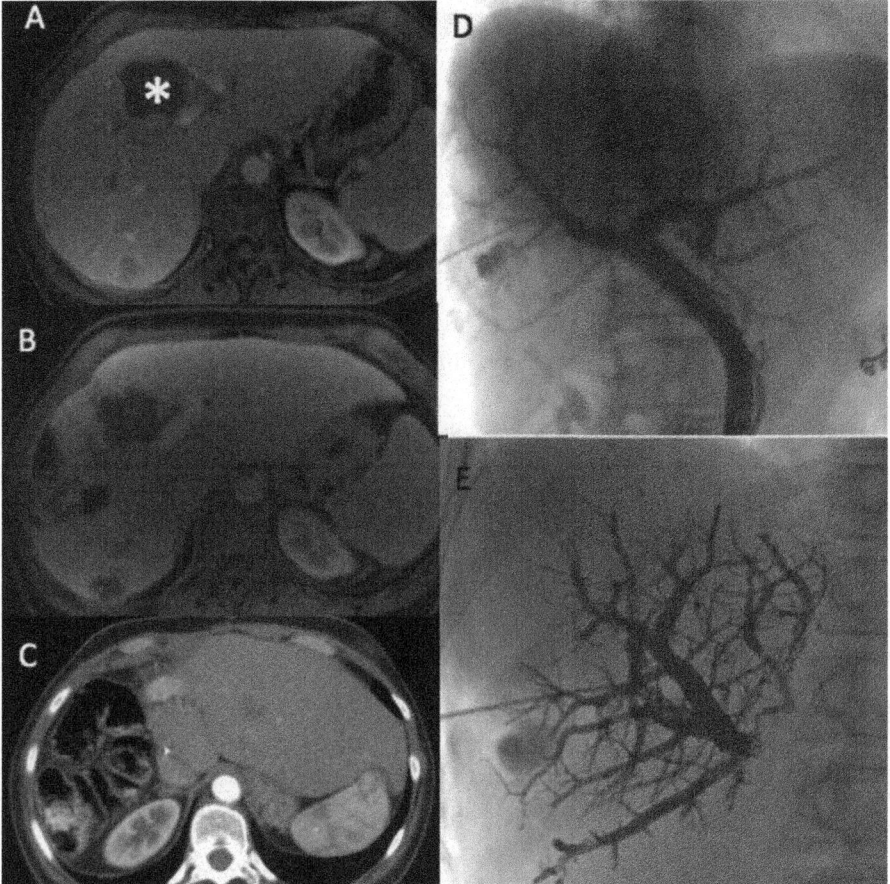

Fig. 4.3 A 49-year-old woman with metastatic colorectal carcinoma (**a**–*white asterisk*). Post-contrast transverse MR images (**a**–**b**) show pre- and post-portal vein embolization features of the liver. Note on image B that the left liver has hypertrophied compared to image A. Images (**a**–**e**) show the portal vein embolization procedure with demonstration of the entire portal system (**d**) and subsequent ipsilateral glue embolization of the right portal system (**e**). The embolization procedure resulted in an increase in the functional liver reserve volume of approximately 15%. The patient underwent right trisectionectomy (**c**)

only 6 of which could be related to access route and none precluded liver resection [52]. Site of portal vein access can also change depending on the choice of embolic material selected which can include glue, Gelfoam, n-butyl-cyanoacrylate (NBC), different types and sizes of beads, alcohol, and nitinol plus. All agents have similar efficacy and there are no official recommendations for a particular type of agent. However, some materials can be hard to manipulate from the ipsilateral side (e.g., glue), while large embolic agents like plugs require larger-diameter access needles which can add to overall risk of procedure especially if done from the side of the FLR [51, 53–58].

To ensure a good hypertrophic response after PVE, it is imperative that the embolization of the selected PV branches be as complete as possible. The reasons for this are twofold: complete PVE avoids recanalization of occluded portal system, and secondly intrahepatic porto-portal shunting can be minimized which can limit regeneration. Complete embolization also reduces the risk of diversion of portal flow to the tumor-containing potion of the liver which can hypothetically lead to accelerated tumor growth [59]. Proponents of PVE believe that there should be very little or no tumor progression during the 4–6 week wait period for regeneration after PVE [43, 47, 56].

Rapid growth of the FLR can be expected within the first 3–4 weeks after PVE and can continue till 6–8 weeks [51]. Results from multiple studies suggest that 8–30% hypertrophy over 2–6 weeks can be expected with slower rates in cirrhotic patients [53].

Most studies comparing outcomes after major hepatectomy with and without preoperative PVE report superior outcomes with PVE [55]. Farges et al. demonstrated significantly less risk of postoperative complications, duration of intensive care unit, and hospital stay in patients with cirrhosis who underwent right hepatectomy after PVE compared to those who did not have preoperative PVE. The authors also reported no benefit of PVE in patients with a normal liver and FLR >30% [60].

Abulkhir et al. reported results from a meta-analysis of 1088 patients undergoing PVE and showed a markedly lower incidence of PHLF and death compared to series reporting outcomes after major hepatectomy in patients who did not undergo PVE. All patients had FLR volume increase, and 85% went on to have liver resection after PVE with a PHLF incidence of 2.5% and a surgical mortality of 0.8% [55]. Several studies looking at the effect of systemic neoadjuvant chemotherapy on the degree of hypertrophy after PVE show no significant impact on liver regeneration and growth [61–63].

The volumetric response to PVE is also a very important factor in understanding the regenerative capacity of a patient's liver and when used together with FLR volume can help identify patients at risk of poor postsurgical outcome [43, 51]. Ribero et al. demonstrated that the risk of PHLF was significantly higher not only in patients with FLR $\leq$ 20% but also in patients with normal liver who demonstrated $\leq$5% of FLR hypertrophy after PVE. The authors concluded that the degree of hypertrophy >10% in patients with severe underlying liver disease and >5% in patients with normal liver predicts a low risk of PHLF and post-resection mortality [54]. Many authors do not routinely offer resection to patients with borderline FLR who demonstrate $\leq$5% hypertrophy after PVE [43, 51, 53, 54, 58].

Yttrium-90 (Y90) Radioembolization

There have been recent reports describing the use of Yttrium-90 (Y90) radioembolization in HCC patients being considered for resection as an effective way to induce hypertrophy of FLR while simultaneously providing tumor control [64, 65]. Lewandowski et al. recently described their experience with neoadjuvant Y90 radioembolization in 13 patients (10 HCC, 2 cholangiocarcinoma, 1 colorectal metastases) being considered for major hepatectomy with inadequate FLR. The authors described a median FLR hypertrophy of 30% (4–105%) after a median of 40 days. Moreover, 92% of the patients with resected tumors had >50% necrosis on pathologic analysis [65]. The antitumor effects of this modality might help address some of the concerns with PVE in patients at a high risk for disease progression in the 4–6-week waiting period prior to resection.

Two-Stage Hepatectomy with Portal Vein Ligation (PVL)

Two-stage hepatectomy with PVL is usually reserved for patients with bilobar tumor involvement and requires two separate surgeries. In the first stage, the FLR is cleared of tumor and opposite side portal vein (side being considered for resection) is ligated. Parenchymal transection is not performed during the first stage. In the case of synchronous colorectal metastatic disease, the first-stage surgery can be performed at the same time as surgery for colorectal primary. Repeat imaging is performed at 4–6 weeks to assess post-PVL hypertrophy of the FLR after which the second-stage laparotomy is planned usually at 6–8 weeks after the first surgery. During the second stage, the parenchyma is transected and the liver on the side of PVL is removed. The two-stage procedure has been found in some studies to be as effective as PVE; however, it requires two surgeries and poses the risk of adhesion formation in the hilum, which can add to the complexity of the second-stage operation [51]. Studies looking at outcomes after PVL and two-stage hepatectomies have shown a median FLR increase of 30–43% after a median of 37–57.9 days, with 62.5–87% patients able to undergo resection in the second stage with a surgical mortality of 5.3–10% [66–68].

Associating Liver Partition and Portal Vein Ligation (ALPPS) in Staged Hepatectomy

ALPPS is a relatively recent technique to aid hepatic resection in patients with small FLRs and has shown to induce more rapid FLR hypertrophy as compared to that seen after PVE or PVL [69]. It is a two-stage procedure with the first stage involving in situ portal vein ligation on the side of the planned resection along with parenchymal transection down to the vena cava without typically dividing the hepatic artery or bile duct. During the second stage, the hepatic artery and bile duct are transected and the diseased liver is excised. The procedure was first described by Schlitt [69] who was attempting an extended right hepatectomy for hilar cholangiocarcinoma. The procedure was converted to a palliative left hepaticojejunostomy as the FLR was felt to be too small; however, the liver parenchyma had already been divided along the falciform ligament in addition to ligation of the right portal vein. CT scan performed 8 days later surprisingly showed a significant increase in the size of the left lateral section, which allowed for subsequent removal of the diseased and partially resected right liver [69]. Since then several authors have shown ALPPS to be a viable strategy for performing liver resection in patients with high tumor burden and small-sized FLRs [70–72]. ALPPS has shown to induce hypertrophy of the FLR up to 80% in a matter of days as compared to 4–6 weeks after PVE and PVL [71, 72]. ALPPS addresses intrahepatic portal collaterals between the FLR and the portal-occluded part of the liver, which have been implicated as the main reason for failure of FLR to hypertrophy after PVE and PVL [72]. In addition, work on mice has shown that growth factor release after the first step in ALPPS also plays a pivotal role in inducing rapid hypertrophy of FLR [73]. The rapid hypertrophy seen after ALPPS generated a lot of enthusiasm initially and was felt to be the answer to the problem of potential dropout of up to 35% in patients undergoing PVE or PVL due to either insufficient FLR hypertrophy or tumor progression within the 4–6-week period of waiting between PVE/PVL and resection [55, 59, 66, 71]. However, several recent reviews have indicated considerably higher morbidity and mortality after ALPPS compared to other portal vein occlusion techniques [48, 71, 72]. There are no randomized control trials comparing ALPPS to other techniques of portal vein occlusion (PVE or PVL), and most of the data available is retrospective raising concerns for selection bias. A recent meta-analysis looking at 90 studies involving 4352 patients (including 320 from the ALPPS registry) showed that in the comparison between ALPPS and PVE, although ALPPS was associated with a greater increase in the FLR (76% vs 37%), and more frequent completion of stage 2 (100% vs 77%), it had a higher morbidity (73% vs 59%) and mortality (14% vs 7%) [72] which has dampened some of the initial enthusiasm. The exact role of ALPPS in management of patients with small FLRs has yet to be established. ALPPS might be an extremely suitable option for patients who demonstrate insufficient growth of FLR after PVE or PVL (salvage ALPPS) and might also be an option for patients with extremely low FLRs who are unlikely to generate enough hypertrophy after PVE or PVL to be candidates for resection [48].

Treatment of PHLF

There are no clear-cut guidelines for the management of PHLF, and treatment strategies are similar to those applied in the management of patients with acute (fulminant) liver failure, acute-on-chronic liver failure, and/or sepsis. These strategies focus more on support of liver and end-organ function rather than therapeutic interventions [1, 4]. Rescue hepatectomy and liver transplantation can be an option in a select group of PHLF patients who otherwise meet criteria for transplantation. Liver transplant is generally not indicated in patients with metastatic hepatic disease [1, 4].

Conclusion

Medical advances in the last couple of decades now allow more and more patients to undergo liver resection for primary and secondary malignancies with increasing safety. However, despite these advancements, PHLF remains a major cause of morbidity and mortality after major liver resections. Though PHLF is impacted by a number of factors, an inadequate liver remnant (FLR) is felt to be the most important modifiable predictor of PHLF. Preoperative evaluation of FLR function and volume is of paramount importance before any major liver resection, and resection should only be considered if FLR is >20% of the TLV in an otherwise healthy liver. Patients with inadequate or borderline FLRs can be considered for liver volume optimization strategies such as PVE, PVL, and ALPPS. The choice of strategy varies by patient to patient and is dictated by patient factors, extent and location of disease, overall surgical plan, and institution preference. Future advancements in preoperative optimization of liver function, perioperative liver support with liver-assist devices, and strategies to enhance liver regeneration will allow major liver resections to be done with an even greater safety profile and decreased incidence of PHLF.

References

1. Hammond JS, Guha IN, Beckingham IJ, et al. Prediction, prevention and management of postresection liver failure. Br J Surg. 2011;98:1188–200.
2. Helling TS. Liver failure following partial hepatectomy. HPB (Oxford). 2006;8:165–74.
3. Guglielmi A, Ruzzenente A, Conci S. How much remnant is enough in liver resection. Dig Surg. 2012;29:6–17.
4. van den Broek MA, Olde Damink SW, Dejong CH. Liver failure after partial hepatic resections: definition, pathophysiology, risk factors and treatment. Liver Int. 2008;28:767–80.
5. Tanabe G, Sakamoto M, Akazawa K, et al. Intraoperative risk factors associated with hepatic resection. Br J Surg. 1995;82:1262–5.
6. Pulitano C, Crawford M, Joseph D, et al. Preoperative assessment of post-operative liver function: the importance of residual liver volume. J Surg Oncol. 2014;110:445–50.
7. Farges O, Malassagne B, Flejou JF, et al. Risk of major liver resection in patients with underlying chronic liver disease: a reappraisal. Ann Surg. 1999;229:210–5.
8. Belghiti J, Hiramatsu K, Benoist S, et al. Seven hundred forty-seven hepatectomies in the 1990's: an update to evaluate the actual risk of liver resection. J Am Coll Surg. 2000;191:38–46.
9. Cherqui D, Benoist S, Malassagne B, et al. Major liver resection for carcinoma in jaundiced patients without preoperative biliary drainage. Arch Surg. 2000;135:302–8.
10. Jarnagin WR, Gonen M, Fong Y, et al. Improvement in perioperative outcome after hepatic resection: an analysis of 1,803 consecutive cases over the past decade. Ann Surg. 2002;236:397–406.
11. Balzan S, Belghiti J, Farges O, et al. The '50-50 criteria' on post operative day 5: an accurate predictor of liver failure and death after hepatectomy. Ann Surg. 2005;242:824–8.
12. Mullen JT, Ribero D, Reddy SK, et al. Hepatic insufficiency and mortality in 1,059 non cirrhotic patients undergoing major hepatectomy. J Am Coll Surg. 2007;204:854–62.
13. Rahbari NN, Garden OJ, Padbury R, et al. Post hepatectomy liver failure: a definition and grading by the International Study Group of Liver Surgery (ISGLS). Surgery. 2011;149:713–24.
14. Michalopoulos GK, DeFrances MC. Liver regeneration. Science. 1997;276:60–6.
15. Nadalin S, Testa G, Malago M, et al. Volumetric and functional recovery of the liver after right hepatectomy for living donation. Liver Transpl. 2004;10:1024–9.
16. Jaeschke H. Molecular mechanisms of hepatic ischemia-reperfusion injury and preconditioning. Am J Physiol Gastrointest Liver Physiol. 2003;284:G15–26.
17. Little SA, Jarnagin WR, DeMatteo RP, et al. Diabetes is associated with increased perioperative mortality but equivalent long-term outcome after hepatic resection for colorectal cancer. J Gastrointest Surg. 2002;6:88–94.

18. Balzan S, Nagarajan G, Farges O, et al. Safety of liver resection in obese and overweight patients. World J Surg. 2010;34:2960–8.
19. Behrns KE, Tsiotos GG, DeSouza NF, et al. Hepatic steatosis is a potential risk factor for major hepatic resection. J Gastrointest Surg. 1998;2:292–8.
20. Kennedy TJ, Yopp A, Qin Y, et al. Role of preoperative biliary drainage of liver remnant prior to extended liver resection for hilar cholangiocarcinoma. HPB (Oxford). 2009;11:445–51.
21. Vauthey JN, Pawlik TM, Ribero D, et al. Chemotherapy regimen predicts steato-hepatitis and in increase 90-day mortality after surgery for hepatic colo-rectal metastases. J Clin Oncol. 2006;24:2065–72.
22. Demetris AJ, Kelly DM, Eghtesad B, et al. Pathophysiologic observations and histopathologic recognition of the portal hyperperfusion or small-for-size syndrome. Am J Surg Pathol. 2006;30:986–93.
23. Hemming AW, Reed AI, Howard RJ, et al. Preoperative portal vein embolization for extended hepatectomy. Ann Surg. 2003;237(5):686–93.
24. House MG, Ito H, Gonen M, et al. Survival after hepatic resection for metastatic colorectal cancer: trends in outcomes for 1600 patients during two decades at a single institution. J Am Coll Surg. 2010;210:744–52.
25. Poon RT, Fan ST, Lo CM, et al. Improving perioperative outcome expands the role of hepatectomy in management of benign and malignant hepatobiliary diseases: analysis of 1222 consecutive patients from a prospective database. Ann Surg. 2004;240:698–708.
26. Schindl M, Redhead D, Fearon K, et al. Edinburgh Liver Surgery and Transplantation Experimental Research Group (eLISTER). The value of residual volume as a predictor of hepatic dysfunction and infection after major liver resection. Gut. 2005;54:289–96.
27. Abdalla EK, Barnett CC, Doherty D. Extended hepatectomy in patients with hepatobiliary malignancies with and without preoperative portal vein embolization. Arch Surg. 2002;137:675–80.
28. Kishi Y, Abdaka EK, Chun YS, et al. Three hundred and one consecutive extended right hepatectomies: evaluation of outcome based on systematic liver volumetry. Ann Surg. 2009;250:540–8.
29. Abdalla EK, Adam R, Bilchik AJ, et al. Improving resectability of hepatic colorectal metastases: expert consensus statement. Ann Surg Oncol. 2006;13:1271–80.
30. Shirabe K, Shimada M, Gion T, et al. Post operative liver failure after major hepatic resection for hepatocellular carcinoma in the modern era with special reference to remnant liver volume. J Am Coll Surg. 1999;188:304–9.
31. Miyagawa S, Makuuchi M, Kawasaki S. Criteria for safe hepatic resection. Am J Surg. 1995;169:589–94.
32. Schroeder RA, Marroquin CE, Bute BP. Predictive indices of morbidity and mortality after liver resection. Ann Surg. 2006;243:373–9.
33. Cucchetti A, Ercolani G, Vivarelli M, et al. Impact of model for end-stage liver disease (MELD) score on prognosis after hepatectomy for hepatocellular carcinoma in cirrhosis. Liver Transpl. 2006;12:966–71.
34. Poon RT, Fan ST. Assessment of hepatic reserve for indication of hepatic resection: how I do it. J Hepato-Biliary-Pancreat Surg. 2005;12:31–7.
35. Abdalla EK, Denys A, Chevalier P, et al. Total and segmental liver volume variations: implications for liver surgery. Surgery. 2004;135:404–10.
36. Lamade W, Glombitza G, Fischer L, et al. The impact of 3-dimensional reconstructions on operation planning in liver surgery. Arch Surg. 2000;135:1256–61.
37. Vauthey JN, Abdalla EK, Doherty DA. Body surface area and body weight predict total liver volume in Western adults. Liver Transpl. 2002;8:233–40.
38. Kubota K, Makuuchi M, Kusaka K, et al. Measurement of liver volume and hepatic functional reserve as a guide to decision-making in resectional surgery for hepatic tumors. Hepatology. 1997;26:1176–81.
39. Ogasawara K, Une Y, Nakajima Y, et al. The significance of measuring liver volume using computer tomographic images before and after hepatectomy. Surg Today. 1995;25:43–8.

40. Dinant S, de Graaaf W, Verwer BJ, et al. Risk assessment of post hepatectomy liver volume using hepatobiliary scintigraphy and CT volumetry. J Nucl Med. 2007;48:685–92.
41. Fan ST, Lai EC, Lo CM, et al. Hospital mortality of major hepatectomy for hepatocellular carcinoma associated with cirrhosis. Arch Surg. 1995;130:198–203.
42. Gazzaniga GM, Cappato S, Belli FE, et al. Assessment of hepatic reserve for the indication of hepatic resection: how I do it. J Hepato-Biliary-Pancreat Surg. 2005;12:27–30.
43. Abdalla E. Portal vein embolization (prior to major hepatectomy) effects on regeneration, resectability and outcome. J Surg Oncol. 2010;102:960–7.
44. Kinoshita H, Sakai K, Hirohashi K, et al. Preoperative portal vein embolization for hepatocellular carcinoma. World J Surg. 1986;10:803–8.
45. Makuuchi M, Thai BL, Takayasu K, et al. Preoperative portal embolization to increase safety of major hepatectomy for hilar bile duct carcinoma: a preliminary report. Surgery. 1990;107:521–7.
46. Madoff DC, Abdalla EK, Gupta S, et al. Transhepatic ipsilateral right portal vein embolization extended to segment IV: Improving hypertrophy and resection outcomes with spherical particles and coils. J Vasc Interv Radiol. 2005;16:215–25.
47. Denys AL, Abehsera M, Sauvanet A, et al. Failure of right portal vein ligation to induce left lobe hypertrophy due to intrahepatic portoportal collaterals: successful treatment with portal vein embolization. Am J Roentgenol. 1999;173:633–5.
48. Hasselgren K, Sandstrom P, Bjornsson B. Role of associating liver partition and portal vein ligation for staged hepatectomy in colorectal liver metastases: a review. World J Gastroenterol. 2015;21(15):4491–8.
49. Worni M, Shah KN, Clary BM. Colorectal cancer with potentially resectable hepatic metastases: optimizing treatment. Curr Oncol Rep. 2014;16:407.
50. Shindoh J, Vauthey JN, Zimmitti G. Analysis of the efficacy of portal vein embolization for patients with extensive liver malignancy and very low future liver remnant volume, including a comparison with the associating liver partition with portal vein ligation for stated hepatectomy approach. J Am Coll Surg. 2013;217:126–33.
51. She WH, Chok KS. Strategies to increase the resectability of hepatocellular carcinoma. World J Hepatol. 2015;7(18):2147–54.
52. Di Stefano DR, de Baere T, Denys A, et al. Preoperative percutaneous portal vein embolization: evaluation of adverse events in 188 patients. Radiology. 2005;234:625–30.
53. Loffroy R, Favelier S, Chevallier O, et al. Preoperative portal vein embolization in liver cancer: indications, techniques and outcomes. Quant Imaging Med Surg. 2015;5(5):730–9.
54. Ribero D, Abdalla EK, Madoff DC, et al. Portal vein embolization before major hepatectomy and its effect on regeneration, resectability and outcome. Br J Surg. 2007;94:1386–94.
55. Abulkhir A, Limongelli P, Healey AJ, et al. Preoperative portal vein embolization for major liver resection: a meta-analysis. Ann Surg. 2008;247:49–57.
56. Elias D, De Baere T, Roche A, et al. During liver regeneration following right portal embolization, the growth rate of liver metastases is more rapid than that of liver parenchyma. Br J Surg. 1999;86:784–8.
57. Palavecino M, Chun YS, Madoff DC, et al. Major hepatic resection for hepatocellular carcinoma with or without portal vein embolization: perioperative outcome and survival. Surgery. 2009;145:399–405.
58. Ribero D, Curley SA, Imamura H. Selection for resection of hepatocellular carcinoma and surgical strategy: indications for resection, evaluation of liver function, portal vein embolization and resection. Ann Surg Oncol. 2008;15:986–92.
59. Hayashi S, Baba Y, Ueno K, et al. Acceleration of primary liver tumor growth rate in embolized hepatic lobe after portal vein embolization. Acta Radiol. 2007;48:721–7.
60. Farges O, Belghiti J, Kianmanesh R, et al. Portal vein embolization before right hepatectomy: prospective clinical trial. Ann Surg. 2003;237:208–17.
61. Simoneau E, Alanazi R, Alshenaifi J, et al. Neoadjuvant chemotherapy does not impair liver regeneration following hepatectomy or portal vein embolization for colorectal cancer liver metastases. J Surg Oncol. 2016;113(4):449–55.

62. Chun YS, Vauthey JN, Ribero D, et al. Systemic chemotherapy and two-stage hepatectomy for extensive bilateral colorectal liver metastases: perioperative safety and survival. J Gastrointest Surg. 2007;11:1498–504.
63. Zorzi D, Chun YS, Madoff DC, et al. Chemotherapy with bevacizumab does not affect liver regeneration after portal vein embolization. Ann Surg Oncol. 2008;15:2765–72.
64. Salem R, Thurston KG. Radioembolization with 90Yttrium microspheres: a state-of-the-art brachytherapy treatment for primary and secondary liver malignancies. Part 1: technical and methodologic considerations. J Vasc Interv Radiol. 2006;17(8):1251–78.
65. Lewandowski RJ, Donahue L, Chokechanachaisakul A, et al. Y90 radiation lobectomy: outcomes following surgical resection in patients with hepatic tumors and small future remnant volumes. J Surg Oncol. 2016;114(1):99–105.
66. Homayounfar K, Liersch T, Schuetze G, et al. Two-stage hepatectomy (R0) with portal vein ligation – towards curing patients with extended bilobar colorectal liver metastases. Int J Color Dis. 2009;24:409–18.
67. Robles R, Marin C, Lopez-Conesa A, et al. Comparative study of right portal vein ligation versus embolization for induction of hypertrophy in two-stage hepatectomy for multiple bilateral colorectal liver metastases. Eur J Surg Oncol. 2012;38:586–93.
68. Capussotti L, Muratore A, Baraachi F, et al. Portal vein ligation is an efficient method of increasing the future liver remnant volume in the surgical treatment of colorectal metastases. Arch Surg. 2008;143:978–82.
69. Schnitzbauer AA, Lang SA, Goessman H. Right portal vein ligation combined with in situ splitting induces rapid left lateral liver hypertrophy enabling 2-staged extended right hepatic resection in small-for-size settings. Ann Surg. 2012;255:405–14.
70. De Santibanes E, Clavien PA. Playing Play-Doh to prevent postoperative liver failure: the "ALPPS" approach. Ann Surg. 2012;255:415–7.
71. Broering DC, Hillert C, Krupski G, et al. Portal vein embolization versus portal vein ligation for induction of hypertrophy of the future liver remnant. J Gastrointest Surg. 2002;6:905–13.
72. Eshmuminov D, Raptis DA, Linecker M, et al. Meta-analysis of associating liver partition with portal vein ligation and portal vein occlusion for two-stage hepatectomy. Br J Surg. 2016;103(13):1768–82.
73. Schlegel A, Lesurtel M, Melloul E, et al. ALPPS: from human to mice highlighting accelerated and novel mechanisms of liver regeneration. Ann Surg. 2014;260:839–46.

Techniques to Minimize Blood Loss During Hepatectomy

5

Justin T. Huntington and Carl R. Schmidt

Introduction

The liver has such a rich blood supply and significant bleeding risk that it was thought by many including Galen, one of the most famous ancient Greek physicians, to be the source of venous blood [1]. Dr. Carl Langenbuch reported the first successful elective hepatectomy in 1888 with the first performed in the United States by Dr. William Keen in 1892 [2, 3]. A major advance in understanding operative liver anatomy came in 1953 when Dr. John Healey defined the liver into eight segments based upon the hepatic arterial and biliary system [4]. Subsequently in 1954 Dr. Claude Couinaud defined the liver in eight segments based upon the portal venous system and is the foundation for the current surgical hepatic anatomy classification system [5]. These advances laid the foundation for the first anatomic hepatectomy in 1952 by Dr. Lortat-Jacob [6]. Outcomes from hepatectomy operations have seen dramatic improvements since the original descriptions of these operations. In the 1970s observed operative mortality rates from hepatectomy procedures ranged from 17% to 24% [7]. Comparatively, modern series show rates of mortality after hepatectomy of around 5% or significantly less [8, 9]. Risk factors associated with operative mortality after partial hepatectomy include operative blood loss and transfusion requirement [10–17]. Bleeding and blood transfusions may even increase the risk of recurrence after hepatectomy for malignant diseases [18, 19]. Thus, reducing operative blood loss is of paramount importance. Risk factors for blood transfusion requirement in hepatectomy include female gender, preoperative anemia, longer operative time, and higher intraoperative central venous pressure (CVP) [20]. Patient factors may or may not be modifiable and surgeon skill and experience may be variable, but other factors can be optimized to reduce blood loss and transfusion

J.T. Huntington, MD, MS • C.R. Schmidt, MD, MS (✉)
Department of Surgery, The Ohio State University Wexner Medical Center,
Columbus, OH, USA
e-mail: Carl.schmidt@osumc.edu

© Springer International Publishing AG 2018
F.G. Rocha, P. Shen (eds.), *Optimizing Outcomes for Liver and Pancreas Surgery*, DOI 10.1007/978-3-319-62624-6_5

requirements. Many techniques exist for attempting to reduce operative blood loss during partial hepatectomy; however, the best techniques to reduce blood loss have been difficult to determine and great controversy persists [21, 22]. This chapter will focus on the current techniques to reduce blood loss during hepatectomy and provide recommendations.

Methods to Reduce Blood Loss

Hepatic Inflow Occlusion

The liver vascular inflow consists of the portal vein and hepatic artery. The portal system delivers approximately 75% of the estimated 16.7 mL/kg/min of hepatic blood flow and 50% of hepatic oxygen content [23–25]. The average blood loss for partial hepatectomy is approximately 300 mL [26]. Not surprisingly, surgeon experience and type of resection result in significant variation in estimated blood loss. Inflow occlusion of hepatic vasculature involves either the individual or combined control of the portal venous or hepatic arterial systems. Temporary total hepatic inflow occlusion is defined as the control of all branches of both the portal venous and hepatic arterial systems. First described by J.H. Pringle in 1908 and thus frequently referred to as the Pringle maneuver, this technique traditionally involves identification of the hepatoduodenal ligament and complete occlusion of the vessels contained within using a tourniquet or clamp (Fig. 5.1) [28]. A further classification of the technique is whether occlusion is continuous, intermittent, or preconditioned followed by continuous occlusion.

For the method originally described by Dr. Pringle, continuous total hepatic inflow occlusion has been shown to neither increase mortality nor alter postoperative liver regeneration for ischemic times of at least 60 min and potentially longer regardless of existing liver damage [28, 29]. Intermittent total hepatic inflow occlusion has been described in many variations, but in most institutions involves inflow occlusion for 15-min intervals alternating with 5-min rest periods of hepatic reperfusion (Table 5.1) [34, 35, 42, 43]. The interest in intermittent occlusion stems from concerns with prolonged ischemia time with continuous occlusion. However, studies have had difficulty demonstrating utility of intermittent over continuous occlusion and could be related to ischemia-reperfusion-type injury mechanisms [44]. In fact, intermittent occlusion ischemic time of longer than 120 min is associated with increased risk of blood loss and transfusion requirements with a trend toward increased morbidity and mortality [43]. One study has shown that compared to continuous occlusion, intermittent occlusion has been shown to lead to increased transection blood loss with no difference in total operative blood loss or transfusion requirements as well as an increased risk of liver damage and liver failure in patients with any degree of preexisting liver damage [42]. One additional study showed reduced blood loss when using intermittent occlusion in both senior and junior surgeons; however, others have demonstrated no difference in operative blood loss with significant increased postoperative transfusion requirements in those undergoing intermittent occlusion [35, 41].

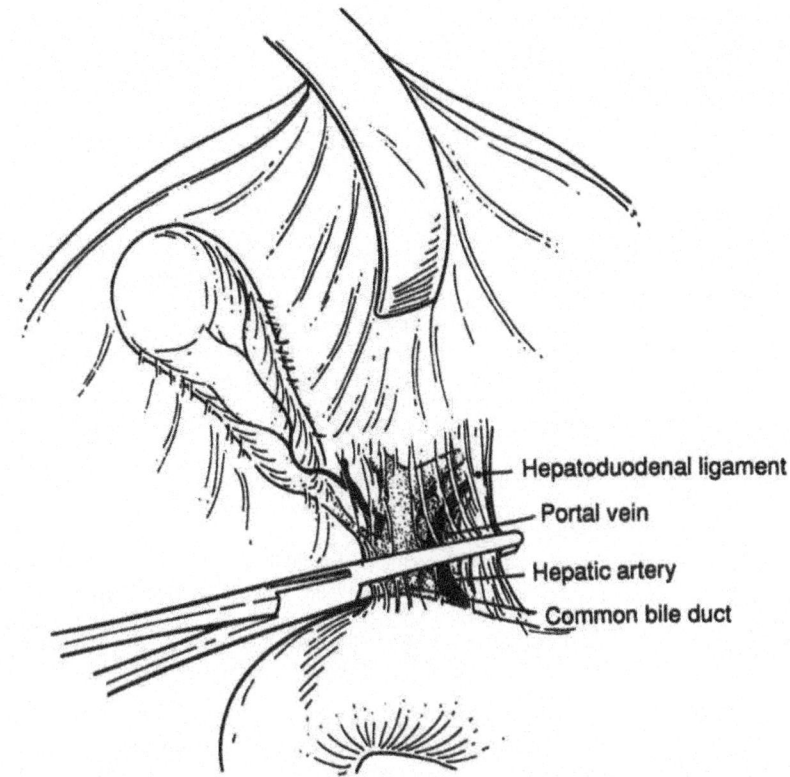

Hepatoduodenal ligament

Portal vein

Hepatic artery

Common bile duct

Fig. 5.1 Pringle maneuver applied by using a non-crushing clamp or other atraumatic techniques by encircling the hepatoduodenal ligament [27]

A recent well-designed, randomized control trial showed no benefit to intermittent hepatic inflow occlusion and a higher complication rate when compared to no inflow occlusion [31]. This study showed no difference during any point in liver transection with regards to blood loss even when taking into account surface area of resection. The authors did find a higher postoperative transaminitis and complication rate in the intermittent Pringle maneuver group. This points to the use of caution and selectivity when applying intermittent Pringle.

The ischemic preconditioning technique utilizes total hepatic inflow occlusion for 10 min followed by 10 min of reperfusion prior to transection followed by continuous occlusion during parenchymal transection [34]. Although there are no studies assessing the safe duration of occlusion for ischemic preconditioning, this method has been found to decrease operative blood loss and may decrease transfusion requirements when compared to intermittent occlusion when used for no longer than 75 min of ischemia time [34].

Hemi-hepatic inflow is the occlusion of either the right or left inflow portal venous and hepatic artery depending on the side of resection [31–33]. The purpose of controlling individual hepatic lobar inflow vessels is to potentially prevent ischemia to the

Table 5.1 Summary of important randomized studies evaluating hepatectomy vascular control methods

Author	Year	N	Method(s) tested	Control	Blood loss	Complications
Zhang [30]	2016	79	Laparoscopic Pringle maneuver versus half-Pringle maneuver, intermittent	Total hepatic inflow occlusion, intermittent	Less in half-Pringle maneuver	Increased in Pringle maneuver
Lee [31]	2012	126	Total hepatic inflow occlusion, intermittent	No inflow occlusion	No difference	Increased
Si-Yuan [32]	2011	180	Hemi-hepatic inflow occlusion, continuousmain portal vein occlusion, continuous	Total hepatic inflow occlusion, continuous AND total hepatic inflow occlusion, intermittent	No difference	Decreased
Liang [33]	2009	80	Hemi-hepatic inflow occlusion, continuous	Total hepatic inflow occlusion, intermittent	No difference	No difference
Petrowsky [34]	2006	73	Total hepatic inflow occlusion, ischemic preconditioning	Total hepatic inflow occlusion, continuous	No difference	No difference
Capussotti [35]	2006	126	Total hepatic inflow occlusion, intermittent	No inflow occlusion	No difference	No difference
Azoulav [36]	2006	60	Selective hepatic vascular exclusion, ischemic preconditioning	Selective hepatic vascular exclusion, continuous	No difference	No difference
Figueras [37]	2005	80	Hemi-hepatic inflow occlusion, intermittent	Total hepatic inflow occlusion, intermittent	No difference	No difference
Smyrniotis [38]	2003	110	Selective hepatic vascular exclusion	Total hepatic inflow occlusion, continuous	Decreased	Increased
Smyrniotis [39]	2002	38	Selective hepatic vascular exclusion	Total hepatic vascular exclusion	No difference	No difference
Belghiti [40]	1999	86	Total hepatic inflow occlusion, continuous	Total hepatic inflow occlusion, intermittent	No difference	Increased (steatosis/cirrhosis)no difference (overall)
Man [41]	1997	100	Total hepatic inflow occlusion, intermittent	No inflow occlusion	Decreased	No difference
Belghiti [42]	1996	52	Total hepatic vascular exclusion	Total hepatic inflow occlusion, continuous	No difference	No difference

non-resected liver. Multiple studies show no difference in operative blood loss or transfusion requirements when comparing hemi-hepatic inflow occlusion to total hepatic inflow occlusion. Main portal vein occlusion is an additional selective inflow occlusion method that requires isolation of the portal vein while preserving flow in the hepatic arterial system. In the sole prospective study evaluating main portal vein occlusion, there was no effect on operative or total blood loss and transfusion requirement [32]. Selective hepatic inflow occlusion has been shown to be feasible using laparoscopic approaches, and one group has shown reduced bleeding and complications compared to complete Pringle using intermittent occlusion [30]. Overall, selective hepatic inflow occlusion is technically more challenging and does not appear to have any utility in terms of operative blood loss, and this is likely explained by the expected compensatory increased flow in hepatic lobar vasculature upon occlusion of the opposite lobar inflow vasculature. Additional studies evaluating hemi-hepatic inflow occlusion are needed prior to making a strong argument for routine use.

Hepatic Outflow Exclusion

Hepatic blood outflow occurs through the inferior vena cava (IVC). Post-sinusoid blood enters the hepatic veins and then predominately collects into the left, middle, and right hepatic veins that drain directly to the IVC posterior to the liver. There are also numerous short retro-hepatic veins draining directly to the IVC (most importantly for the caudate lobe). Outflow hepatic vascular occlusion is attractive given that this should be the only source of significant bleeding not controlled by the Pringle maneuver. Although hepatic inflow vascular occlusion originated in 1908, the first description of hepatic vascular outflow occlusion did not come until 1966 by Dr. John Heaney [45]. The total hepatic vascular exclusion (THVE) technique, later modified by Dr. Huguet in 1978, involves control of the hepatic vascular outflow through clamping of the infra-hepatic and supra-hepatic IVC in addition to total hepatic inflow occlusion (Fig. 5.2) [46]. In the sole study evaluating THVE,

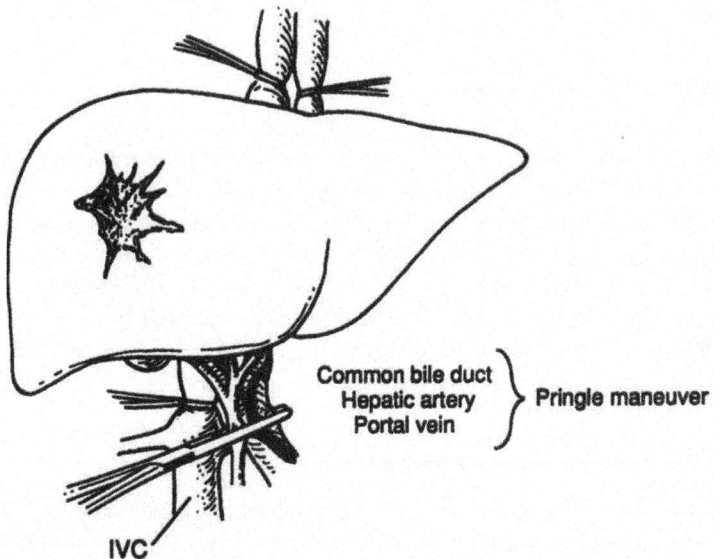

Fig. 5.2 Caval control in addition to Pringle maneuver to help achieve hemostasis [27]

there was no effect found on operative or total blood loss and transfusion requirement when compared to total hepatic inflow occlusion alone [42]. The study did however find a significant increase in operative hemodynamic instability, ischemic duration, operative time, and hospital stay in the THVE group with a trend toward a higher complication rate (particularly a higher risk of symptomatic pulmonary emboli) [42]. These results do not seem surprising given the technical difficulties of THVE as well as manipulation and complete occlusion of the IVC.

In order to address concerns associated with increased operative risk, Dr. Elias introduced selective hepatic vascular exclusion (SHVE) in 1995 [47]. SHVE involves control of the hepatic inflow and outflow with preservation of caval flow and elimination of caval manipulation by dissecting and occluding hepatic veins prior to their drainage into the IVC, thus diminishing adverse hemodynamic issues [39, 47]. SHVE has been shown to decrease operative blood loss and transfusion requirements in major hepatectomy patients with and without existing liver damage compared to total hepatic inflow occlusion alone [38]. Additionally SHVE was shown to be associated with decreased hospital stay and no difference in overall complication rates, although postoperatively SHVE was associated with higher bleeding risk [38]. In a separate study, SHVE was shown to have no difference in operative blood loss or complications compared to THVE, although there was an associated decreased transfusion requirement in the SHVE group [39]. THVE and SHVE are technically more difficult and require increased dissection time due to the need to isolate the infra-hepatic IVC with confirmation of the location distal to the right adrenal vein and the left renal vein in addition to isolation of the supra-hepatic IVC distal to the junction of the right hepatic vein. In summary, given the complex surgical technique involved in THVE and the even more complex SHVE technique with the known increased risk of emboli secondary to vena caval manipulation, these techniques may have a limited role in experienced hands only.

Parenchymal Transection

The risk of blood loss during parenchymal transection is significant compared to other tissues due to the lack of mechanisms preventing operative fluid losses such as the lack of vasoconstriction within hepatic sinusoids and the tissue consistency of the liver. The development of anatomical hepatectomy procedures aided in the safety and efficacy of parenchymal transection by taking into account the underlying hepatic vasculature; additionally there has been considerable research by surgeons and the industry into transection method, transection device, and the use of hemostatic agents.

Transection Method

Sharp transection is the traditional technique for hepatic parenchymal transection and refers to the use of a sequential transection of parenchyma [48]. Sharp parenchymal transection can be challenging due to the need to identify and suture ligate major intrahepatic vascular structures without subsequent significant blood loss.

The advent of intraoperative ultrasound has aided in the identification of hepatic vasculature, thereby becoming an important tool in reducing blood loss [48]. Ultrasound has thus become a commonly used tool by surgeons today.

The first alternative technique to sharp transection described was finger fracture by Dr. Tien-Yu Lin in 1958 [49]. Finger fracture or digitoclassy refers to insertion of the fingers to effectively compress and release the liver parenchyma allowing better identification of vascular structures during transection. Early retrospective analyses of the finger-fracture method in the 1970s and 1980s showed significant decrease in operative blood loss and reduced mortality in hepatectomy procedures [50, 51]. Despite evidence of improved operative blood loss and mortality, adoption of the finger-fracture method was slow within America due to a perceived risk of damage to the hepatic parenchyma by this technique [51]. A further modification of the finger facture technique was developed by Dr. Lin in 1974 and is called the clamp-crush technique. The clamp-crush technique is performed using a surgical clamp such as a hemostat or Kelly clamp to compress liver parenchyma proximal to the transection line and then releasing and resecting just distal to the crushed parenchyma [52]. This helps in identification of major vascular structures during transection. In a retrospective analysis, Lin demonstrated decreased operative blood loss when using the clamp-crush technique compared to previous studies [52]. However, in the sole prospective randomized study evaluating parenchymal transection techniques, no significant difference in blood loss or transfusion requirement as well as morbidity or operative time when using the clamp-crush technique compared to sharp transection were found [48].

Stapling Devices

Recently, stapling devices have been developed which are capable of transecting hepatic tissue and vessels. Vascular staplers are able to crush hepatic parenchyma and immediately transect the parenchyma and ligate vessels simultaneously. One study describes a 50% reduction in blood loss using vascular staplers during hepatectomy compared to the clamp-crush technique, even when the stapler cohort had patients with larger tumors and more major resections [53]. Further, the stapling technique was associated with less use of vascular control. There is a lack of robust data for stapling devices compared to other techniques, but they certainly have a role in vascular division.

Transection Devices

Device development has been of particular interest recently with the development of various instruments aimed to improve operative blood loss, operative speed, and resections margins (Table 5.2). Vessel-sealing devices such as LigaSure® (Covidien, Colorado, USA) and Enseal® (Ethicon, Cincinnati, OH, USA) have become popular because of their availability, ease of use, and their ability to compress, transect, and coagulate hepatic parenchymal tissue simultaneously [64]. However, early work has shown mixed

Table 5.2 Summary of important randomized studies evaluating hepatectomy transection methods

Author	Year	N	Method(s) tested	Control	Blood loss	Complications
Gotohda [54]	2015	211	Energy device (ultrasonically activated device [Harmonic®] or bipolar [LigaSure®])	No energy device	No difference	Decreased operative time and decreased bile leak with energy device
Guo [55]	2014	380	Bipolar or bipolar and CUSA®	Clamp-crush transection	Decreased in bipolar and bipolar and CUSA® (similar)	Increased in clamp-crush transection
Rahbari [56]	2014	130	Stapler transection	Clamp-crush transection	No difference	No difference
Kaibori [57]	2013	109	CUSA® with bipolar sealer (Aquamantys®)	CUSA® with standard bipolar cautery	Decreased in CUSA® and bipolar sealer	Decreased operative time in CUSA® and bipolar sealer
Muratore [58]	2013	100	Radiofrequency vessel-sealing (LigaSure® small jaw, LF1212)	Clamp-crush transection	No difference	No difference, diminished operative times with radiofrequency vessel-sealing
Savlid [59]	2013	100	Endoscopic vascular staplers	Cavitron ultrasonic surgical aspirator® (CUSA®)	No difference	No difference
Li [60]	2013	75	Radiofrequency transection	Clamp-crush transection, Pringle maneuver or hemi-hepatic vascular occlusion	Decreased	Decreased
Richter [61]	2009	96	Radiofrequency dissector Water-jet dissector Ultrasonic dissector	None	No difference	No difference
Ikeda [62]	2009	120	Vessel-sealing dissector	Clamp-crush transection	No difference	No difference
Lupo [63]	2007	50	RF dissector	Clamp-crush transection	No difference	Increased
Campagnacci [64]	2007	24	Vessel-sealing dissector	Ultrasonic dissector	Decreased	Decreased

(continued)

Table 5.2 (continued)

Author	Year	N	Method(s) tested	Control	Blood loss	Complications
Saiura [65]	2006	60	Vessel-sealing dissector	Clamp-crush transection	Decreased (minor) no difference (major)	No difference
Smyrniotis [48]	2005	82	Sharp transection	Clamp-crush transection	No difference	No difference
Lesurtel [66]	2005	100	RF dissector Water-jet dissector Ultrasonic dissector	Clamp-crush transection	Increased (all groups)	No difference
Takayama [67]	2001	132	Ultrasonic dissector	Clamp-crush transection	No difference	No difference

results in terms of operative blood loss, transfusion requirement, morbidity, and mortality compared to the clamp-crush technique alone [62, 65, 68]. One meta-analysis recently showed vessel-sealing devices to offer reduced blood loss, decreased incidence of postoperative bile leak, and shorter hospital stays when compared to traditional clamp-crush techniques [69].

Radiofrequency devices, which utilize various designs to coagulate tissue with electromechanical waves, are generally the slowest dissecting of the devices available [61, 66]. One randomized prospective study by two surgeons comparing radiofrequency-assisted hepatectomy compared to the clamp-crush technique and vascular inflow occlusion showed decreased blood loss and less morbidity in the radiofrequency group [60]. However, these results have not been replicated with other studies finding no difference in blood loss or even greater blood loss and no difference in transfusion requirement or tumor recurrence with a radiofrequency device compared to the clamp-crush technique alone [60, 66]. Water-jet devices utilize pressurized water combined with electrothermal coagulation and are generally faster dissecting devices compared to traditional methods [61]. The sole prospective study evaluating water-jet devices demonstrated an increased operative blood loss utilizing a water-jet device compared to the clamp-crush technique and a radiofrequency device [66]. Ultrasonic devices in contrast to radiofrequency employ mechanical wave energy to coagulate tissue and are generally the least expensive of the transection devices [61]. However, this technology has shown no improvement in operative and total blood loss, morbidity, or mortality compared to the clamp-crush technique alone [66, 67]. A prospective trial did show that the Harmonic® scalpel (Ethicon, Cincinnati, OH, USA) was safe for small veins (less than or equal to 2 mm) and actually safer than conventional control using suture material [70]. Combination techniques, such as clamp-crush and energy device together are also possible. Surgeon preference is a large factor in what devices are used, how they are used, and their effectiveness, thus making steadfast conclusions difficult.

The Aquamantys® (Medtronic, Minneapolis, MN, USA) is a relatively new device that uses a saline-coupled bipolar sealing device. This system delivers radio-frequency energy and saline simultaneously, thereby heating tissue to around 100 °C resulting in collagen shrinkage within blood vessels and subsequent hemostasis while preventing eschar formation [71]. Early work has shown this device to be feasible and safe with minimal blood loss (5–80 mL in one study of 12 Child-Pugh A cirrhotic patients with hepatocellular carcinoma undergoing partial hepatecto-mies with Aquamantys® and suture ligation or clips for vessels larger than 6 mm without Pringle maneuver) [72]. A number of parenchymal transection tools such as the Cavitron ultrasonic aspirator® (CUSA®, Integra Lifesciences Corporation, NJ, USA), saline-linked radiofrequency precoagulation, Harmonic® scalpel, bipolar scissors, LigaSure® device, hydrodissectors, or monopolar floating ball can be used with the Aquamantys® system [71]. Combining CUSA® with Aquamantys® is one technique that has shown increased operative efficiency with decreased blood loss [57]. The Aquamantys® is very appealing given its ability to coagulate nearby tis-sue, allow for minimal blood loss, and aide in transection for hepatectomy.

Topical Agents

Hemostatic topical agents are a group of synthetic and biological products designed to improve hemostasis through coagulation techniques (Table 5.3). The three classes of agents are collagens, cyanoacrylates, and fibrins. Cyanoacrylate polymers have been shown to produce tissue necrosis and inflammatory mediator release, therefore preventing use in hepatic parenchymal hemostasis [70]. Some products include both collagen and fibrin agents in varying concentrations.

Collagen agents are typically sheets (referred to as collagen fleece) of collagen-based material and can be coated with additional components in an attempt to improve the hemostatic effect. There are numerous brands of collagen agents, and each product uses a proprietary mixture of components. They include Antema® (Opocrin, Modena, Italy), Avitene™ (Bard, New Jersey, USA), Gelfoam® (Pfizer, New York, NY, USA), and TachoSil® (Takeda Pharma A/S, Roskilde, Denmark). Agents that can be added in varying concentrations to improve the hemostatic effect include coagulation factors (typically thrombin) and anti-thrombolytic agents (typi-cally proteins C and S). The potential benefit of collagen agents is a moderately more rapid time to hemostasis, which has been suggested to be true in some pro-spective studies [85]. In a study evaluating the addition of a collagen agent, TachoSil® (Nycomed Pharma SA, Madrid, Spain), there was no difference in opera-tive blood loss; however, a significant increase in postoperative transfusion require-ment was found in the control group compared to those patients in which the collagen agent was used [80]. This study did find a decreased hospital stay, lower readmission rate, and decreased overall morbidity in the collagen agent group. However, these results appeared limited to the major hepatectomy subgroup [80]. In another study evaluating the difference between two collagen agents, there was no significant difference noted in blood loss, transfusion requirement, and mortality or morbidity [83].

Table 5.3 Summary of important randomized studies evaluating topical agents in hepatectomy procedures

Author	Year	N	Method(s) tested	Control	Blood loss	Complications
Kobayashi [73]	2016	786	Fibrin sealant with polyglycolic acid felt (PGA-FS)	Fibrinogen-based collagen fleece (CF)	No difference	Less surgical site infection/effusion around the liver in the PGA-FS group
Moench [74]	2014	128	Collagen hemostat	Carrier-bound fibrin sealant	No difference	No difference
Bektas [75]	2014	70	Fibrin sealant	Manual compression	Decreased	No difference
Kakaei [76]	2013	45	TachoSil®, Surgicel® (Ethicon, Somerville, NJ, USA), Glubran® (GEM Srl, Viareggio, Italy)	Comparison of topical agents	Less bleeding in TachoSil® group	Higher complications in Surgicel® group
Ollinger [77]	2012	50	Veriset™ hemostatic patch (Covidien, Mansfield, MA, USA)	TachoSil® hemostatic patch	Faster hemostasis with Veriset™	No difference
Koea [26, 78]	2012, 2015	102	Fibrin pad	Manual compression, cellulose	Decreased	Decreased
de Boer [79]	2012	310	Fibrin sealant	No topical agent	No difference	No difference
Briceno [80]	2010	115	Collagen sponge	No topical agent	No difference	Decreased
Figueras [81]	2007	300	Fibrin sealantcollagen sponge	No topical agent	No difference	No difference
Schwartz [82]	2004	112	Fibrin sealant	Collagen sponge, collagen powder, fibrin sealant, thrombin sealant	No difference	Not evaluated
Chapman [83]	2000	67	Collagen/thrombin composite	Collagen sponge	No difference	No difference
Kohno [84]	1992	62	Collagen powder	Fibrin sealant	No difference	No difference

Fibrin agents are typically prepared intraoperatively and subsequently applied. Similar to other topical agents, fibrin agents are numerous, contain varying concentrations of components, and include FloSeal® (Baxter Healthcare Corporation, Deerfield, IL, USA), Tisseel® (Baxter Healthcare Corporation, Deerfield, IL, USA), Tissucol® (Baxter, Warsaw, Poland), and Vitagel™ (Orthovita, Malvern, PA, USA). Fibrin agents are typically comprised of fibrinogen and activating agents such as calcium chloride and thrombin. This necessitates on site preparation and immediate application. A randomized prospective trial of fibrin sealant versus no topical agent found no difference in blood loss and complication rate [35, 79]. An additional study using a combination of a fibrin agent (Tissucol®) with a collagen agent for major and minor hepatectomy procedures demonstrated no difference in operative blood loss, transfusion requirement, or morbidity and mortality compared to traditional techniques; however, operative times were increased by the use of fibrin and collagen agents [79]. Comparing a fibrin agent (Beriplast®, Aventis Behring, King of Prussia, PA, USA) to a collagen agent (Avitene™) additionally found no significant difference in operative blood loss or transfusion requirement, although a trend toward improved morbidity and mortality was present without significance in the fibrin agent group [84]. An additional comparative study showed no difference in blood loss when using a fibrin agent (Crosseal™, OMRIX biopharmaceuticals Ltd., Kiryat Ono, Israel) and multiple collagen agents across minor and major hepatectomy procedures [82]. A recent randomized prospective trial found decreased blood loss and complication rate with prophylactic use of a fibrin pad compared to manual compression and cellulose application at the resection site [78]. An additional single-center randomized controlled trial study comparing fibrin sealant (Tisseel®) with synthetic aprotinin as a fibrinolysis inhibitor with manual compression for oozing once major artery and venous bleeding was controlled showed improvement in hemostasis at 4, 6, 8, and 10 min [75].

The multitude of studies provides evidence that while there are numerous available compositions of collagen and fibrin agents, there does not appear to be superior products in terms of efficacy. More importantly, there is no evidence that topical agents yield a significant difference in operative blood loss or transfusion requirement during minor hepatectomy procedures. There may be some benefit in postoperative transfusion requirement and overall complication rates during major hepatectomy. The limited data would not at this time support the routine use of any specific topical agent for hepatectomy, but specific cases may benefit from application of topical agents.

Non-operative Methods

Despite advances in surgical methods since the introduction of hepatectomy procedures, there continues to be an associated estimated blood loss for major hepatectomy of up to one liter [11]. Hepatectomy is a major operation and good outcomes require a team effort in the operating room. The role of non-operative methods to reduce blood loss highlights this important concept.

Low Central Venous Pressure

Low central venous pressure (CVP) is a mechanism whereby operative blood loss is reduced based on the premise that this physiologic state should reduce the impedance for blood flow through the hepatic venous system into the IVC. The subsequent decrease in hepatic venous pressure allows for reduced retrograde venous bleeding during transection and improved coagulative effects of any surgical technique being used [26]. Based on multiple studies, the target operative CVP during transection is less than 5 mmHg. This level has been shown to reduce operative blood loss, transfusion requirements, length of operation, and associated morbidity and mortality in hepatectomy procedures (Table 5.4) [90, 93–96]. Potential harmful consequences of maintaining a low CVP include air embolism and unnecessary hypoperfusion with end-organ dysfunction [93, 94]. The most common and easiest method for reducing CVP intraoperatively is decreased intravenous fluid volume. Other methods include morphine and nitroglycerin infusions and reducing mechanical ventilation tidal volume [90, 91, 93–95, 97]. Decreased tidal volumes have been shown to have no significant effect on blood loss or transfusion requirement due to the small change produced in CVP of only about 0.5 mmHg [91]. An operative technique for reducing CVP is through infra-hepatic IVC occlusion, although this technique is associated with an increased risk of symptomatic pulmonary emboli as discussed previously [86–88].

Various patient factors often determine what methods should be used to induce low CVP. One simple method to reduce CVP is to place the patient in a head-down

Table 5.4 Summary of important randomized studies evaluating physiologic variable manipulation in hepatectomy procedures

Author	Year	N	Method(s) tested	Control	Blood Loss	Complications
Zhu [86]	2012	192	Low CVP, IVC clamp induced	Low CVP, anesthetic induced	Decreased	No difference
Rahbari [87]	2011	128	Low CVP, IVC clamp induced	Low CVP, anesthetic induced	Decreased	No difference (increased pulmonary emboli)
Kato [88]	2008	85	Low CVP, clamp induced	Uncontrolled CVP	No difference	No difference
Jarnagin [89]	2008	130	Acute normovolemic hemodilution	Allogenic transfusion	No difference	No difference (decreased allogenic transfusion)
Wang [90]	2006	50	Low CVP, anesthetic induced	Uncontrolled CVP	Decreased	No difference
Hasegawa [91]	2002	80	Low CVP, hypoventilation induced	Uncontrolled CVP	No difference	No difference
Matot [92]	2002	78	Acute normovolemic hemodilution	Allogenic transfusion	No difference	No difference (decreased allogenic transfusion)

(Trendelenburg) position with the angle of the body at least 15°, thus resulting in decreased flow of venous blood in the superior to inferior direction, permitting lower pressures in the IVC [95]. A simple reduction of the intravenous fluids to near 75 mL/hr. can yield a reduced CVP in many patients without clinically impairing renal function or mortality while yielding a statistically significant reduction in operative blood loss and transfusion requirement [90]. When low-volume intravenous fluids are unable to accomplish the goal of CVP, pharmacologic methods may be necessary [90, 93, 94]. Agents that have been successfully used include systemic nitroglycerin, furosemide, and morphine. Nitroglycerin decreases CVP by providing systemic vasodilation. Morphine is likewise believed to produce venodilation through the release of histamine and μ3-receptor activation. Experienced anesthesiologists are crucial when maintaining low CVP as reducing the CVP overaggressively creates a potential need for vasopressor agents to maintain adequate arterial perfusion pressures [90, 93–95]. Typically once parenchymal transection is complete and hemostasis is achieved, CVP can be returned to normal with fluid resuscitation to improve global perfusion and reduce risks of under-resuscitation in the operating room and postoperatively; detrimental effects of low CVP on liver or renal function are overall rare [90, 94, 96]. Mild elevations in creatinine are common following low CVP anesthesia but clinically relevant renal dysfunction is very uncommon, especially in patients with normal preoperative kidney function [98]. Decreased CVP is clearly effective in decreasing operative blood loss and transfusion requirement in hepatectomy procedures and should be considered standard of care. Necessity of direct CVP monitoring is clinician dependent, and for most hepatectomies judicious use of fluids can be used as a substitute for measures of CVP, thereby eliminating the time and potential complications of central venous catheter placement. Communication between the anesthesia and surgical teams is important, and once the resection is complete, fluid resuscitation can then be initiated.

Hemodilution

Acute normovolemic hemodilution (ANH) is a concept that has been attempted in surgical procedures with significant blood loss. The purpose of which is based upon the inherent risks associated with allogenic blood transfusion such as viral transmission, transfusion reactions, clerical error, cost of blood banks, and national shortages in blood products. The method involves immediate preoperative removal of a calculated volume of the patient's blood and storage of the blood during the procedure; the volume is then replaced appropriately with mixtures of colloid and crystalloid solutions [89, 92, 99]. The maximal blood volume to be removed can be estimated using

the established formula: $V_L = EBV \times \left(\dfrac{H_O - H_F}{H_{AV}} \right)$, where V_L represents the volume

to be removed, EBV is the estimated blood volume of the patient, H_O is the patient initial hemoglobin concentration, H_F is the minimum desired hemoglobin concentration, and HAV is the average of the H_O and H_F [100]. In one study, the proposed value for minimum hemoglobin concentration was 8.0 g/dL (or a hematocrit of approximately 24%) [89, 92]. The removed autologous volume is then replaced as needed if transfusion is necessary during the operation or upon completion of the procedure. A study comparing ANH to normal management demonstrated a 50% reduction in intraoperative red blood cell transfusion requirements [89]. Additional studies have also reported similar reductions in allogenic red blood cell transfusions with an estimated reduction of 71% overall for patients undergoing major hepatectomy procedures and decreased hospital stay among patients undergoing ANH [92, 99]. Postoperative hemoglobin concentration in patients undergoing ANH has consistently been higher and with more rapid correction compared to traditionally managed patients [89, 92]. ANH has been shown to be associated with lower initial systolic blood pressure although this difference is only transient and not present upon completion of the procedure [89, 92].

An important factor in selection of patients who may benefit from ANH is predictably the likely operative blood loss. The operative blood loss must be at least 0.7 of the patient's estimated blood volume to prevent transfusion of one unit of red blood cells and at least 0.5 to have any reduction in autologous red blood cell volume [101]. Using this calculation the estimated blood loss to prevent allogenic transfusion would be approximately 3500 mL in a standard patient with a blood volume of 5000 mL. Additional studies have shown that the threshold for utilizing ANH may likely be closer to a predicted blood loss of 0.2 of the patient's estimated total blood volume [89, 92]. Therefore, utilizing ANH must be selective and reserved for those cases where substantial blood losses are expected.

Special Considerations

Laparoscopy and robotic-assisted approaches are increasingly being used for hepatectomy. In experienced hands, minimally invasive techniques are completely acceptable and lead to good outcomes with improved cosmesis [102]. The same considerations to open surgery should be followed, and surgeons should be facile using these techniques including intracorporeal suturing if needed to control bleeding. Additionally, pneumoperitoneum of 10–14 mmHg assists in hemostasis and maintains hemodynamics of the patient [103]. Low CVP anesthesia should still be used, vascular inflow control is feasible, and precoagulation with radiofrequency ablation and use of previously described transection devices and topical hemostatic agents may be used [30, 103, 104]. Due to the heterogeneity of studies, surgeon preferences, and patient factors, determining efficacy of one transection device compared to others has been difficult, and surgeon experience in minimally invasive liver surgery is probably the most important factor in reducing blood loss using these advanced techniques and when deciding between minimally invasive approaches and open techniques [105–107].

Summary

Major hepatectomy procedures (three or more segments resected) are independently associated with increased operative blood loss, and surgeons should consider methods to reduce blood loss in these patients, particularly low central venous pressure (CVP) anesthesia and vascular inflow occlusion. Low CVP is recommended for parenchymal transection in major hepatectomy procedures maintaining a pressure between 2 and 5 mmHg. Infra-hepatic IVC occlusion is not commonly needed and is associated with increased risk of clinically significant pulmonary emboli and is technically challenging. Ultrasound assistance is an important instrument that can aide the surgeon intraoperatively in performing anatomic resections by identifying major vascular structures.

Depending on surgeon preference and experience, vascular occlusion may be considered for major hepatectomy procedures with continuous total hepatic inflow occlusion for up to 60 min or intermittent occlusion for up to 120 min. Use of topical agents after major hepatectomy parenchyma transection may reduce postoperative transfusion requirements, but there is a lack of strong evidence to support this. Topical agent selection is at the discretion of the surgeon as collagen and fibrin agents appear to have similar efficacy. The parenchymal transection technique chosen should be at the discretion of the surgeon. Technology will likely continue to advance to create even better instruments. Acute normovolemic hemodilution (ANH) can be beneficial for major hepatectomy procedures if the estimated operative blood loss is at least 20% of the estimated blood volume.

Acknowledgments None.

Disclosures None.

References

1. Pasipoularides A. Galen, father of systematic medicine. An essay on the evolution of modern medicine and cardiology. Int J Cardiol. 2014;172(1):47–58.
2. Langenbuch C. Ein fall von resection eines linksseitigen schnurlappens der leber. Heilung Klin Wochenschr. 1888;25:37–8.
3. Keen WW. On resection of the liver, especially for hepatic Tumors. Bosn Med Surg J. 1892;126:405–9.
4. Healey JE Jr, Schroy PC. Anatomy of the biliary ducts within the human liver; analysis of the prevailing pattern of branchings and the major variations of the biliary ducts. AMA Arch Surg. 1953;66:599–616.
5. Couinaud C. Anatomic principles of left and right regulated hepatectomy: technics. J Chir (Paris). 1954;70:933–66.
6. Lortat-Jacob JL, Robert HG, Henry C. Case of right segmental hepatectomy. Mem Acad Chir (Paris). 1952;78:244–51.
7. Foster JH. Survival after liver resection for cancer. Cancer. 1970;26:493–502.
8. Asiyanbola B, Chang D, Gleisner AL, et al. Operative mortality after hepatic resection: are literature-based rates broadly applicable? J Gastrointest Surg. 2008;12:842–51.
9. Day RW, Brudvik KW, Vauthey JN, et al. Advances in hepatectomy technique: toward zero transfusions in the modern era of liver surgery. Surgery. 2016;159(3):793–801.
10. Kooby DA, Stockman J, Ben-Porat L, et al. Influence of transfusions on perioperative and long-term outcome in patients following hepatic resection for colorectal metastases. Ann Surg. 2003;237:860–9; discussion 869–70.
11. Fan ST, Mau Lo C, Poon RT, et al. Continuous improvement of survival outcomes of resection of hepatocellular carcinoma: a 20-year experience. Ann Surg. 2011;253:745–58.
12. Yeh CN, Chen MF, Lee WC, Jeng LB. Prognostic factors of hepatic resection for hepatocellular carcinoma with cirrhosis: univariate and multivariate analysis. J Surg Oncol. 2002;81:195–202.

13. Sitzmann JV, Greene PS. Perioperative predictors of morbidity following hepatic resection for neoplasm. A multivariate analysis of a single surgeon experience with 105 patients. Ann Surg. 1994;219:13–7.
14. Shimada M, Takenaka K, Fujiwara Y, et al. Risk factors linked to postoperative morbidity in patients with hepatocellular carcinoma. Br J Surg. 1998;85:195–8.
15. Ibrahim S, Chen CL, Lin CC, et al. Intraoperative blood loss is a risk factor for complications in donors after living donor hepatectomy. Liver Transpl. 2006;12:950–7.
16. Jarnagin WR, Gonen M, Fong Y, et al. Improvement in perioperative outcome after hepatic resection: analysis of 1,803 consecutive cases over the past decade. Ann Surg. 2002;236:397–406; discussion 406–7.
17. Pathak S, Hakeem A, Pike T, et al. Anaesthetic and pharmacological techniques to decrease blood loss in liver surgery: a systematic review. ANZ J Surg. 2015;85(12):923–30.
18. Yamamoto J, Kosuge T, Takayama T, et al. Perioperative blood transfusion promotes recurrence of hepatocellular carcinoma after hepatectomy. Surgery. 1994;115:303–9.
19. De Boer MT, Molenaar IQ, Porte RJ. Impact of blood loss on outcome after liver resection. Dig Surg. 2007;24:259–64.
20. Cheng ES, Hallet J, Hanna SS, et al. Is central venous pressure still relevant in the contemporary era of liver resection? J Surg Res. 2016;200(1):139–46.
21. Huntington JT, Royall NA, Schmidt CR. Minimizing blood loss during hepatectomy: a literature review. J Surg Oncol. 2014;109(2):81–8.
22. Simillis C, Li T, Vaughan J, et al. Methods to decrease blood loss during liver resection: a network meta-analysis. Cochrane Database Syst Rev. 2014;4:CD010683.
23. Tygstrup N, Winkler K, Mellemgaard K, Andreassen M. Determination of the hepatic arterial blood flow and oxygen supply in man by clamping the hepatic artery during surgery. J Clin Invest. 1962;41:447–54.
24. Schenk WG Jr, JC MD, McDonald K, Drapanas T. Direct measurement of hepatic blood flow in surgical patients: with related observations on hepatic flow dynamics in experimental animals. Ann Surg. 1962;156:463–71.
25. Ternberg JL, Butcher HR Jr. Blood-flow relation between hepatic artery and portal vein. Science. 1965;150:1030–1.
26. Koea JB, Batiller J, Patel B, et al. A phase III, randomized, controlled, superiority trial evaluating the fibrin pad versus standard of care in controlling parenchymal bleeding during elective hepatic surgery. HPB. 2013;15:61–70.
27. Skandalakis LJ, Skandalakis JE, Skandalakis PN. Surgical Anatomy and Technique: a pocket manual. 3rd ed. New York: Springer; 2009.
28. Pringle JHV. Notes on the arrest of hepatic Hemorrhage due to trauma. Ann Surg. 1908;48:541–9.
29. Huguet C, Gavelli A, Chieco PA, et al. Liver ischemia for hepatic resection: where is the limit? Surgery. 1992;111:251–9.
30. Zhang Y, Yang H, Deng X, et al. Intermittent Pringle maneuver versus continuous hemihepatic vascular inflow occlusion using extra-glissonian approach in laparoscopic liver resection. Surg Endosc. 2016;30(3):961–70.
31. Lee KF, Cheung YS, Wong J, et al. Randomized clinical trial of open hepatectomy with or without intermittent Pringle manoeuvre. Br J Surg. 2012;99:1203–9.
32. Si-Yuan FU, Yee LW, Guang-Gang L, et al. A prospective randomized controlled trial to compare Pringle maneuver, hemihepatic vascular inflow occlusion, and main portal vein inflow occlusion in partial hepatectomy. Am J Surg. 2011;201:62–9.
33. Liang G, Wen T, Yan L, et al. A prospective randomized comparison of continuous hemihepatic with intermittent total hepatic inflow occlusion in hepatectomy for liver tumors. Hepato-Gastroenterology. 2009;56:745–50.
34. Petrowsky H, McCormack L, Trujillo M, et al. A prospective, randomized, controlled trial comparing intermittent portal triad clamping versus ischemic preconditioning with continuous clamping for major liver resection. Ann Surg. 2006;244:921–8; discussion 928–30.
35. Capussotti L, Muratore A, Ferrero A, et al. Randomized clinical trial of liver resection with and without hepatic pedicle clamping. Br J Surg. 2006;93:685–9.

36. Azoulay D, Lucidi V, Andreani P, et al. Ischemic preconditioning for major liver resection under vascular exclusion of the liver preserving the caval flow: a randomized prospective study. J Am Coll Surg. 2006;202:203–11.
37. Figueras J, Llado L, Ruiz D, et al. Complete versus selective portal triad clamping for minor liver resections: a prospective randomized trial. Ann Surg. 2005;241:582–90.
38. Smyrniotis VE, Kostopanagiotou GG, Contis JC, et al. Selective hepatic vascular exclusion versus Pringle maneuver in major liver resections: prospective study. World J Surg. 2003;27:765–9.
39. Smyrniotis VE, Kostopanagiotou GG, Gamaletsos EL, et al. Total versus selective hepatic vascular exclusion in major liver resections. Am J Surg. 2002;183:173–8.
40. Belghiti J, Noun R, Malafosse R, et al. Continuous versus intermittent portal triad clamping for liver resection: a controlled study. Ann Surg. 1999;229:369–75.
41. Man K, Fan ST, Ng IO, et al. Prospective evaluation of Pringle maneuver in hepatectomy for liver tumors by a randomized study. Ann Surg. 1997;226:704–11; discussion 711–3.
42. Belghiti J, Noun R, Zante E, et al. Portal triad clamping or hepatic vascular exclusion for major liver resection controlled study. Ann Surg. 1996;224:155–61.
43. Ishizaki Y, Yoshimoto J, Miwa K, et al. Safety of prolonged intermittent pringle maneuver during hepatic resection. Arch Surg. 2006;141:649–53; discussion 654.
44. Sanjay P, Ong I, Bartlett A, et al. Meta-analysis of intermittent Pringle manoeuvre versus no Pringle manoeuvre in elective liver surgery. ANZ J Surg. 2013;83(10):719–23.
45. Heaney JP, Stanton WK, Halbert DS, et al. An improved technic for vascular isolation of the liver: experimental study and case reports. Ann Surg. 1966;163:237–41.
46. Huguet C, Nordlinger B, Galopin JJ, et al. Normothermic hepatic vascular exclusion for extensive hepatectomy. Surg Gynecol Obstet. 1978;147:689–93.
47. Elias D, Lasser P, Debaene B, et al. Intermittent vascular exclusion of the liver (without vena cava clamping) during major hepatectomy. Br J Surg. 1995;82:1535–9.
48. Smyrniotis V, Arkadopoulos N, Kostopanagiotou G, et al. Sharp liver transection versus clamp crushing technique in liver resections: a prospective study. Surgery. 2005;137:306–11.
49. Lin TY, Chen KM, Lin TK. Study on lobectomy of the liver: a new technical suggestion on hemihepatectomy and reports of three cases of primary hepatoma treated with total left lobectomy of the liver. J Formos Med Assoc. 1958;57:742–61.
50. Lin TY. Results in 107 hepatic lobectomies with a preliminary report on the use of a clamp to reduce blood loss. Ann Surg. 1973;177:413–21.
51. Pachter HL, Spencer FC, Hofstetter SR, Coppa GF. Experience with the finger fracture technique to achieve intra-hepatic hemostasis in 75 patients with severe injuries of the liver. Ann Surg. 1983;197:771–8.
52. Lin TYA. Simplified technique for hepatic resection: the crush method. Ann Surg. 1974;180:285–90.
53. Reddy SK, Barbas AS, Gan TJ, et al. Hepatic parenchymal transection with vascular staplers: a comparative analysis with the crush-clamp technique. Am J Surg. 2008;196:760–7.
54. Gotohda N, Yamanaka T, Saiura A, et al. Impact of energy devices during liver parenchymal transection: a multicenter randomized controlled trial. World J Surg. 2015;39(6):1543–9.
55. Guo JY, Li DW, Liao R, et al. Outcomes of simple saline-coupled bipolar electrocautery for hepatic resection. World J Gastroenterol. 2014;20(26):8638–45.
56. Rahbari NN, Elbers H, Koch M, et al. Randomized clinical trial of stapler versus clamp-crushing transection in elective liver resection. Br J Surg. 2014;101(3):200–7.
57. Kaibori M, Matsui K, Ishizaki M, et al. A prospective randomized controlled trial of hemostasis with bipolar sealer during hepatic transection for liver surgery. Surgery. 2013;154(5):1046–52.
58. Muratore A, Mellano A, Tarantino G, et al. Radiofrequency vessel-sealing system versus the clamp-crushing technique in liver resection: results of a prospective randomized study on 100 consecutive patients. HPB (Oxford). 2014;16(8):707–12.
59. Savlid M, Strand AH, Jansson A, et al. Transection of the liver parenchyma with an ultrasound dissector or a stapler device: results of a randomized clinical study. World J Surg. 2013;37(4):799–805.

60. Li M, Zhang Y, Li Y, et al. Radiofrequency-assisted versus clamp-crushing parenchyma transection in cirrhotic patients with hepatocellular carcinoma: a randomized clinical trial. Dig Dis Sci. 2013;58:835–40.
61. Richter S, Kollmar O, Schuld J, et al. Randomized clinical trial of efficacy and costs of three dissection devices in liver resection. Br J Surg. 2009;96:593–601.
62. Ikeda M, Hasegawa K, Sano K, et al. The vessel sealing system (LigaSure) in hepatic resection: a randomized controlled trial. Ann Surg. 2009;250:199–203.
63. Lupo L, Gallerani A, Panzera P, et al. Randomized clinical trial of radiofrequency-assisted versus clamp-crushing liver resection. Br J Surg. 2007;94:287–91.
64. Campagnacci R, De Sanctis A, Baldarelli M, et al. Hepatic resections by means of electrothermal bipolar vessel device (EBVS) LigaSure V: early experience. Surg Endosc. 2007;21:2280–4.
65. Saiura A, Yamamoto J, Koga R, et al. Usefulness of LigaSure for liver resection: analysis by randomized clinical trial. Am J Surg. 2006;192:41–5.
66. Lesurtel M, Selzner M, Petrowsky H, et al. How should transection of the liver be performed? A prospective randomized study in 100 consecutive patients: comparing four different transection strategies. Ann Surg. 2005;242:814–22; discussion 822–3.
67. Takayama T, Makuuchi M, Kubota K, et al. Randomized comparison of ultrasonic vs clamp transection of the liver. Arch Surg. 2001;136:922–8.
68. Nanashima A, Abo T, Arai J, et al. Usefulness of vessel-sealing devices combined with crush clamping method for hepatectomy: a retrospective cohort study. Int J Surg. 2013;11(9):891–7.
69. Alexiou VG, Tsitsias T, Mavros MN, et al. Technology-assisted versus clamp-crush liver resection: a systematic review and meta-analysis. Surg Innov. 2013;20(4):414–28.
70. Olmez A, Karabulut K, Aydin C, et al. Comparison of harmonic scalpel versus conventional knot tying for transection of short hepatic veins at liver transplantation: prospective randomized study. Transplant Proc. 2012;44:1717–9.
71. Felekouras E, Petrou A, Neofytou K, et al. Combined ultrasonic aspiration and saline-linked radiofrequency precoagulation: a steptoward bloodless liver resection without the need of liver inflow occlusion: analysis of 313 consecutive patients. World J Surg Oncol. 2014;12:357.
72. Curro G, Lazzara S, Barbera A, et al. The Aquamantys system as alternative for parenchymal division and hemostasis in liver resection for hepatocellular carcinoma: a preliminary study. Eur Rev Med Pharmacol Sci. 2014;18(2 Suppl):2–5.
73. Kobayashi S, Takeda Y, Nakahira S, et al. Fibrin sealant with polyglycolic acid felt vs fibrinogen-based collagen fleece at the liver cut surface for prevention of postoperative bile leakage and hemorrhage: a prospective, randomized, controlled study. J Am Coll Surg. 2016;222(1):59–64.
74. Moench C, Mihaljevic AL, Hermanutz V, et al. Randomized controlled multicenter trial on the effectiveness of the collagen hemostat Sangustop compared with a carrier-bound fibrin sealant during liver resection (ESSCALIVER study, NCT00918619). Langenbeck's Arch Surg. 2014;399(6):725–33.
75. Bektas H, Nadalin S, Szabo I, et al. Hemostatic efficacy of latest-generation fibrin sealant after hepatic resection: a randomized controlled clinical study. Langenbeck's Arch Surg. 2014;399(7):837–47.
76. Kakaei F, Seyyed Sadeghi MS, Sanei B, et al. A randomized clinical trial comparing the effect of different haemostatic agents for haemostasis of the liver after hepatic resection. HPB Surg. 2013;2013:587608.
77. Ollinger R, Mihaljevic AL, Schuhmacher C, et al. A multicentre, randomized clinical trial comparing the Veriset haemostatic patch with fibrin sealant for the management of bleeding during hepatic surgery. HPB (Oxford). 2013;15(7):548–58.
78. Koea JB, Batiller J, Aguirre N, et al. A multicenter, prospective, randomized, controlled trial comparing EVARREST fibrin sealant patch to standard of care in controlling bleeding following elective hepatectomy: anatomic versus non-anatomic resection. HPB (Oxford). 2016;18(3):221–8.
79. de Boer MT, Klaase JM, Verhoef C, et al. Fibrin sealant for prevention of resection surface-related complications after liver resection: a randomized controlled trial. Ann Surg. 2012;256:229–34.
80. Briceno J, Naranjo A, Ciria R, et al. A prospective study of the efficacy of clinical application of a new carrier-bound fibrin sealant after liver resection. Arch Surg. 2010;145:482–8.

81. Figueras J, Llado L, Miro M, et al. Application of fibrin glue sealant after hepatectomy does not seem justified: results of a randomized study in 300 patients. Ann Surg. 2007;245:536–42.
82. Schwartz M, Madariaga J, Hirose R, et al. Comparison of a new fibrin sealant with standard topical hemostatic agents. Arch Surg. 2004;139:1148–54.
83. Chapman WC, Clavien PA, Fung J, et al. Effective control of hepatic bleeding with a novel collagen-based composite combined with autologous plasma: results of a randomized controlled trial. Arch Surg. 2000;135:1200–4; discussion 1205.
84. Kohno H, Nagasue N, Chang YC, et al. Comparison of topical hemostatic agents in elective hepatic resection: a clinical prospective randomized trial. World J Surg. 1992;16:966–9; discussion 970.
85. Fischer L, Seiler CM, Broelsch CE, et al. Hemostatic efficacy of TachoSil in liver resection compared with argon beam coagulator treatment: an open, randomized, prospective, multi-center, parallel-group trial. Surgery. 2011;149:48–55.
86. Zhu P, Lau WY, Chen YF, et al. Randomized clinical trial comparing infrahepatic inferior vena cava clamping with low central venous pressure in complex liver resections involving the Pringle manoeuvre. Br J Surg. 2012;99:781–8.
87. Rahbari NN, Koch M, Zimmermann JB, et al. Infrahepatic inferior vena cava clamping for reduction of central venous pressure and blood loss during hepatic resection: a randomized controlled trial. Ann Surg. 2011;253:1102–10.
88. Kato M, Kubota K, Kita J, et al. Effect of infra-hepatic inferior vena cava clamping on bleeding during hepatic dissection: a prospective, randomized, controlled study. World J Surg. 2008;32:1082–7.
89. Jarnagin WR, Gonen M, Maithel SK, et al. A prospective randomized trial of acute normovolemic hemodilution compared to standard intraoperative management in patients undergoing major hepatic resection. Ann Surg. 2008;248:360–9.
90. Wang WD, Liang LJ, Huang XQ, Yin XY. Low central venous pressure reduces blood loss in hepatectomy. World J Gastroenterol. 2006;12:935–9.
91. Hasegawa K, Takayama T, Orii R, et al. Effect of hypoventilation on bleeding during hepatic resection: a randomized controlled trial. Arch Surg. 2002;137:311–5.
92. Matot I, Scheinin O, Jurim O, Eid A. Effectiveness of acute normovolemic hemodilution to minimize allogeneic blood transfusion in major liver resections. Anesthesiology. 2002;97:794–800.
93. Smyrniotis V, Kostopanagiotou G, Theodoraki K, et al. The role of central venous pressure and type of vascular control in blood loss during major liver resections. Am J Surg. 2004;187:398–402.
94. Melendez JA, Arslan V, Fischer ME, et al. Perioperative outcomes of major hepatic resections under low central venous pressure anesthesia: blood loss, blood transfusion, and the risk of postoperative renal dysfunction. J Am Coll Surg. 1998;187:620–5.
95. Jones RM, Moulton CE, Hardy KJ. Central venous pressure and its effect on blood loss during liver resection. Br J Surg. 1998;85:1058–60.
96. Li Z, Sun YM, FX W, et al. Controlled low central venous pressure reduces blood loss and transfusion requirements in hepatectomy. World J Gastroenterol. 2014;20(1):303–9.
97. Neuschwander A, Futier E, Jaber S, et al. The effects of intraoperative lung protective ventilation with positive end-expiratory pressure on blood loss during hepatic resection surgery: a secondary analysis of data from a published randomised control trial (IMPROVE). Eur J Anaesthesiol. 2016;33(4):292–8.
98. Correa-Gallego C, Berman A, Denis SC, et al. Renal function after low central venous pressure-assisted liver resection: assessment of 2116 cases. HPB (Oxford). 2015;17(3):258–64.
99. Johnson LB, Plotkin JS, Kuo PC. Reduced transfusion requirements during major hepatic resection with use of intraoperative isovolemic hemodilution. Am J Surg. 1998;176:608–11.
100. Gross JB. Estimating allowable blood loss: corrected for dilution. Anesthesiology. 1983;58:277–80.
101. Weiskopf RB. Efficacy of acute normovolemic hemodilution assessed as a function of fraction of blood volume lost. Anesthesiology. 2001;94:439–4.
102. Meguro M, Mizuguchi T, Kawamoto M, et al. Clinical comparison of laparoscopic and open liver resection after propensity matching selection. Surgery. 2015;158(3):573–87.

103. Tranchart H, O'Rourke N, Van Dam R, et al. Bleeding control during laparoscopic liver resection: a review of literature. J Hepatobiliary Pancreat Sci. 2015;22(5):371–8.
104. Dua MM, Worhunsky DJ, Hwa K, et al. Extracorporeal Pringle for laparoscopic liver resection. Surg Endosc. 2015;29(6):1348–55.
105. Scatton O, Brustia R, Belli G, et al. What kind of energy devices should be used for laparoscopic liver resection? Recommendations from a systematic review. J Hepatobiliary Pancreat Sci. 2015;22(5):327–34.
106. Kawaguchi Y, Nomi T, Fuks D, et al. Hemorrhage control for laparoscopic hepatectomy: technical details and predictive factors for intraoperative blood loss. Surg Endosc. 2015;30(6):2543–51.
107. Itano O, Ikoma N, Takei H, et al. The superficial precoagulation, sealing, and transection method: a "bloodless" and "ecofriendly" laparoscopic liver transection technique. Surg Laparosc Endosc Percutan Tech. 2015;25(1):e33–6.

Minimally Invasive Hepatic Resection

6

Iswanto Sucandy and Allan Tsung

Introduction

The field of hepatobiliary surgery has evolved dramatically in the past few decades, with improved understanding of the segmental anatomy of the liver, advancements in modern imaging techniques, better operative instrumentation, and improved perioperative anesthesia care. At the same time, minimally invasive surgery technique has become an integral part of each surgical subspecialty. The laparoscopic approach has become standard of care in colorectal resection, bariatric surgery, hernia repair, and many urogynecology procedures. In liver operation, however, the adoption of minimally invasive techniques has been slow, and it is still far from being a standard technique for most liver surgeons, even at major academic centers in the United States. This reluctance stems in part from the technical complexity of liver operations, concern for significant intraoperative bleeding or gas embolism, and lack of formal training in minimally invasive techniques. In addition to the laparoscopic approach for liver resection, the current minimally invasive approach also includes robotic liver resections [1, 2].

An important principle of minimally invasive surgery is that the availability of this technique does not alter the indication. A laparoscopic or robotic liver resection should be considered only for lesions that would otherwise be treated with open hepatic surgery. Malignant primary and metastatic liver lesions, symptomatic hemangioma or focal nodular hyperplasia (FNH), and hepatic adenomas larger than 4 cm should be resected. The recently published International Survey on Technical Aspects of Laparoscopic Liver Resection (INSTALL) study demonstrated an

I. Sucandy, MD
Digestive Health Institute, Florida Hospital Tampa, Tampa, FL, USA

A. Tsung, MD (✉)
Division of Hepatobiliary and Pancreatic Surgery, University of Pittsburgh Medical Center, Pittsburgh, PA, USA
e-mail: tsunga@upmc.edu

© Springer International Publishing AG 2018
F.G. Rocha, P. Shen (eds.), *Optimizing Outcomes for Liver and Pancreas Surgery*, DOI 10.1007/978-3-319-62624-6_6

expanding indication for LLR which includes higher tumor size, number, and lesion in difficult locations [3]. While approximately 36% of laparoscopic liver resections are performed in patients with background liver cirrhosis, postoperative liver insufficiency has always been an important factor in deciding extent of hepatic resection, whether in open or minimally invasive technique. In order to avoid postoperative liver failure, for minor liver resection (≤2 segments), majority of liver surgeons set the upper limit of a total bilirubin at 2.0 mg/dl, whereas for major resection (≥3 segments), the threshold is lowered to 1.5 mg/dl or less [3]. While extended hepatectomies, which remove up to 70–80% of liver parenchyma, are safe in noncirrhotic patients, a more conservative resection must be performed when the background liver has cirrhotic changes. In a multi-institutional Japanese study, Takahara et al. reported that the incidence of postoperative liver failure after laparoscopic liver resection and open liver resection was about 0.5% and 1.8%, respectively [4]. The INSTALL study reported that over 80% of surgeons set the cutoff at 40% volume for future liver remnant when the liver is found to be cirrhotic.

In liver resection, the main differences between benign and malignant lesions are related to achieving adequate margins and avoidance of tumor rupture intraoperatively. For malignant liver tumors, lesions abutting major vasculature or tumors that are too large to be manipulated with minimally invasive technique should be resected using an open approach. Perihilar cholangiocarcinomas (Klatskin tumor) are often very challenging even by an open approach and generally should not be done using the minimally invasive technique. The presence of dense adhesions that prevent safe dissection, unexpected difficulty in manipulating the liver, and failure to make progress are indications for conversion to an open technique. Such a decision is never considered a failure but rather a good judgment call, employed in order to prevent unnecessary complications. Finally, only about 5% of laparoscopic liver resection around the world is performed in the context of live donor liver transplantation [3, 5–8]. Laparoscopic live donor hepatectomy has been described for left lateral sectionectomy and adult-to-adult right hepatectomy [5, 7]. Caution is noted in that these operations should only be done by transplant teams with extensive open live donor liver transplantation expertise, as well as minimally invasive liver resection experience.

Clinical Advantages of Minimally Invasive Hepatic Resection

More than 150 publications have shown the safety and efficacy of laparoscopic liver resection. In the world review of laparoscopic liver resection in 2804 patients by Nguyen et al., overall mortality was 0.3% (9/2804 patients) and morbidity was 10.5% [9]. Two relatively recent studies reviewed the clinical benefits of laparoscopic versus open liver resection. The first study is a critical appraisal of 31 publications that compared laparoscopic with open liver resection in 2473 patients [10]. In case-cohort studies of well-matched patients, laparoscopic group was associated with less blood loss, less packed red blood cell transfusion, quicker resumption of oral intake, less pain medication requirement, and shorter length of stay, as compared to the open group. Further, seven publications in this analysis reported a lower morbidity (complication rates) in laparoscopic liver resection group, while the remaining studies found no statistical difference in complication rates [4]. Other potential advantages include better cosmetic result and potentially a lesser physiologic stress response, which includes lower frequency of postoperative liver insufficiency, which was mentioned earlier [11]. This result might be explained by less destruction of the collateral blood vessels/lymphatic channels with minimally invasive approach during abdominal access and liver mobilization. In those patients undergoing laparoscopic hepatic resection for cancer, there was no difference in 3- or 5-year overall survival when compared with well-matched open hepatic resection cases [11].

The subsequent review is a meta-analysis of 26 articles comparing laparoscopic to open liver resection from 1998 to 2009 [12]. In this study, the laparoscopic liver resection group had a lower operative blood loss, shorter hospital stay, less intravenous narcotic use, fewer days until oral intake, and lower relative risk of postoperative complications compared to the open group. Further, the hazards ratio for recurrence of malignant tumors was not significantly different between the two groups (HR = 0.79, $P = 0.37$). In another study, Martin et al. reported on 90 laparoscopic versus 360 open formal hepatic lobectomies [13]. Patients in the two arms were matched in a 1:4 ratio for age, American Society of Anesthesiology (ASA) class, tumor size, histology, and tumor location. Benign tumors were more common in the laparoscopic group. Estimated intraoperative blood loss, Pringle time, total and pulmonary complication rates, and hospital length of stay were significantly lower for the laparoscopic group.

Oncologic Outcomes of Minimally Invasive Hepatic Resection

To date, there is no evidence in the literature that documents compromise of tumor margins or worse oncologic outcomes using 5-year overall or disease-free survival with minimally invasive liver resection when compared with traditional open liver resection. The most recent large study on long-term outcomes of laparoscopic versus open liver resection for colorectal liver metastases by Beppu et al. is a 1:2 propensity score matched multi-institutional study from 32 Japanese centers between 2005 and 2010 [14]. Five-year recurrence-free survival (53.4% vs 51.2%), overall survival (70.1% vs 68%), and disease-specific survival (73.2% vs 69.8%) did not differ significantly between laparoscopic and open liver resection groups, respectively. Several meta-analyses have also shown comparable oncologic outcomes and survival between open and laparoscopic liver resections [15–19].

Patient Assessment and Operative Strategy

The indications and preoperative evaluation for minimally invasive (laparoscopic and robotic) liver resections are similar to those of open liver resections. Imaging of the liver is best obtained with triphasic liver computed tomography (CT) scan or magnetic resonance imaging (MRI). Biopsy of liver mass is generally reserved only for diagnostic uncertainty, despite high-quality imaging. Evaluation of future liver remnant and patient general health performance are similar to what is done for open resection. The decision to perform minimally invasive liver resection is mainly influenced by the tumor location, size, vicinity to the vital structures, and the experience of the surgical team. For robotic liver resection, both console surgeon and his/her bedside assistant should be ideally proficient in open and robotic hepatectomy. They should be interchangeable throughout the entire case. Central and high posterior lesions provide challenges and require significant minimally invasive experience. The technical challenges with liver mobilization, hilar dissection, parenchymal transection, and hemostasis can be minimized by optimal port placement, good patient positioning, and an efficient operating room team. Difficult dissections which require significantly prolonged operative time, failure to progress, and significant intraoperative bleeding should prompt a consideration for conversion to the open approach. The anesthesia team should also understand that a low central venous pressure should always be maintained during any liver operation, regardless of the operative approach. A transjugular central line should be placed prior to starting a major liver resection (resection of >2 segments). In a minor liver resection, the use of central line should be based on surgeon's discretion. Temporary inflow occlusion with Pringle maneuver is sometimes necessary. In our institution, we use a flat rubber vascular loop tape, which is placed around the hepatoduodenal ligament via the foramen of Winslow using a blunt laparoscopic or robotic grasper. The rubber tape is placed in a Potts fashion, tightened by pulling its two ends together, and subsequently held in place by a laparoscopic or robotic clip. When Pringle maneuver is necessary, a gentle anterior traction can be immediately applied to the ends of the rubber tape with a robotic or a laparoscopic grasper.

Techniques in Minimizing Blood Loss During Hepatectomy

Despite established advantages of minimally invasive technique, hemorrhage during laparoscopic or robotic liver resection remains a major concern. The initial slow development of minimally invasive liver resection is partly explained by the fear of inability to control bleeding. This important question was discussed among a panel of 34 experts covering 5 continents during the Second International Conference on Laparoscopic Liver Resection Surgery in Morioka, Iwate, Japan, in October 2014. Several studies have been designed to elucidate potential factors responsible for reduced blood loss during minimally invasive liver resection. It is widely accepted that the main reasons for reduced blood loss are the positive pressure of the carbon dioxide pneumoperitoneum (10–15 mmHg), low central venous pressure

(≤5 mmHg), the emergence of new transection devices, and the facilitation of inflow and outflow controls [20]. Experts who were present in Morioka agreed that low central venous pressure and pneumoperitoneum act in a synergistic manner to reduce bleeding. Image magnification provided by a laparoscope or robotic camera allows more precise dissections and theoretically facilitates good control of segmental or subsegmental portal pedicles. In cases of severe bleeding, increasing the pneumoperitoneum pressure and decreasing the airway pressure by a brief pause in the artificial ventilation are maneuvers that can be used to decrease back bleeding [3]. Decailliot et al. demonstrated in a nonrandomized study that Pringle maneuver during laparoscopic liver resection is as efficient as Pringle maneuver during open liver surgery in decreasing intraoperative blood loss [21]. Type of instruments by energy sources and technique used in parenchymal transection vary among each surgeon and institution. We recommend that liver surgeons should select techniques and instruments based on their familiarity and complete understanding of the system for each specific case. There have been no randomized controlled trials which answer the question of the best technique or device for laparoscopic hepatic parenchymal transection. All studies on this subject have been case controls, case series, case reports, experimental studies, and reviews [22]. In addition to the use of multiple hemostatic methods such as bipolar cautery (for vessels ≤2 mm), vessel sealing device or clips (for vessels 3–7 mm), locked clips or staplers (for vessels ≥7 mm), thermofusion, radio-frequency coagulation, bipolar precoagulation, and many others, experts advocate that liver surgeons should master intracorporeal suturing techniques when performing laparoscopic liver resection. With the robotic system, intracorporeal suturing is greatly facilitated. The commonly described technical difficulty with suturing becomes no longer an issue, especially for surgeons without prior advanced laparoscopic skills/training. Careful inspection of the transection surface for bleeding and bile leak after decreasing the pneumoperitoneal pressure should be performed routinely prior to completion of the liver resection.

Technical Approaches to Laparoscopic Liver Resection

There are two main approaches for performing laparoscopic liver resection—pure laparoscopic and hand assisted. A third option is using the laparoscopic technique for mobilization of the liver before making an incision to complete parenchymal resection through a relatively small minilaparotomy opening (so-called hybrid technique) [23]. Some authors use a hand port for all cases, while others use it selectively, and some never use it at all. The benefits of the hand-assisted technique are the relative ease of manipulation of the liver, direct palpation for improved tactile sensation, and the ability to quickly control significant bleeding in the case of a major vascular injury. Because most specimens mandate a utility incision for intact specimen extraction, the main difference between hand-assisted and pure laparoscopy is the position of the incision. There have been no comparative studies to support the benefit or inferiority of the three techniques, and the choice is strictly surgeon's preference. The hand-assisted and the hybrid methods are claimed by their proponents to be beneficial for larger lesions, posteriorly located lesions, donor hepatectomy, and for training of surgeons in major laparoscopic liver resection techniques [1, 7, 23, 24]. In a large review of more than 2800 laparoscopic liver resections by Nguyen et al., the majority of minimally invasive liver resections were pure laparoscopic (75%), followed by hand-assisted approach (17%). The hybrid technique was used rarely, only in 2% of patients. The remainder of the cases were performed using gasless laparoscopic (1.8%) and thoracoscopic approach (0.2%). Four percent of patients required conversion to traditional open approach [9].

In the operating room, the patient is placed in supine position with both arms extended. Some authors favor the French lithotomy position. The preparation is similar to that of major liver resection, including line placement, bladder catheterization, and orogastric tube insertion. We use a footboard and strapping that allow for steep rotational manipulations of the operating table during laparoscopic liver resection. In the case of a planned major hepatectomy, we use a hand port and place it at the beginning of the procedure, as a supraumbilical midline incision. In the case of a small patient (e.g., less than 5'8" in height), the incision can be infraumbilical. The initial pneumoperitoneum is established via a trocar inserted through the hand port. The hand port incision may be used for a rapid conversion, by extending it to a longer midline cephalad if needed.

Laparoscopic Right Hepatectomy

After inserting the hand port and establishing the pneumoperitoneum to a pressure limit of 14 mm Hg, four additional trocars are placed. Trocar positioning is shown in Fig. 6.1. The falciform ligament is divided with endoshears, and the round ligament is divided using a linear stapler or LigaSure™ vessel sealing device (Covidien, Norwalk, CT, USA). The falciform ligament is left long on the liver side to facilitate later retraction. Intraoperative ultrasound is performed to identify the lesion and mark the parenchymal transection line. After taking down the right coronary and triangular ligaments, the right lobe is gradually rotated off the retroperitoneum and lifted off the inferior vena cava (IVC). Short hepatic veins are clipped with 5-mm Hemolocks. Small veins can be divided with the LigaSure™ vessel sealing device. At that stage, the right hepatic vein is exposed and can be divided with a vascular stapler. If the exposure of the right hepatic vein is not optimal, it can be divided inside the liver at the end of the parenchymal transection. The next step is the hilar dissection. It is started with the cholecystectomy and exposure of the right hepatic artery, right portal vein, and bile duct. The right hepatic artery is doubly secured with locking clips. A clamping test must be performed to ensure an intact arterial flow in the left hepatic artery prior to division. The right portal vein is dissected and encircled. It can be transected with a linear vascular stapler; however, if the angle precludes safe stapling, it can be left to the end of the procedure and controlled with a small bulldog clamp inserted through the hand port to allow for an ipsilateral Pringle maneuver. Next, superficial parenchymal transection is started with an ultrasonic dissector or LigaSure™ to a depth of approximately 2 cm. The deeper liver

Fig. 6.1 Trocar
positioning for
laparoscopic right liver
resection

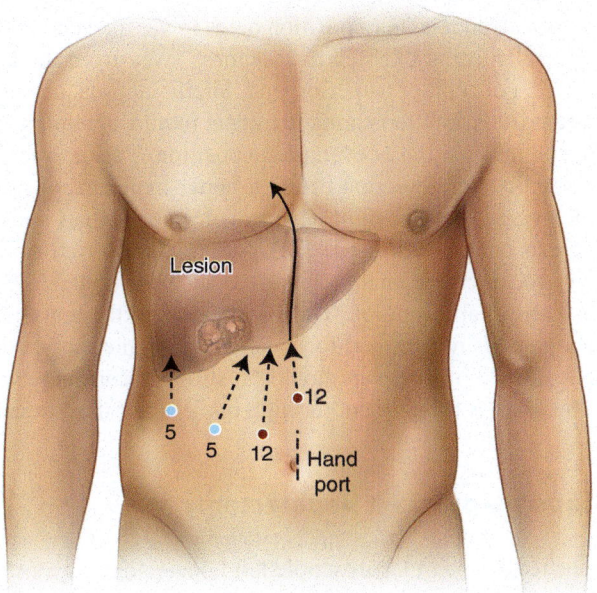

parenchyma, which contains crossing middle hepatic vein branches, is divided with vascular staplers. Some surgeons utilize a bipolar pinching forceps and/or cavitron ultrasonic surgical aspirator (CUSA) or hydrojet to help divide the parenchyma. During the parenchymal transection, as in an open hepatic resection, the central venous pressure is kept low in order to minimize blood loss. If not already done, the right portal vein and right hepatic veins are divided as the parenchymal transection is deepened, along with the right hepatic duct inside the liver. If a hand port is utilized, the hand can provide a laparoscopic "hanging maneuver" to facilitate exposure and transection. Wakabayashi et al. and Soubrane et al. advocated a limited liver mobilization before transection, as a potential technique to decrease bleeding during a laparoscopic liver resection [25, 26]. The anterior approach provides the advantage of performing minimally invasive liver resection without having to mobilize the liver before transection, which is not always easy and safe to accomplish minimally invasively, particularly in case of heavy liver weight or a large-sized tumor.

The caudal approach is the main conceptual change in laparoscopic liver resection. The caudal approach, which relies on visual magnification, offers improved exposure around the right adrenal gland and the inferior vena cava. This approach also greatly facilitates identification of the Glissonian pedicles at the hilar plate. Using this technique, the inferior vena cava from caudal to cranial can be efficiently exposed, which is then followed by division of the short hepatic veins before parenchymal transection [26]. A meticulous caudal to cranial parenchymal transection with laparoscopic magnification results in better identification of intraparenchymal structures for optimal liver parenchymal division. Placement of patients in slight reverse Trendelenburg position helps lower the venous pressure and improves gravitational shifting of visceral structures away from the liver hilum. A recently introduced concept of superior and lateral approaches with or without the use of intercostals and transthoracic trocars requires patients to be placed in the left lateral decubitus position or even prone position. This new technical advancement in laparoscopic liver resection offers a better exposure of the right posterosuperior segments and lifts the right hepatic vein higher than the vena cava to reduce hepatic venous back bleeding [27, 28]. Any oozing from the cut edge is controlled with an electrocautery or energy sealing device. Any visible bile leaks are oversewn with 4-0 absorbable sutures. The specimen is extracted through the hand port, and the abdomen is reinspected for bleeding. Placement of a closed suction drain about the cut surface of the liver should be strongly considered after major liver resections. The drain is brought out through one of the 5-mm trocar sites.

Laparoscopic Left Hepatectomy

The technique of laparoscopic left hepatectomy is mostly similar to that of the right lobe. Trocar positioning for the laparoscopic left hepatectomy is shown in Fig. 6.2. Often laparoscopic left lateral sectionectomy and left formal lobectomy can be done using pure laparoscopic approach, with the hand port being reserved for a large tumor or difficult case. Care must be given to avoid injury to the left phrenic and left hepatic veins when taking down the left triangular ligament. The gastrohepatic ligament is divided (watching for a replaced left hepatic artery), and the left hilum is dissected at the base of the falciform ligament after opening the liver bridge between segment III and segment IVB. The left hepatic artery is doubly clipped and divided, followed by dissection of the left portal vein. The left portal vein can be controlled/divided in a manner similar to that of the right portal vein. The left hepatic duct is transected laterally at the base of the umbilical fissure to avoid injury to a not infrequently seen right posterior (or right anterior) duct coming off the proximal end of the left hepatic duct. This is seen in about 10% of patients. A hepatotomy is made in segment IVB, and a linear stapler is insinuated into the hepatotomy in order to divide the left hepatic duct. Parenchymal transection is performed using a LigaSure™ vessel sealing device or an ultrasonic dissector, followed by application of linear vascular staplers to divide the left hepatic vein intrahepatically toward the end of the transection.

Robotic Liver Resection

The most recent development in minimally invasive liver resection is robotic hepatectomy. The first report of robotic-assisted liver resection was published in 2006 by Ryska et al. [29]. The known advantages of robotic platform include improved precision, dexterity, degree of movement, superior visual magnification, as well as

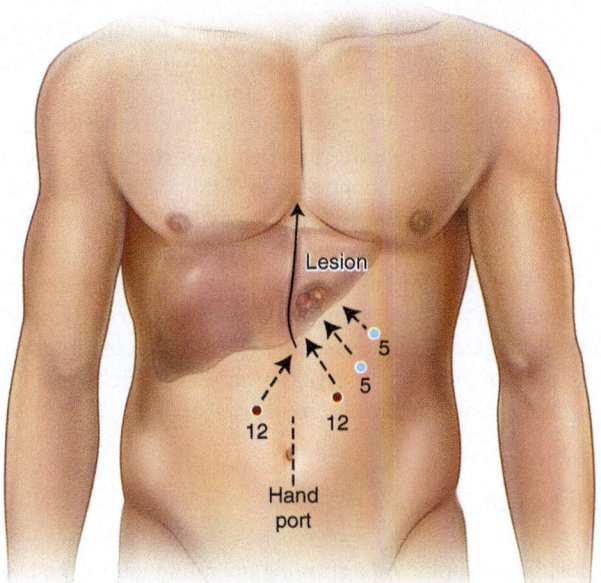

Fig. 6.2   Trocar positioning for laparoscopic left liver resection

decreased surgeon tremor and fatigue. Robotic liver resection has gained significant popularity in recent years because of its potential to overcome limitations of conventional laparoscopy. Over the last 5 years, many case reports and single institutional case series of robotic liver resections have emerged. In 2014, Tsung et al. reported our institutional experience of robotic versus laparoscopic hepatectomy with a 1:2 matched analysis [2]. The patients were matched for the presence of background liver disease, extent of hepatic resection, diagnosis, body mass index (BMI), age, gender, and ASA class. With the exception of higher operative time and overall room time in the robotic group, there were no significant differences between perioperative outcomes of robotic and laparoscopic groups. R0 negative margin status was also comparable, which indicates that the oncologic outcome is not compromised by either approach. The technical advantages associated with robotic approach, however, allow completion of a greater percentage of minor and major hepatectomies using the purely minimally invasive technique. Ninety-three percent of the robotic liver resections were accomplished without the need for hand-assisted ports or the hybrid technique, while only 49.1% of those in the laparoscopic group were performed without these adjuncts [30]. This finding suggests the robotic system offers greater technical ease for liver surgeons in accomplishing purely minimally invasive liver resections. The robotic approach may also facilitate better vascular control during major liver resections when compared to its laparoscopic counterpart. Pretransection extrahepatic inflow and outflow control is more easily achieved with the robot. Laparoscopic stapling of the portal vein extrahepatically is sometimes difficult to accomplish with the laparoscopic approach due to a poor stapler angle. Increased degree of freedom with the robotic instrumentation mitigates this problem by allowing control of the portal vein extrahepatically using suture ligation or placement of locking clips. Similar issues apply to the hepatic vein outflow control. During hepatic parenchymal transection, superior three-dimensional magnification provided by the robotic camera allows surgeon to identify individual vessels more clearly for precise control and ligation/clipping. The downside of robotic approach is added costs for the robotic system and slightly longer operative time [31]. The overall perioperative outcomes are comparable between the laparoscopic and robotic liver resections. A future larger-scale prospective multicenter study is needed to objectively determine the ultimate superiority of robotic over the traditional laparoscopic technique. Based on the most recent international consensus in Morioka, Japan, major robotic liver surgery is still recommended to be done within an institutional review board-approved registry [1].

Robotic Right Hepatectomy

The patient is positioned supine on a split leg operating table. The bedside assistant stands between the patient legs. Operating room setup and robotic system docking position are shown in Fig. 6.3. We utilize 6 port techniques with a goal to achieve adequate triangulation around the target anatomy (Fig. 6.4). The operation begins with division of the round and falciform ligaments using a 5-mm LigaSure™ vessel sealing device. Attachments between the liver and retroperitoneum are taken down using a robotic hook electrocautery. The third robotic arm is positioned to provide upward and medial retraction to the right liver in order to expose the right triangular ligament laterally and short hepatic veins medially. Appropriate adjustment is made by the third arm as the dissection proceeds cranially toward the hepatic hilum. The right side of the inferior vena cava is dissected carefully off the posterior aspect of the liver. The short hepatic veins are individually isolated and divided between clips and silk ties. Small short hepatic veins can be taken with robotic vessel sealer.

Portal dissection is started by appropriately lifting the inferior aspect of the liver cranially using the third robotic arm. Gallbladder when still presents can be used as a natural grasping handle by the third arm. The proper hepatic artery which leads to the right hepatic artery is identified. The right hepatic artery branch is dissected and isolated using a hook electrocautery. A robotic Maryland dissector can be used to facilitate isolation of the right hepatic artery. Ultrasound over the left hepatic artery must be performed to ensure intact arterial flow in the left hepatic artery prior to division. Silk ties with placement of metal clips or Hemolock clips are commonly used for this step. Close attention must be exercised to identify and control a replaced or accessory right hepatic artery which is present in up to 25% of patients. The right portal vein is then carefully dissected and isolated prior to division using a linear vascular stapler. Small branches to the caudate lobe often need to be divided in order to provide an adequate space for division. Finally the right hepatic duct is

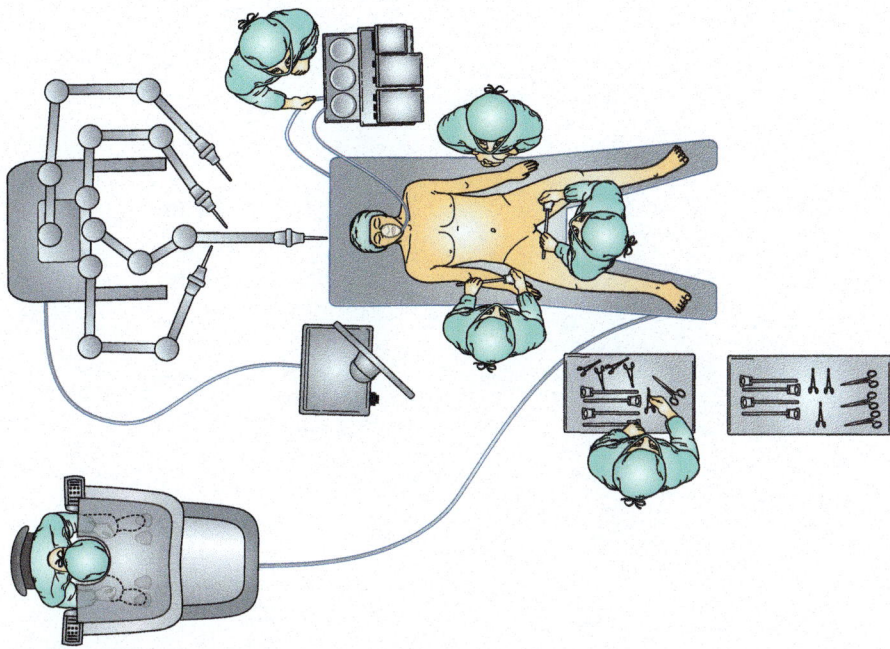

Fig. 6.3 Operating room setup and robotic system docking position

isolated, ligated, and divided after an intraoperative cholangiogram confirming the presence of an intact contralateral hepatic duct.

The right hepatic vein is then isolated and encircled with a vessel loop. A linear vascular stapler is used to divide the right hepatic vein by the bedside assistant, which safely secures the outflow control. Line of parenchymal transection is then marked with the hook electrocautery, which follows a demarcation line on the liver surface. Placement of figure of eight silk sutures on both sides of the transection plane can be helpful for lateral retraction. Intraoperative ultrasonography is performed to confirm adequate tumor margins and to anticipate any large underlying crossing vessels. The TilePro® feature of da Vinci system is helpful in transferring the ultrasonographic images to the console. The liver parenchymal transection is started using a combination of a robotic vessel sealer, a Maryland bipolar forceps, clips, and ties. Medium- and large-sized crossing vessels/branches found intrahepatically are individually secured using ties and clips before division. Alternatively, they can also be handled using linear vascular stapler, fired by the bedside surgeon. Use of rubber bands for lateral traction of the liver in minimally invasive hepatectomy was introduced by Choi et al. [32, 33]. As the parenchymal transection progresses, self-retraction created by each rubber band opens up the plane of transection. The bedside surgeon should help with tissue hemostasis and dynamic exposure of the plane of transection. Thorough hemostasis and meticulous search for bile leak are performed along the cut surface prior to considering placement of an abdominal

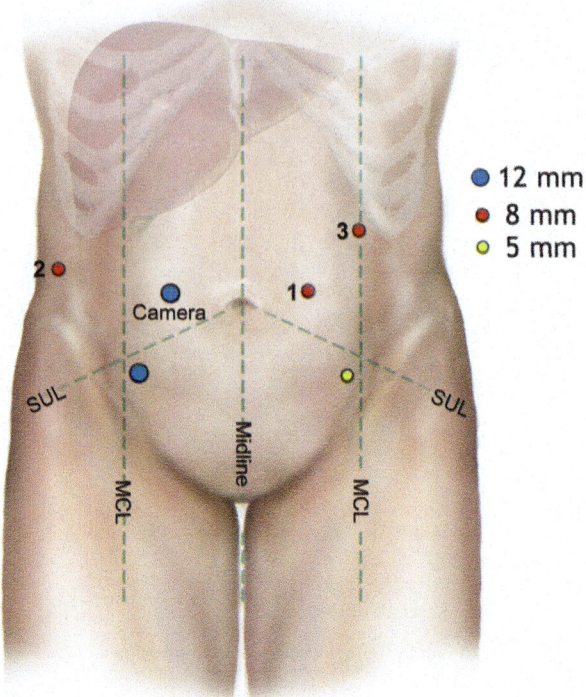

Fig. 6.4 Trocar positioning for robotic right liver resection

drain. The resected specimen is placed in a large endo bag retrieval system and removed via either enlarged camera port at the umbilical location or via a Pfannenstiel incision.

Robotic Left Hepatectomy

Patient positioning, operating room setup, and robotic system docking position are similar to the right hepatectomy. Trocar placement for left hepatectomy is slightly different than for the right hepatectomy, and it is shown in Fig. 6.5. The round and falciform ligaments are taken using similar technique as the right liver resection. A complete stomach decompression via a naso-/orogastric tube is important at the beginning of the case. The left triangular ligament is divided using the hook electrocautery. It is important to not injure the branch of the phrenic vein often located nearby. Access into the lesser sac is obtained by dividing the gastrohepatic ligament. An accessory or replaced left hepatic artery is ligated and clipped prior to division when present (about 10–15% of patients).

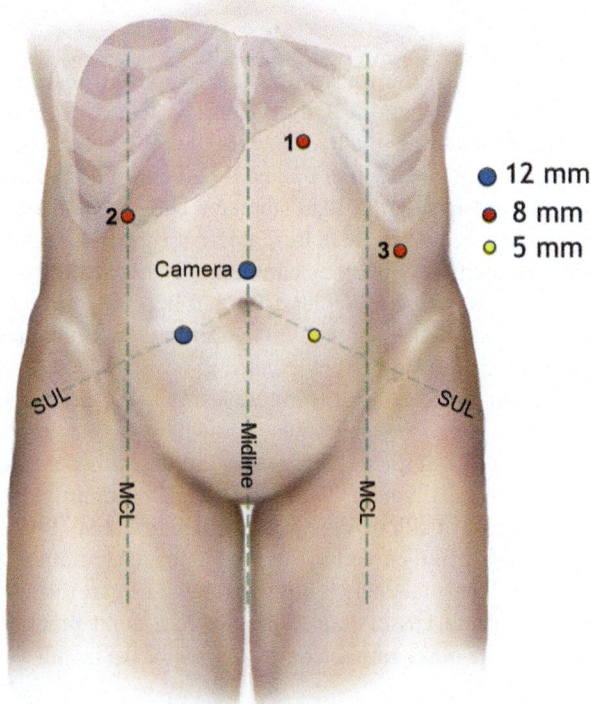

Fig. 6.5 Trocar positioning for robotic left liver resection

The lesser sac is medially opened all the way cephalad, toward the origin of the left hepatic vein. The goal is to obtain a complete mobilization of the left hemiliver. The portal dissection and parenchymal transection are performed using similar techniques as the right liver resection. The transverse portion of the left portal inflow allows a technically safer dissection, close to the junction between the transverse and ascending portion of the left portal vein. Outflow dissection is subsequently performed after the division of the Arantius ligament. With the left lobe reflected toward the right, the origin of the left and middle hepatic veins is carefully dissected. In majority of patients, the left and middle hepatic veins create a common trunk before entering the inferior vena cava. A linear vascular stapler is used to divide the hepatic vein after encirclement using a vessel loop. If a safe outflow dissection cannot be achieved extrahepatically, the hepatic veins can also be divided intrahepatically as the parenchymal transection proceeds cephalad. Hemostasis and bile stasis are meticulously ensured prior to completion.

Robotic Left Lateral Sectionectomy and Nonanatomic Liver Resection

In left lateral sectionectomy, the transection line is located just to the left of the falciform ligament after left hemiliver mobilization. The divided round ligament can be used as a handle to elevate the liver toward the right anterior direction, which opens up the transection plane. Segment 2 and 3 pedicles are taken (either together or individually) with linear vascular load staplers. The parenchymal transection is performed using similar steps to those in formal left or right hepatectomies. Crossing vessels are usually encountered, but they can be easily managed with either robotic vessel sealer device, clips, or linear staplers. The left hepatic vein is divided intrahepatically toward the end of the parenchymal transection. For nonanatomic liver resection, intraoperative ultrasonography is used to ensure adequate margins and to detect underlying major vessels to and from the lesions. Adequate planning for vascular control of medium/large vessel branches shown by the ultrasound should be in place prior to transection. Complete hemostasis and detection of bile leak must be ensured after parenchymal division. When bile leak is identified from a biliary branch, careful placement of silk or Vicryl sutures are effective. For hemostasis, we recommend the use of saline-cooled radio-frequency coagulation device, which gives excellent results. Thermal energy, however, must be carefully applied in areas near the hepatic hilum and vessel staple lines. It is a good practice to lower the pneumoperitoneum while observing the liver cut surface for occult bleeding prior to closure [34].

It is very critical to have a skilled bedside assistant surgeon when performing this type of advanced liver operation. Intraoperative bleeding during parenchymal transection is primary reason for conversion to open surgery during major minimally invasive liver resection, both laparoscopic and robotic. Conversion rates in laparoscopic major hepatectomy range from 33% in the early experience of Dulucq et al. [35] to a lower rate of 14% reported more recently by Gayet et al. [36]. In the totally robotic right hepatectomy of 24 patients reported by Giulianotti et al. [37], open conversion only occurred in 1/24 patients, which was related to oncologic concerns (inability to carefully evaluate the resection margins) .

Management of Postoperative Liver Failure

Prevention with proper surgical planning is the best strategy to limit incidence of postoperative liver failure, even though it is sometimes unavoidable in certain patients. There are only limited publications on the management of postoperative liver failure, and there have been no comparative studies in this regard [38]. Treatment strategies vary among institutions and hepatobiliary surgeons; however, in general the management of liver failure after hepatic resection is guided by organ systems. An intensive care unit should be available for optimal supportive care of patients with liver failure. Early management is key to avoid the downstream vicious cycle of sequelae associated with postoperative liver failure.

Postoperative liver failure manifests in encephalopathy secondary to reduced ammonia clearance, hypoglycemia due to reduced gluconeogenesis, lactic acidosis due to reduced lactic acid clearance, hypotension due to inadequate glucocorticoid secretion, acute respiratory distress syndrome, impaired innate immunologic function with associated sepsis, intracerebral hypertension, cerebral edema, and acute kidney injury/failure. Patients who appear jaundice after extended hepatectomy should be investigated in order to rule out obstructive causes. The generous use of albumin (instead of crystalloids) should be instituted for patients who need hemodynamic support. Early continuous renal replacement therapy rather than hemodialysis should be started when acute renal injury/failure is encountered. Fresh frozen plasma should be used appropriately to manage coagulopathy. In patients where infection or early sepsis is suspected, antibiotics should be initiated. Development of ascites is also commonly seen in patients with postoperative liver failure. Patients with ascites should be first managed with Lasix and spironolactone. Intermittent paracentesis is used for symptomatic relieve. Patients who develop encephalopathy should be started on rifaximin and lactulose. In terms of nutritional support during the liver failure period, even though the enteral route is preferred, it must be used with caution in order to avoid aspiration. Parenteral nutrition should be used when enteral routes are not practical or unsafe. Branched chain amino acids (leucine, isoleucine, and valine) as amino acid solutions should be used preferentially over whole protein formulations in patients with worsening encephalopathy.

Hepatic support via plasma exchange, molecular absorbent recirculating system, and the extracorporeal liver assist device are newer therapeutic strategies that have been described recently. Even though there may be theoretical benefits, there has been no survival advantage recorded from the use of these modalities, despite effective detoxification and symptomatic clinical improvement of liver failure sequelae [39, 40]. In the setting of worsening and persistent postoperative liver failure when all available therapies have been exhausted, there may be a role for orthotopic liver transplantation as a last resort. However, the underlying malignant diseases for which the liver resection was originally indicated often disqualify such patients for this approach. Therefore, this last option can only be offered for patients who have initially been considered a transplant candidate prior to the hepatectomy (e.g., hepatocellular carcinoma within Milan criteria).

Early Recovery After Surgery Pathways for Hepatic Surgery

Enhanced recovery after surgery (ERAS) was first introduced by Kehlet in 1997 and was shown to reduce the complication rate and hospital stay duration after colorectal surgery [41, 42]. During the past decade, ERAS protocols have rapidly evolved with the application of various effective components, which included perioperative education, improved anesthetic and analgesic methods (less narcotic use), early resumption of oral intake (postoperative day 0–1), and early postoperative mobilization. Patients are planned for discharge on postoperative day 4 after colectomy when postsurgical recovery is uneventful. Because of its proven benefits in gastrointestinal surgery, ERAS protocols are now being implemented in other fields of surgery including pancreaticoduodenectomy and hepatic resection. He et al. reported a study of 86 patients managed with ERAS protocol after laparoscopic liver resection [43]. Postoperative length of stay was significantly reduced in the ERAS group when compared with the control group (6 versus 10 days, $p = 0.04$). First flatus occurrence was seen earlier in the ERAS group (2 versus 3 days, $p = 0.02$). Because of shorter hospitalization, postoperative costs were significantly less in the ERAS group, with no differences in readmission rate, blood loss, conversions to open surgery, mortality, or surgical complications. A similar study by Liang et al. demonstrated an enhanced recovery protocol after surgery for laparoscopic liver resection led to a shorter duration of hospital stay, fewer complications, and lower overall hospital costs [44]. Rate of readmission was not affected by an ERAS protocol.

Summary

Minimally invasive liver resection is an evolving discipline in the field of hepatobiliary surgery. Multiple studies have shown that laparoscopic and robotic liver resections are safe and effective in the hands of experienced surgeons in selected patients. Clinical benefits to the patients include reduced blood loss, postoperative pain, narcotic use, and earlier discharge. From the oncologic standpoint, minimally invasive liver resections have been shown to yield equivalent cancer outcomes. Proper planning with appropriate presurgical evaluation of liver function is the best method in preventing postoperative liver failure. When it occurs, maximum supportive care in an intensive care unit with early intervention of failing organ systems is crucial for patient survival. Finally, ERAS protocols have been used after liver resections with favorable perioperative outcomes. Further data is needed to draw more definitive conclusions about the effectiveness of enhanced recovery protocols after minimally invasive liver resections.

References

1. Wakabayashi G, Cherqui D, Geller DA, et al. Recommendations for laparoscopic liver resection: a report from the second international consensus conference held in Morioka. Ann Surg. 2015;261(4):619–29.
2. Tsung A, Geller DA, Sukato DC, et al. Robotic versus laparoscopic hepatectomy: a matched comparison. Ann Surg. 2014;259(3):549–55.
3. Hibi T, Cherqui D, Geller DA, et al. Expanding indications and regional diversity in laparoscopic liver resection unveiled by the International Survey on Technical Aspects of Laparoscopic Liver Resection (INSTALL) study. Surg Endosc. 2016 Jul;30(7):2975–83.
4. Takahara T, Wakabayashi G, Beppu T, et al. Long-term and perioperative outcomes of laparoscopic versus open liver resection for hepatocellular carcinoma with propensity score matching: a multi-institutional Japanese study. J Hepatobiliary Pancreat Sci. 2015;22(10):721–7.
5. Soubrane O, Cherqui D, Scatton O, et al. Laparoscopic left lateral sectionectomy in living donors: safety and reproducibility of the technique in a single center. Ann Surg. 2006;244:815.

6. Kurosaki I, Yamamoto S, Kitami C, et al. Video-assisted living donor hemihepatectomy through a 12-cm incision for adult-to-adult liver transplantation. Surgery. 2006;139:695.
7. Koffron AJ, Kung R, Baker T, et al. Laparoscopic-assisted right lobe donor hepatectomy. Am J Transplant. 2006;6:2522.
8. Soubrane O, de Rougemont O, Kim KH, et al. Laparoscopic living donor left lateral sectionectomy: a new standard practice for donor hepatectomy. Ann Surg. 2015;262(5):757–63.
9. Nguyen KT, Gamblin TC, Geller DA. World review of laparoscopic liver resection—2804 patients. Ann Surg. 2009;250:831.
10. Nguyen KT, Marsh JW, Tsung A, et al. Comparative benefits of laparoscopic versus open hepatic resection: a critical appraisal. Arch Surg. 2011;146:348.
11. Endo Y, Ohta M, Sasaki A, et al. A comparative study of the long-term outcomes after laparoscopy-assisted and open left lateral hepatectomy for hepatocellular carcinoma. Surg Laparosc Endosc Percutan Tech. 2009;19:171.
12. Kris PC, Michael HY. Laparoscopic vs open hepatic resection for benign and malignant tumors: an updated meta-analysis. Arch Surg. 2010;145:1109.
13. Martin RC, Scoggins CR, McMasters KM. Laparoscopic hepatic lobectomy: advantages of a minimally invasive approach. J Am Coll Surg. 2010;210:627.
14. Beppu T, Wakabayashi G, Hasegawa K, et al. Long-term and perioperative outcomes of laparoscopic versus open liver resection for colorectal liver metastases with propensity score matching: a multi-institutional Japanese study. J Hepatobiliary Pancreat Sci. 2015;22(10):711–20.
15. Schiffman SC, Kim KH, Tsung A, et al. Laparoscopic versus open liver resection for metastatic colorectal cancer: a metaanalysis of 610 patients. Surgery. 2015;157(2):211–22.
16. Parks KR, Kuo YH, Davis JM, et al. Laparoscopic versus open liver resection: a meta-analysis of long-term outcome. HPB (Oxford). 2014;16(2):109–18.
17. Wei M, He Y, Wang J, et al. Laparoscopic versus open hepatectomy with or without synchronous colectomy for colorectal liver metastasis: a meta-analysis. PLoS One. 2014;9(1):e87461.
18. Luo LX, Yu ZY, Bai YN. Laparoscopic hepatectomy for liver metastases from colorectal cancer: a meta-analysis. J Laparoendosc Adv Surg Tech A. 2014;24(4):213–22.
19. Zhou Y, Xiao Y, Wu L, et al. Laparoscopic liver resection as a safe and efficacious alternative to open resection for colorectal liver metastasis: a meta-analysis. BMC Surg. 2013;13:44.
20. Tranchart H, O'Rourke N, Van Dam R, et al. Bleeding control during laparoscopic liver resection: a review of literature. J Hepatobiliary Pancreat Sci. 2015;22(5):371–8.
21. Decailliot F, Streich B, Heurtematte Y, et al. Hemodynamic effects of portal triad clamping with and without pneumoperitoneum: an echocardiographic study. Anesth Analg. 2005;100(3):617–22.
22. Otsuka Y, Kaneko H, Cleary SP, et al. What is the best technique in parenchymal transection in laparoscopic liver resection? Comprehensive review for the clinical question on the 2nd International Consensus Conference on Laparoscopic Liver Resection. J Hepatobiliary Pancreat Sci. 2015;22(5):363–70.
23. Koffron AJ, Kung RD, Auffenberg GB, et al. Laparoscopic liver surgery for everyone: the hybrid method. Surgery. 2007;142:463.
24. Cardinal JS, Reddy SK, Tsung A, Marsh JW, Geller DA. Laparoscopic major hepatectomy: pure laparoscopic approach versus hand-assisted technique. J Hepatobiliary Pancreat Sci. 2013;20(2):114–9.
25. Wakabayashi G, Nitta H, Takahara T, et al. Standardization of basic skills for laparoscopic liver surgery towards laparoscopic donor hepatectomy. J Hepato-Biliary-Pancreat Surg. 2009;16(4):439–44.
26. Soubrane O, Schwarz L, Cauchy F, et al. A conceptual technique for laparoscopic right hepatectomy based on facts and oncologic principles: the caudal approach. Ann Surg. 2015;261(6):1226–31.
27. Wakabayashi G, Cherqui D, Geller DA, et al. Laparoscopic hepatectomy is theoretically better than open hepatectomy: preparing for the 2nd International Consensus Conference on Laparoscopic Liver Resection. J Hepatobiliary Pancreat Sci. 2014;21(10):723–31.

28. Ikeda T, Mano Y, Morita K, et al. Pure laparoscopic hepatectomy in semiprone position for right hepatic major resection. J Hepatobiliary Pancreat Sci. 2013;20(2):145–50.
29. Ryska M, Fronek J, Rudis J, et al. Manual and robotic laparoscopic liver resection. Two case-reviews. Rozhl Chir. 2006;85(10):511–6.
30. Tsung A, Geller DA. Reply to letter: "Does the robot provide an advantage over laparoscopic liver resection?". Ann Surg. 2015;262(2):e70–1.
31. Packiam V, Bartlett DL, Tohme S, et al. Minimally invasive liver resection: robotic versus laparoscopic left lateral sectionectomy. J Gastrointest Surg. 2012;16(12):2233–8.
32. Gigot JF, Glineur D, Santiago Azagra J, et al. Laparoscopic liver resection for malignant liver tumors: preliminary results of a multicenter European study. Ann Surg. 2002;236:90.
33. Laurent A, Cherqui D, Lesurtel M, et al. Laparoscopic liver resection for subcapsular hepato-cellular carcinoma complicating chronic liver disease. Arch Surg. 2003;138:763.
34. Dagher I, O'Rourke N, Geller DA, et al. Laparoscopic major hepatectomy: an evolution in standard of care. Ann Surg. 2009;250:856.
35. Dulucq JL, Wintringer P, Stabilini C, et al. Laparoscopic liver resections: a single center experience. Surg Endosc. 2005;19(7):886–91.
36. Gayet B, Cavaliere D, Vibert E, et al. Totally laparoscopic right hepatectomy. Am J Surg. 2007;194:685.
37. Giulianotti PC, Sbrana F, Coratti A, et al. Totally robotic right hepatectomy: surgical technique and outcomes. Arch Surg. 2011;146(7):844–50.
38. Qadan M, Garden OJ, Corvera CU, Visser BC. Management of postoperative hepatic failure. J Am Coll Surg. 2016;222(2):195–208.
39. Arroyo V, Fernandez J, Mas A, Escorsell A. Molecular adsorbents recirculating system (MARS) and the failing liver: a negative editorial for a positive trial? Hepatology. 2008;47(6):2143–4.
40. Schmidt LE, Tofteng F, Strauss GI, Larsen FS. Effect of treatment with the molecular adsor-bents recirculating system on arterial amino acid levels and cerebral amino acid metabolism in patients with hepatic encephalopathy. Scand J Gastroenterol. 2004;39(10):974–80.
41. Kehlet H. Multimodal approach to control postoperative pathophysiology and rehabilitation. Br J Anaesth. 1997;78:606–17.
42. Varadhan KK, Neal KR, Dejong CH, et al. The enhanced recovery after surgery (ERAS) path-way for patients undergoing major elective open colorectal surgery: a meta-analysis of ran-domized controlled trials. Clin Nutr. 2010;29:434–40.
43. He F, Lin X, Xie F, Huang Y, Yuan R. The effect of enhanced recovery program for patients undergoing partial laparoscopic hepatectomy of liver cancer. Clin Transl Oncol. 2015;17(9):694–701.
44. Liang X, Ying H, Wang H, et al. Enhanced recovery program versus traditional care in laparo-scopic hepatectomy. Medicine (Baltimore). 2016;95(8):e2835.

Post-hepatectomy Liver Failure

7

Gaya Spolverato, Fabio Bagante, and Timothy M. Pawlik

Definition and Epidemiology

Among postoperative complications associated with liver surgery, such as infections, fluid collections, deep venous thrombosis, bleeding, and bile leak, liver insufficiency/failure is typically the most life-threatening condition. In fact, post-hepatectomy liver failure (PHLF) can be the cause of serious morbidity and mortality after liver resection, especially among patients with fibrosis or cirrhosis of the underlying liver [1, 2]. The incidence of PHLF varies between 0.7% and 34% due in part to the wide variability in the definition of PHLF, making comparison of data from various studies challenging. Differences in the type and extent of hepatic resection, as well as varied patient-specific characteristics, such as age and comorbidities, also contribute to the large variability in the incidence of PHLF reported in the literature [3–9].

PHLF is determined by several patient-specific and perioperative factors that affect the regenerative ability of the remaining liver following hepatic resection. Dysfunctional or insufficient regeneration of the hepatic mass can lead to failure of the synthetic, metabolic, and/or excretory function of the liver and in turn to specific signs, such as hyperbilirubinemia, hypoalbuminemia, prolonged prothrombin time, elevated serum lactate, and/or hepatic encephalopathy [10].

G. Spolverato, MD • F. Bagante, MD
Department of Surgery, The Ohio State University Comprehensive Cancer Center, Columbus, OH, USA

Department of Surgery, University of Verona, Verona, Italy

T.M. Pawlik, MD, MPH, PhD (✉)
Department of Surgery, The Ohio State University Comprehensive Cancer Center, Columbus, OH, USA
e-mail: tpawlik1@jhmi.edu

© Springer International Publishing AG 2018   119
F.G. Rocha, P. Shen (eds.), *Optimizing Outcomes for Liver and Pancreas Surgery*, DOI 10.1007/978-3-319-62624-6_7

Predictive Factors for PHLF

Several risk factors for PHLF have been described, including patient characteristics, liver quality and volume, as well as intraoperative variables.

Patient-Related Factors

Age, male sex, malnutrition/low albumin levels, diabetes (either alone or in combination with metabolic syndrome), obesity, and higher American Society of Anesthesiology (ASA) score have been described as predictors of PHLF [11, 12]. While some studies have reported age over 65 years as an independent predictor of death among patients undergoing liver surgery [13], several studies have failed to confirm this finding, noting that both minor and major liver resections were safe procedures in elderly patients [13–17]. Other investigators have demonstrated a correlation between malnutrition and PHLF due to the poor regenerative ability of the hepatocytes and the weak immune response of malnourish patients [18, 19]. Indeed, malnourishment has been confirmed as a predictor of PHLF in a prospective study by Fan et al. [18] Specifically, among patients undergoing a hepatectomy, there was a reduction in overall postoperative morbidity and a lower deterioration of liver function (determined by rate of clearance of indocyanine green) among patients who received perioperative nutritional support [18]. Other clinical factors associated with an increased risk of PHLF include renal insufficiency, pulmonary diseases, as well as liver-specific factors that suggest preoperative liver insufficiency (e.g., hyperbilirubinemia) or portal hypertension (e.g., thrombocytopenia) [20–23].

Liver-Related Factors

Both quality and quantity of the remaining liver are risk factors for PHLF. In particular diseases of the underlying hepatic parenchyma, such as cirrhosis, steatosis, steatohepatitis, and chemotherapy-induced liver injury, all can affect the regenerative capacity of the liver and correlate with PHLF. Cirrhosis has been historically described as the most frequent cause of impaired liver regeneration among patients undergoing liver surgery [24–26]. The degree of cirrhosis, defined by the Child-Pugh classification, also is associated with PHLF-associated mortality; specifically, Child-Pugh class A patients have a lower in-hospital mortality after liver resection compared with Child-Pugh class B or C patients [27]. The Model for End-Stage Liver Disease (MELD) score, initially used for patients undergoing transjugular intrahepatic portosystemic shunt and subsequently widely accepted to prioritize candidates for liver transplantation, has a direct correlation with postoperative mortality related to PHLF [28, 29].

The underlying physiopathological process around PHLF has been studied in animal models. In particular, lower levels of hepatocyte growth factor, impaired transcription factors, and reduced DNA synthesis have all been reported as leading causes of poor regenerative ability of the remaining parenchyma [30–32]. In addition, steatosis and steatohepatitis can affect liver function and regeneration following hepatic resection and, in turn, increase risk of perioperative death and complications [33, 34]. Patients with 30% or more steatosis have been reported to be at higher risk of postoperative morbidity and mortality compared with patients without steatosis. Thus, the "safe" lower limit of the future liver remnant (FLR) in mild and severe steatosis is typically 30–35% and 40%, respectively [35–38]. Steatohepatitis (i.e., steatosis with signs of active inflammation) further increases the risk of worse short- and long-term outcomes after liver surgery, and a larger FLR is warranted to avoid PHLF [39, 40]. With modern chemotherapeutic and biologic agents, including 5-fluorouracil, irinotecan, oxaliplatin, cetuximab, and bevacizumab, chemotherapy-associated steatohepatitis (CASH) has also been recognized as a risk factor for PHLF [41–44]. Due to potential hepatic parenchymal damage including sinusoidal dilatation, steatosis, and steatohepatitis that may affect the function and regenerative ability of the remaining liver, a FLR of at least 30% is typically desired when operating on patients who have been extensively treated with preoperative chemotherapy [40, 45, 46]. Cholestasis also needs to be considered as a potential risk factor for PHLF. Major hepatectomy in the setting of severe hyperbilirubinemia can be dangerous and can inhibit the growth of the small liver remnant postoperatively. Thus, when planning an extended liver resection, cholestasis should be resolved (e.g., bilirubin <7.0 ng/ml) and an adequate (e.g., 30–35%) FLR maintained [47, 48].

As noted, the volume of the FLR is critical in maintaining liver function and avoiding PHLR after hepatic resection. The needed volume of the FLR depends on the quality of liver with the typical goal of FLR being 20–30% for patients with a normal underlying liver versus 30–40% for patients with steatosis, steatohepatitis, or CASH. However, the exact FLR size required to minimize the likelihood of PHLF among patients has yet to be determined [49–52]. Most data regarding FLR and PHLF derive from the living donor liver transplant literature, where small size of the graft was noted to be associated with a higher risk of severe graft dysfunction. Similarly, following resection, an insufficient FLR can result in an inadequate hepatic parenchymal mass, as well as damage to the small remaining FLR, which in turn can contribute to PHLF.

Surgery-Related Factors

In addition to the extension of liver resection and the corresponding FLR, several intraoperative factors are associated with risk of PHLF, such as blood loss, use of transfusion, as well as major vascular resection, operative time > 240 min, and duration of the Pringle maneuver [43, 53–56]. In particular blood loss >1 l has been correlated with postoperative complications, including PHLF, as a result of fluid shifts, bacterial translocation, and systemic inflammation [4]. Coagulopathy can also be a consequence of excessive blood loss, with an increasing risk of intra-abdominal hematomas and infection [4]. Blood transfusion has historically been correlated with an increased risk of postoperative morbidity, in particular infectious complications. Indeed, while transfusion can improve tissue perfusion and oxygen delivery, it can also result in a diminished immune response and in transfusion-related acute lung injury [57–60]. Other postoperative factors, including deep infections, fluid collections, postoperative hemorrhage, and bile leak, can also increase the risk of PHLF.

Preoperative Evaluation of the Liver

Considering the high mortality associated with PHLF, preoperative identification of patients at high risk for hepatic dysfunction and PHLF is critical. Preoperative evaluation of the liver consists on both functional and volumetric assessment. Several functional measures have been proposed to access hepatic reserve including the Child-Pugh criteria, the indocyanine green clearance (ICG) test, measurements to assess the degree of hepatic steatosis, as well as cross-sectional volumetry to calculate FLR.

Serum laboratory values including alanine aminotransferase (ALT), aspartate aminotransferase (ALT), alkaline phosphatase (ALP), gamma-glutamyl transpeptidase (GGT), lactate dehydrogenase (LDH), albumin, and prothrombin time (PT) have not been reported to accurately risk-stratify patients with regard to PHLF [61–68]. However, aggregate risk scores that incorporate laboratory values such as the Child-Pugh and MELD scores have been widely accepted as tools to stratify patient PHLF risk. The Child-Pugh classification is based on bilirubin, albumin, international normalized ratio (INR), ascites, and hepatic encephalopathy [69]. The MELD score includes biochemical variables such as creatinine, bilirubin, and INR [70]. Proposed as tools to evaluate liver transplant candidates, these aggregate scores can be helpful to predict the risk of PHLF [69, 71, 72]. Both Child-Pugh and MELD classifications correlate with the risk of PHLF, with MELD also strongly predictive of postoperative 30- and 90-day mortality [26]. In particular, Child-Pugh B or C patients, as well as patients with MELD >10–12, should be considered at very high risk of PHLF and therefore should typically not be considered candidates for elective liver surgery [4, 73].

Techniques, such as ICG clearance and ICG retention rate (ICG R15), have also been utilized to estimate liver function and the risk of PHLF [74–76]. ICG is an injectable water-soluble, nontoxic fluorescent organic anion that binds to albumin. Since ICG hepatocyte uptake is followed by its biliary excretion without enterohepatic circulation, ICG clearance is a reflection of hepatocytes function and intrahepatic blood flow. Based on the percentage of retention at 15 min, the ICG can be used to help calculate the needed remnant liver volume after hepatic resection. There is no clear consensus, however, on the cutoff value for ICG R15 that would be safe for hepatic surgery. ICG R15 has been criticized as costly and time-consuming and thus is not widely adopted in Western countries [11, 13]. Several other liver function tests based on the principle of hepatic clearance and on the synthetic ability of the liver have been proposed; however, high complexity and

Table 7.1 Formulas to calculate future liver remnant

Reference	Year	Formula	Threshold for hepatectomy
Yamanaka et al. [100]	1994	−84.6 + 0.933 × PHRR + 1.11 × ICG-R15 + 0.999 × age	45
Kubota et al. [101]	1997	(resected volume-tumor volume)/(TLV-tumor volume)	40% non-tumorous parenchyma
Vauthey et al. [102]	2000	(CT FLR)/(706 × BSA + 2.4)	20% in normal livers
Ribero et al. [103]	2008	(CT FLR)/(−794 + 1267 × BSA)	20% in normal livers
Uchiyama et al. [104]	2008	164.8–0.58 × albumin–1.07 × hepaplastin test + 0.062 × glutamate oxaloacetate transaminase–685 × ICG-K–3.57 × oral glucose tolerance test linearity index + 0.074 × weight of resected liver	25
Du et al. [105]	2011	ICG-K × 22.487 + standardized remnant liver volume × 0.02	13.1

Obtained with permission from Lafaro et al. [49]
PHRR parenchymal hepatic resection rate, *ICG R15* indocyanine green dye retention rate 15 min after injection of 0.5 mg/kg, *TLV* total liver volume, *CT* computer tomography, *FLR* future liver remnant, *BSA* body surface area, *ICG-K* K value of indocyanine green clearance test

costs have been barriers to clinical implementation [35, 49]. Liver stiffness measurement, using transient elastography (Fibroscan®, Echosens, Paris, France), has also been proposed as a noninvasive, reproducible, and rapid method to access liver fibrosis and cirrhosis [77]. Few studies have, however, correlated the level of liver stiffness measurement (LSM) with postoperative outcomes; only one recent study by Chong et al. reported a positive correlation between LSM >12 kPa and incidence of high-grade PHLF [77–81].

Cross-sectional imaging with computer tomography (CT) and magnetic resonance imaging (MRI) is the most common way to measure the FLR volume, as well as the ratio of FLR volume to the total functioning liver volume (TLV) (Table 7.1).

Yamanaka et al. used the ICG R15 value and the patient's age to compute the prediction score (PS) that was derived from the multiple regression equation, $Y = -84.6 + 0.933$ PHRR $+1.11$ ICG R15 $+ 0.999$ age, where PHRR is the parenchymal hepatic resection rate. A PS of 50 points was used to discriminate between survivors and nonsurvivors, a PS >55 was classified as risky, a PS between 45 and 55 was considered borderline, and a PS <45 was considered safe. Kubota et al. used resected liver volume and tumor volume to guide the decision making in resectional surgery for liver tumors, concluding that patients can undergo resection of up to 40% of the non-tumorous parenchyma. Vauthey et al. provided a simple method of measurement to assess the liver remnant before resection. The total liver volume was estimated on the basis of the body surface area with the formula: liver volume $(\text{cm}^3) = 706 \times$ body surface area $(\text{m}^2) + 2.4$. The ratio of future FLR volume to absolute liver volume as estimated by this formula was also obtained. The authors showed that complications were more frequent among patients with a FLR volume of ≤25%. Ribero et al. described the rationale for FLR measurement, methods of measuring FLR volume, and standardization to the total estimated liver volume, while using the same variables proposed by the same group in the study by Vauthey et al. Uchiyama et al. proposed a formula for liver functional evaluation, constructed from preoperative hepatic function parameters including hepaplastin (HPT), albumin, K value of indocyanine green clearance test (K. ICG), linearity index of oral glucose tolerance test (OGTT), and weight of resected liver (RW). A score below 25 was considered safe for hepatectomy. Du et al. assessed the liver function compensatory (LFC) value to predict liver dysfunction of the patients after hepatectomy, defined as the preoperative K(ICG) value × 22.487 + standard remnant liver volume (SRLV) × 0.020. An expected LFC value of 13.01 was found to be a safe limit for liver resection.

The percentage of the remaining liver, as determined by the semiautomated contouring of the liver, has been reported to be predictive of PHLF. The attenuation of the liver, compared with the attenuation of the spleen, can also assist in the diagnosis of steatosis, while indirect signs, such as splenomegaly, varices, and ascites, can support the diagnosis of cirrhosis [49]. MRI can potentially provide both qualitative and quantitative information of liver function, which is critical for surgical candidates with liver parenchymal disease [82]. Hepatocyte-specific contrast mediums, such as gadoxetic acid [83], have been developed to improve morphological assessment as well as provide functional information [84], due to the temporary accumulation in the liver and subsequent enhancement of the normal liver parenchyma [85]. Preoperative gadoxetic acid-enhanced 3-T MRI, which can provide a comprehensive overview of liver anatomy, as well as identify of any underlying liver disease, has been reported to be superior than the use of laboratory values alone in predicting PHLF [86].

Clinical Manifestation of PHLF

Signs and symptoms of PHLF include jaundice, coagulopathy, ascites, edema, and/or hepatic encephalopathy (HE). HE is caused by high level of serum ammonium and is graded from I to IV in severity. Grade I HE is characterized by mild confusion and changes in behavior with minimal changes in the level of consciousness; Grade II is characterized by drowsiness, gross disorientation, and inappropriate behavior; Grade III is characterized by marked confusion, incoherent speech, and arousable somnolence; Grade IV is characterized by coma [87]. The effects of hepatic failure on the circulatory system can resemble septic shock with progressive hypotension, peripheral vasodilation, and disseminated intravascular coagulopathy [39]. The effects on the kidney can lead to renal failure as a consequence of hypovolemic shock and hepatorenal syndrome. Finally pulmonary edema, acute lung injury, and acute respiratory distress syndrome can also be a result of liver failure [10].

Postoperative Models to Assess PHLF

Several clinical tools have been proposed to precisely define, predict, and grade the severity of PHLF. The three clinical tools that are probably the most widely adopted include the 50–50 criteria [13], peak bilirubin >7 mg/dL [15], and the ISGLS criteria [88]. In addition, a clinical risk score to identify PHLF early has been proposed by our own group [73].

The 50–50 criteria, initially proposed by Balzan et al. and defined as a prothrombin time (PT) <50% (corresponding to INR > 1.7) and serum bilirubin (SB) >50 µml/L (corresponding to >2.9 mg/dL) on postoperative day (POD) 5, was advocated as a simple, early, and accurate estimation of PHLF, which predicted a 59% mortality after liver resection (Fig. 7.1) [13]. While the "50–50" rule has been validated in several studies including a large number of patients undergoing liver surgery [89–91], other reports have failed to find any association between the 50–50 criteria and risk of PHLF [15, 73].

As such, Mullen et al. proposed a revision of the 50–50 criteria that exclude PT and suggested a peak postoperative bilirubin >7 mg/dL [15]. In this study, the authors noted that bilirubin >7 mg/dL was an independent predictor of any complication, major complication, 90-day mortality, and 90-day PHLF-related mortality (Fig. 7.2) [15]. As with the 50–50 criteria, peak bilirubin >7 mg/dL has been validated by some studies [92], while other authors have questioned the ability of bilirubin as a sole parameter to predict accurately PHLF-related mortality [73, 93].

In an effort to standardize the definition of PHLF, the International Study Group of Liver Surgery (ISGLS) proposed an increase in INR combined with hyperbilirubinemia on or after POD 5 as the definition of PHLF [88]. The authors noted that

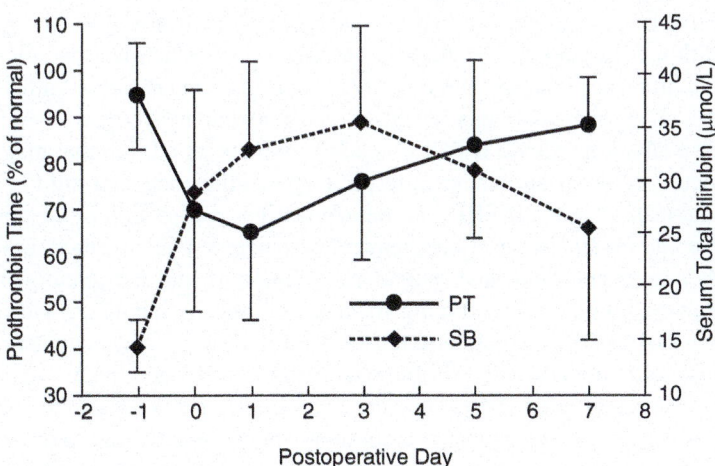

Fig. 7.1 Kinetics of postoperative biologic liver function tests. Means and standard deviation of prothrombin time (PT) and total serum bilirubin (SB) in overall group of hepatectomies. Kinetic of postoperative prothrombin time (PT) and serum total bilirubin level (SB) (Obtained with permission from Balzan et al. [13])

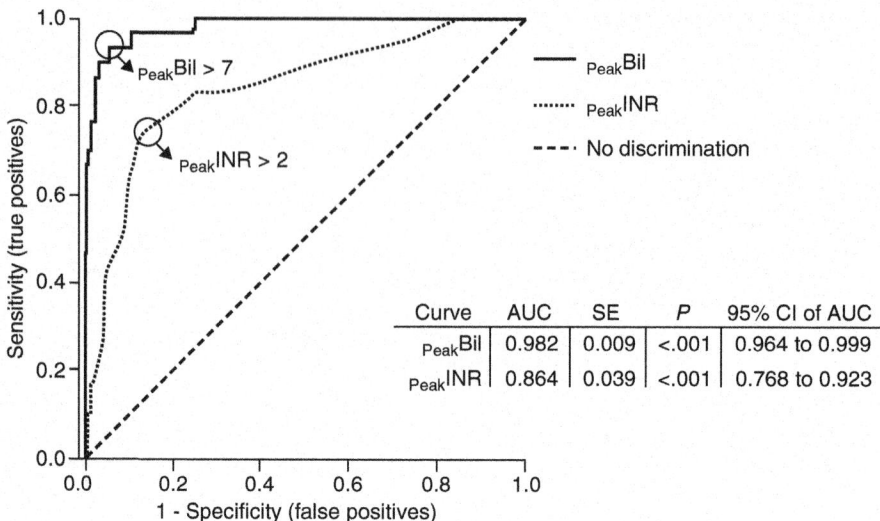

Fig. 7.2 Receiver operating characteristic (ROC) curves demonstrating that the cutoff peak post-operative bilirubin (PeakBil) value to predict liver failure-related death is 7.0 mg/dL (area under the curve (AUC) 0.982; sensitivity 93.3%; specificity 94.3%), and international normalized ratio (PeakINR) cutoff value 2.0 (AUC 0.846; sensitivity 76.7%; and specificity 82.0%) (Obtained with permission from Mullen et al. [15])

these criteria could be used to quantify the impaired ability of the liver and its ability to maintain synthetic, excretory, and detoxifying functions. Since the severity of PHLF can range from a transient impairment of liver function that recovers as the liver regenerates to a potentially life-threatening condition, ISGLS proposed a grading system to better characterize PHLF (Table 7.2). Grade A PHLF is an asymptomatic condition, characterized by the sole deviation in biochemical parameters that does not require any change in the clinical management. Patients with Grade A PHLF have an uninterrupted postoperative course and do not require any additional diagnostic evaluation. Grade B PHLF is a symptomatic condition that may present with clinically relevant ascites, mild respiratory insufficiency, and mild symptoms of encephalopathy. Grade B PHLF is characterized by a deviation in the postoperative course and an alteration in biochemical parameters of liver function. Grade B PHLF often requires additional diagnostic evaluations and is typically managed with noninvasive treatment including fresh-frozen plasma, albumin, and diuretics with transfer to the intermediate or intensive care unit being rare. In contrast, Grade C PHLF is a critical clinical condition that should be managed in an intensive care unit. Patients with Grade C PHLF can present with large-volume ascites, anasarca, hemodynamic instability, advanced respiratory insufficiency, and severe encephalopathy. Infections are also common among these patients. Grade C PHLF results in a profound deviation from regular clinical management and requires significant intervention. The management of patients with Grade C PHLF can include intubation and mechanical ventilation, hemodialysis, vasoactive drugs, extracorporeal liver support, rescue hepatectomy, and transplantation [88].

Table 7.2 Grades of post-hepatectomy liver failure

	Criteria for PHLF Grade A	Criteria for PHLF Grade B	Criteria for PHLF Grade C
Specific treatment	Not required	Fresh-frozen plasma Albumin Daily diuretics Noninvasive ventilation Transfer to intermediate/intensive care unit	Transfer to the intensive care unit Circulatory support (vasoactive drugs) Need for glucose infusion Hemodialysis Intubation and mechanical ventilation Extracorporeal liver support Rescue hepatectomy/liver transplantation
Hepatic function	Adequate coagulation (INR <1.5) No neurological symptoms	Inadequate coagulation (INR ≥1.5 < 2.0) Beginning of neurologic symptoms (i.e., somnolence and confusion)	Inadequate coagulation (INR ≥2.0) Severe neurologic symptoms/hepatic encephalopathy
Renal function	Adequate urine output (>0.5 mL/kg/h) BUN <150 mg/dL No symptoms of uremia	Inadequate urine output (≤0.5 ml/kg/h) BUN <150 mg/dL No symptoms of uremia	Renal dysfunction not manageable with diuretics BUN ≥150 mg/dL Symptoms of uremia
Pulmonary function	Arterial oxygen saturation > 90% May have oxygen supply via nasal cannula or oxygen mask	Arterial oxygen saturation < 90% despite oxygen supply via nasal cannula or oxygen mask	Severe refractory hypoxemia (arterial oxygen saturation ≤ 85% with high fraction of inspired oxygen)
Additional evaluation	Not required	Abdominal ultrasonography/CT Chest radiography Sputum, blood, urine cultures Brain CT	Abdominal ultrasonography/CT Chest radiography/CT Sputum, blood, urine cultures Brain CT ICP monitoring device

Obtained with permission from Rahbari et al. [88]
BUN blood urea nitrogen, *ICP* intracranial pressure
The patient's PHLF is graded by the worst identified criteria in required treatment

There is still no consensus on which definition should be universally applied in clinical practice. Skrzypczyk et al. reported on 680 patients undergoing hepatectomy and failed to demonstrate the superiority of the ISGLS criteria over either the 50–50 criteria or peak bilirubin >7 mg/dL [90]. In this study, the ISGLS definition was less discriminatory than the "50–50" rule and peak bilirubin >7 mg/dL criteria

Table 7.3 Multivariate logistic regression predicting the risk of 90-day mortality among 2056 patients who underwent liver resection

Variable	β	OR	95% CI	p value	Numeric score
Serum INR day 3	2.47	11.87	1.57–89.69	0.02	2.5
Each, complication grade increase	1.63	5.08	3.32–7.78	<0.001	1.5
Serum bilirubin day 3	0.15	1.16	0.80–1.70	0.42	0.15
Serum creatinine day 3	0.62	1.87	1.08–3.25	0.03	0.5

Obtained with permission from Hyder et al. [72]
INR international normalized ratio, *OR* odds ratio

in identifying patients at risk of post-hepatectomy major complications or death. In particular, the ISGLS definition was least able to predict mortality with a positive predictive value (PPV) of only about 20% on POD 5 and POD 10; the PPV to predict morbidity was similarly poor at 50% on POD 5 and POD 10. Of note, the negative predictive value (NPV) was higher, suggesting that patients who did not meet the ISGLS criteria were at very low risk of dying or develop PHLF after liver surgery [90].

Given the varied performance of previous PHLF definitions, Hyder et al. proposed a novel integer-based score for 90-day mortality after liver surgery [73]. Using a large dataset that included 2056 patients who underwent liver resection between 1990 and 2011, factors such as INR on POD3, bilirubin on POD3, serum creatinine on POD3, as well as Clavien-Dindo grade of postoperative complications were independent predictors of 90-day mortality (Table 7.3). The authors assigned an integer value to each of these factors based on the beta coefficient of the multivariable model, which was used to develop a risk model. When patients were stratified according to the number of points derived from the score, there was a proportional increase in the risk of death. For example, patients who had a score < 6 points only had a 0.2% risk of death within 90 days compared with 1.2% for patients who had a score 6–8.9, 34.3% for those with a score of 9–10.9, and 83.3% for patients who had a score ≥ 11. Of note, a score ≥ 11 had a sensitivity of 83.3% and a specificity of 98.9% (Fig. 7.3) [73].

Management of PHLF

Liver and end organs are the main focus of PHLF management. Since the most relevant clinical manifestations of PHLF are coagulopathy, ascites, HE, respiratory, and renal complications, treatments will be varied and depend on the system affected. For example, vasopressor therapy may be necessary to support the circulation, daily diuretics to maintain a urine output of at least 0.5 ml/Kg/h, and ventilator support to preserve adequate oxygen saturation. Platelets and fresh-frozen plasma are administered to manage coagulopathy. In the case of HE, lactulose is the

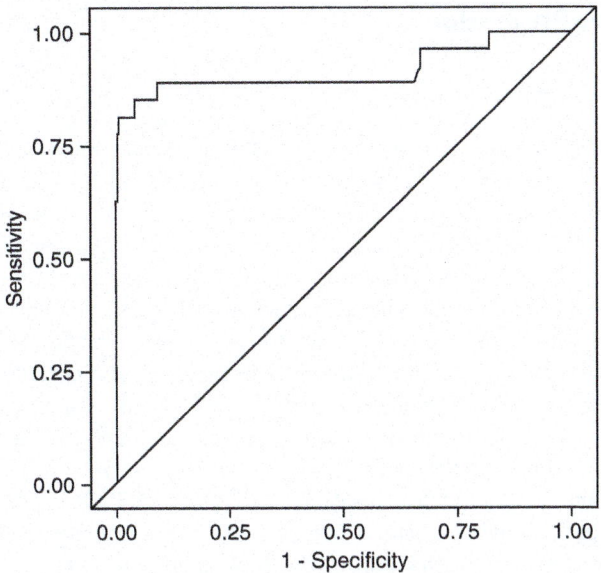

Fig. 7.3 The receiver operating characteristic (ROC) of the proposed composite prediction rule. The composite score consists of weighted values for grade of postoperative complication, as well as international normalized ratio, bilirubin, and creatinine on postoperative day 5. The composite rule performed well on ROC curve analysis (area under the curve (AUC) 0.927), as well as on n-fold cross-fold validation (AUC 0.893) (Obtained with permission from Hyder et al. [72])

treatment of choice, while hyperventilation, hypertonic saline, mannitol, and cooling are considered neuroprotective strategies. Nutritional support, and in particular enteral nutrition, which can preserve the integrity of the gut barrier, can help reduce malnutrition and electrolyte imbalance. Supplements with vitamins and branched-chain amino acids should also be considered, with protein intake not exceeding 60 g/day, especially in patients with HE [10].

While a specific treatment is not required for patients with Grade A PHLF, patients with Grade B PHLF often benefit from fresh-frozen plasma, albumin, diuretics, noninvasive ventilation, and eventually intermediate/intensive care unit management. Grade C PHLF patients typically need to be managed in the intensive care unit, since circulatory support, intubation with mechanical ventilation, glucose infusion, hemodialysis, and eventually extracorporeal liver support, rescue hepatectomy, or liver transplant are needed (Table 7.2) [10].

Strategies to Prevent PHLF

Given the high postoperative mortality associated with PHLF, great effort should be placed into prevention.

Preoperative Prevention

Consider the correlation between quality and quantity of liver volume and risk of PHLF. Increasing the remnant volume and preserving the function of future liver remnant has been the rationale behind several preoperative strategies. In particular portal vein embolization (PVE), while reducing the blood flow to the liver to be resected and increasing the blood flow of the remnant liver, allows for preoperative hypertrophy of the FLR. PVE is typically performed as an ultrasound-guided percutaneous procedure with embolization of the ipsilateral liver with coils, embospheres, foam, or glue. This embolization induces hypertrophy of the contralateral side of the liver, increasing the FLR volume. PVE allows for hypertrophy of the FLR by 30–40% within 4–6 weeks in more than 80% of patients, as reported by CT volumetry usually performed 3–4 weeks after PVE [22]. PVE also stimulates the production of hepatic growth factor and tumor growth factors, along with the redistribution of the portal blood flow to the FLR.

In some cases, a portal vein ligation (PVL) rather than PVE is preferred. In particular, those patients who require a two-stage hepatectomy approach may benefit from PVL that usually occurs during the first operation, when a parenchymal-sparing liver resection is performed [94, 95]. The second stage is usually performed within 3–6 weeks after the first resection and usually consists of an extended hepatectomy.

When PVE is not technically feasible, some surgeons have advocated for the association of liver partition and portal vein ligation for staged hepatectomy (ALPPS) procedure [96]. The rationale behind ALPPS is the clearance of one side of the liver while maintaining the main liver mass to prevent PHLF, combined with portal vein ligation to induce FLR hypertrophy. By portioning the liver at the time of the first operation, ALPPS allows a more rapid hypertrophy of the liver. The results with ALPPS have been mixed, however. A recent meta-analysis noted that ALPPS provided an additional 17% increment hypertrophy of the FLR compared with PVE [97]; however, the high perioperative mortality of ALPPS (12–23% of patients) has prevented it from becoming widely adopted [98].

As previously noted, cholestasis is an important preoperative risk factor for PHLF, and therefore, preoperative endoscopic or percutaneous transhepatic biliary drainage (PTBD) should be strongly considered before extending hepatic resection in those patients who have a bilirubin >7 ng/dL.

Intraoperative Prevention

At the time of surgery, one of the main factors that influence morbidity, mortality, and risk of PHLF is blood loss. As such, surgeons should focus on limiting blood loss at the time of hepatic resection. Several techniques are associated with decreased blood loss, including selective ligation of the right, left, or smaller branches of the portal system supplying the liver portion to be resected; extrahepatic dissection, isolation, and transection of the hepatic artery and portal vein can also be performed in patients undergoing a formal hemihepatectomy. For patients undergoing a non-anatomic resection, continuous or intermittent Pringle maneuver can be considered in certain clinical situations to decrease blood loss. While not often needed, occlusion of both inflow and hepatic outflow (total vascular exclusion) can also be utilized. A central venous pressure (CVP) equal or below 5 mmHg during parenchymal transection is also important to reduce the impedance for blood flow through the hepatic veins into the IVC, thus limiting intraoperative blood loss. To maintain a low CVP, the team should minimize pre-parenchymal transection intravenous fluid volume, as well as reduce mechanical ventilation tidal volume [99].

Postoperative Prevention

Early detection of signs and symptoms of PHLF is crucial in the postoperative setting. In particular, albumin, INR, creatinine, and signs of HE should be monitored. Moreover, a prompt and appropriate antibiotic treatment in case of postoperative infection is important, as well as a timely management of bile leak and postoperative hemorrhage [10].

Conclusions

PHLF is a life-threatening condition that can lead to a cascade of events including coagulopathy, ascites, HE, respiratory, cardiac, and renal complications. An accurate assessment of the anatomy and the FLR reserve, as well as impeccable intraoperative technique and detailed postoperative care, are all critical in avoiding and managing PHLF.

References

1. Paugam-Burtz C, Janny S, Delefosse D, Dahmani S, Dondero F, Mantz J, Belghiti J. Prospective validation of the "fifty-fifty" criteria as an early and accurate predictor of death after liver resection in intensive care unit patients. Ann Surg. 2009;249(1):124–8.
2. Jaeck D, Bachellier P, Oussoultzoglou E, Weber JC, Wolf P. Surgical resection of hepatocellular carcinoma. Post-operative outcome and long-term results in Europe: an overview. Liver Transpl. 2004;10(2 Suppl 1):S58–63.
3. Schreckenbach T, Liese J, Bechstein WO, Moench C. Posthepatectomy liver failure. Dig Surg. 2012;29(1):79–85.
4. van den Broek MA, Olde Damink SW, Dejong CH, Lang H, Malago M, Jalan R, Saner FH. Liver failure after partial hepatic resection: definition, pathophysiology, risk factors and treatment. Liver Int. 2008;28(6):767–80.
5. Ribeiro HS, Costa WL Jr, Diniz AL, Godoy AL, Herman P, Coudry RA, Begnami MD, Mello CA, Silva MJ, Zurstrassen CE, Coimbra FJ. Extended preoperative chemotherapy, extent of liver resection and blood transfusion are predictive factors of liver failure following resection of colorectal liver metastasis. Eur J Surg Oncol. 2013;39(4):380–5.
6. Filicori F, Keutgen XM, Zanello M, Ercolani G, Di Saverio S, Sacchetti F, Pinna AD, Grazi GL. Prognostic criteria for postoperative mortality in 170 patients undergoing major right hepatectomy. Hepatobiliary Pancreat Dis Int. 2012;11(5):507–12.

7. Jiang XB, Ke C, Han ZA, Lin SH, Mou YG, Luo RZ, Wu SX, Chen ZP. Intraparenchymal papillary meningioma of brainstem: case report and literature review. World J Surg Oncol. 2012;10:10.
8. Ren Z, Xu Y, Zhu S. Indocyanine green retention test avoiding liver failure after hepatectomy for hepatolithiasis. Hepato-Gastroenterology. 2012;59(115):782–4.
9. Helling TS. Liver failure following partial hepatectomy. HPB (Oxford). 2006;8(3):165–74.
10. Yadav K, Shrikhande S, Goel M. Post hepatectomy liver failure: concept of management. J Gastrointest Cancer. 2014;45(4):405–13.
11. Timchenko NA. Aging and liver regeneration. Trends Endocrinol Metab. 2009;20(4):171–6.
12. Le Couteur DG, Warren A, Cogger VC, Smedsrod B, Sorensen KK, De Cabo R, Fraser R, McCuskey RS. Old age and the hepatic sinusoid. Anat Rec. 2008;291(6):672–83.
13. Balzan S, Belghiti J, Farges O, Ogata S, Sauvanet A, Delefosse D, Durand F. The "50-50 criteria" on postoperative day 5: an accurate predictor of liver failure and death after hepatectomy. Ann Surg. 2005;242(6):824–8. discussion 828–829
14. Aldrighetti L, Arru M, Caterini R, Finazzi R, Comotti L, Torri G, Ferla G. Impact of advanced age on the outcome of liver resection. World J Surg. 2003;27(10):1149–54.
15. Mullen JT, Ribero D, Reddy SK, Donadon M, Zorzi D, Gautam S, Abdalla EK, Curley SA, Capussotti L, Clary BM, Vauthey JN. Hepatic insufficiency and mortality in 1,059 noncirrhotic patients undergoing major hepatectomy. J Am Coll Surg. 2007;204(5):854–62. discussion 862–854
16. Nanashima A, Abo T, Nonaka T, Fukuoka H, Hidaka S, Takeshita H, Ichikawa T, Sawai T, Yasutake T, Nakao K, Nagayasu T. Prognosis of patients with hepatocellular carcinoma after hepatic resection: are elderly patients suitable for surgery? J Surg Oncol. 2011;104(3):284–91.
17. Kim JM, Cho BI, Kwon CH, Joh JW, Park JB, Lee JH, Kim SJ, Paik SW, Park CK. Hepatectomy is a reasonable option for older patients with hepatocellular carcinoma. Am J Surg. 2015;209(2):391–7.
18. Fan ST, Lo CM, Lai EC, Chu KM, Liu CL, Wong J. Perioperative nutritional support in patients undergoing hepatectomy for hepatocellular carcinoma. N Engl J Med. 1994;331(23):1547–52.
19. Fan ST. Review: nutritional support for patients with cirrhosis. J Gastroenterol Hepatol. 1997;12(4):282–6.
20. Jarnagin WR, Gonen M, Fong Y, DeMatteo RP, Ben-Porat L, Little S, Corvera C, Weber S, Blumgart LH. Improvement in perioperative outcome after hepatic resection: analysis of 1,803 consecutive cases over the past decade. Ann Surg. 2002;236(4):397–406. discussion 406–397
21. Tzeng CW, Cooper AB, Vauthey JN, Curley SA, Aloia TA. Predictors of morbidity and mortality after hepatectomy in elderly patients: analysis of 7621 NSQIP patients. HPB (Oxford). 2014;16(5):459–68.
22. Golse N, Bucur PO, Adam R, Castaing D, Sa Cunha A, Vibert E. New paradigms in posthepatectomy liver failure. J Gastrointest Surg. 2013;17(3):593–605.
23. Aloia TA, Fahy BN, Fischer CP, Jones SL, Duchini A, Galati J, Gaber AO, Ghobrial RM, Bass BL. Predicting poor outcome following hepatectomy: analysis of 2313 hepatectomies in the NSQIP database. HPB (Oxford). 2009;11(6):510–5.
24. Mansour A, Watson W, Shayani V, Pickleman J. Abdominal operations in patients with cirrhosis: still a major surgical challenge. Surgery. 1997;122(4):730–5. discussion 735–736
25. Garrison RN, Cryer HM, Howard DA, Polk HC Jr. Clarification of risk factors for abdominal operations in patients with hepatic cirrhosis. Ann Surg. 1984;199(6):648–55.
26. Teh SH, Nagorney DM, Stevens SR, Offord KP, Therneau TM, Plevak DJ, Talwalkar JA, Kim WR, Kamath PS. Risk factors for mortality after surgery in patients with cirrhosis. Gastroenterology. 2007;132(4):1261–9.
27. Capussotti L, Muratore A, Amisano M, Polastri R, Bouzari H, Massucco P. Liver resection for hepatocellular carcinoma on cirrhosis: analysis of mortality, morbidity and survival--a European single center experience. Eur J Surg Oncol. 2005;31(9):986–93.

28. Teh SH, Christein J, Donohue J, Que F, Kendrick M, Farnell M, Cha S, Kamath P, Kim R, Nagorney DM. Hepatic resection of hepatocellular carcinoma in patients with cirrhosis: Model of End-Stage Liver Disease (MELD) score predicts perioperative mortality. J Gastrointest Surg. 2005;9(9):1207–15. discussion 1215
29. Cucchetti A, Ercolani G, Vivarelli M, Cescon M, Ravaioli M, La Barba G, Zanello M, Grazi GL, Pinna AD. Impact of model for end-stage liver disease (MELD) score on prognosis after hepatectomy for hepatocellular carcinoma on cirrhosis. Liver Transpl. 2006;12(6):966–71.
30. Kaibori M, Inoue T, Sakakura Y, Oda M, Nagahama T, Kwon AH, Kamiyama Y, Miyazawa K, Okumura T. Impairment of activation of hepatocyte growth factor precursor into its mature form in rats with liver cirrhosis. J Surg Res. 2002;106(1):108–14.
31. Zhao G, Nakano K, Chijiiwa K, Ueda J, Tanaka M. Inhibited activities in CCAAT/enhancer-binding protein, activating protein-1 and cyclins after hepatectomy in rats with thioacetamide-induced liver cirrhosis. Biochem Biophys Res Commun. 2002;292(2):474–81.
32. Garcea G, Maddern GJ. Liver failure after major hepatic resection. J Hepato-Biliary-Pancreat Surg. 2009;16(2):145–55.
33. de Meijer VE, Kalish BT, Puder M, Ijzermans JN. Systematic review and meta-analysis of steatosis as a risk factor in major hepatic resection. Br J Surg. 2010;97(9):1331–9.
34. Inaba Y, Furutani T, Kimura K, Watanabe H, Haga S, Kido Y, Matsumoto M, Yamamoto Y, Harada K, Kaneko S, Oyadomari S, Ozaki M, Kasuga M, Inoue H. Growth arrest and DNA damage-inducible 34 regulates liver regeneration in hepatic steatosis in mice. Hepatology. 2015;61(4):1343–56.
35. Hoekstra LT, de Graaf W, Nibourg GA, Heger M, Bennink RJ, Stieger B, van Gulik TM. Physiological and biochemical basis of clinical liver function tests: a review. Ann Surg. 2013;257(1):27–36.
36. Otsuka Y, Duffy JP, Saab S, Farmer DG, Ghobrial RM, Hiatt JR, Busuttil RW. Postresection hepatic failure: successful treatment with liver transplantation. Liver Transpl. 2007;13(5):672–9.
37. Rahman SH, Evans J, Toogood GJ, Lodge PA, Prasad KR. Prognostic utility of postoperative C-reactive protein for posthepatectomy liver failure. Arch Surg. 2008;143(3):247–53. discussion 253
38. Guglielmi A, Ruzzenente A, Conci S, Valdegamberi A, Iacono C. How much remnant is enough in liver resection? Dig Surg. 2012;29(1):6–17.
39. Rivers E, Nguyen B, Havstad S, Ressler J, Muzzin A, Knoblich B, Peterson E, Tomlanovich M. Early goal-directed therapy collaborative G. Early goal-directed therapy in the treatment of severe sepsis and septic shock. N Engl J Med. 2001;345(19):1368–77.
40. Abdalla EK, Adam R, Bilchik AJ, Jaeck D, Vauthey JN, Mahvi D. Improving resectability of hepatic colorectal metastases: expert consensus statement. Ann Surg Oncol. 2006;13(10):1271–80.
41. Fong Y, Bentrem DJ. CASH (chemotherapy-associated steatohepatitis) costs. Ann Surg. 2006;243(1):8–9.
42. Karoui M, Penna C, Amin-Hashem M, Mitry E, Benoist S, Franc B, Rougier P, Nordlinger B. Influence of preoperative chemotherapy on the risk of major hepatectomy for colorectal liver metastases. Ann Surg. 2006;243(1):1–7.
43. Fernandez FG, Ritter J, Goodwin JW, Linehan DC, Hawkins WG, Strasberg SM. Effect of steatohepatitis associated with irinotecan or oxaliplatin pretreatment on resectability of hepatic colorectal metastases. J Am Coll Surg. 2005;200(6):845–53.
44. Peppercorn PD, Reznek RH, Wilson P, Slevin ML, Gupta RK. Demonstration of hepatic steatosis by computerized tomography in patients receiving 5-fluorouracil-based therapy for advanced colorectal cancer. Br J Cancer. 1998;77(11):2008–11.
45. Vauthey JN, Pawlik TM, Ribero D, Wu TT, Zorzi D, Hoff PM, Xiong HQ, Eng C, Lauwers GY, Mino-Kenudson M, Risio M, Muratore A, Capussotti L, Curley SA, Abdalla EK. Chemotherapy regimen predicts steatohepatitis and an increase in 90-day mortality after surgery for hepatic colorectal metastases. J Clin Oncol. 2006;24(13):2065–72.

46. Robinson SM, Wilson CH, Burt AD, Manas DM, White SA. Chemotherapy-associated liver injury in patients with colorectal liver metastases: a systematic review and meta-analysis. Ann Surg Oncol. 2012;19(13):4287–99.
47. Ferrero A, Vigano L, Polastri R, Muratore A, Eminefendic H, Regge D, Capussotti L. Postoperative liver dysfunction and future remnant liver: where is the limit? Results of a prospective study. World J Surg. 2007;31(8):1643–51.
48. Suda K, Ohtsuka M, Ambiru S, Kimura F, Shimizu H, Yoshidome H, Miyazaki M. Risk factors of liver dysfunction after extended hepatic resection in biliary tract malignancies. Am J Surg. 2009;197(6):752–8.
49. Lafaro K, Buettner S, Maqsood H, Wagner D, Bagante F, Spolverato G, Xu L, Kamel I, Pawlik TM. Defining post hepatectomy liver insufficiency: where do we stand? J Gastrointest Surg. 2015;19(11):2079–92.
50. Emond JC, Renz JF, Ferrell LD, Rosenthal P, Lim RC, Roberts JP, Lake JR, Ascher NL. Functional analysis of grafts from living donors. Implications for the treatment of older recipients. Ann Surg. 1996;224(4):544–52. discussion 552–544
51. Kiuchi T, Kasahara M, Uryuhara K, Inomata Y, Uemoto S, Asonuma K, Egawa H, Fujita S, Hayashi M, Tanaka K. Impact of graft size mismatching on graft prognosis in liver transplantation from living donors. Transplantation. 1999;67(2):321–7.
52. Furukawa H, Kishida A, Omura T, Kamiyama T, Suzuki T, Matsushita M, Nakajima Y, Todo S. Indication and strategy for adult living related liver transplantation. Transplant Proc. 1999;31(5):1952.
53. Melendez J, Ferri E, Zwillman M, Fischer M, DeMatteo R, Leung D, Jarnagin W, Fong Y, Blumgart LH. Extended hepatic resection: a 6-year retrospective study of risk factors for perioperative mortality. J Am Coll Surg. 2001;192(1):47–53.
54. Nanashima A, Yamaguchi H, Shibasaki S, Ide N, Morino S, Sumida Y, Tsuji T, Sawai T, Nakagoe T, Nagayasu T. Comparative analysis of postoperative morbidity according to type and extent of hepatectomy. Hepato-Gastroenterology. 2005;52(63):844–8.
55. Fujii Y, Shimada H, Endo I, Morioka D, Nagano Y, Miura Y, Tanaka K, Togo S. Risk factors of posthepatectomy liver failure after portal vein embolization. J Hepato-Biliary-Pancreat Surg. 2003;10(3):226–32.
56. Shoup M, Gonen M, D'Angelica M, Jarnagin WR, DeMatteo RP, Schwartz LH, Tuorto S, Blumgart LH, Fong Y. Volumetric analysis predicts hepatic dysfunction in patients undergoing major liver resection. J Gastrointest Surg. 2003;7(3):325–30.
57. Bueter M, Thalheimer A, Schuster F, Bock M, von Erffa C, Meyer D, Fein M. Transfusion-related acute lung injury (TRALI)--an important, severe transfusion-related complication. Langenbecks Arch Surg. 2006;391(5):489–94.
58. Popovsky MA, Chaplin HC Jr, Moore SB. Transfusion-related acute lung injury: a neglected, serious complication of hemotherapy. Transfusion. 1992;32(6):589–92.
59. Pinheiro de Almeida J, Vincent JL, Barbosa Gomes Galas FR, Marinho de Almeida EP, Fukushima JT, Osawa EA, Bergamin F, Lee Park C, Nakamura RE, Fonseca SM, Cutait G, Inacio Alves J, Bazan M, Vieira S, Vieira Sandrini AC, Palomba H, Ribeiro U Jr, Crippa A, Dalloglio M, Del Pilar Estevez Diz M, Kalil Filho R, Costa Auler JO Jr, Rhodes A, Hajjar LA. Transfusion requirements in surgical oncology patients: a prospective, randomized controlled trial. Anesthesiology. 2015;122(1):29–38.
60. Roberson RS, Bennett-Guerrero E. Impact of red blood cell transfusion on global and regional measures of oxygenation. Mt Sinai J Med. 2012;79(1):66–74.
61. Oussoultzoglou E, Jaeck D, Addeo P, Fuchshuber P, Marzano E, Rosso E, Pessaux P, Bachellier P. Prediction of mortality rate after major hepatectomy in patients without cirrhosis. Arch Surg. 2010;145(11):1075–81.
62. Maeda Y, Nishida M, Takao T, Mori N, Tamesa T, Tangoku A, Oka M. Risk factors for postoperative liver failure after hepatectomy for hepatocellular carcinoma. Hepato-Gastroenterology. 2004;51(60):1792–6.
63. Osada S, Saji S. The clinical significance of monitoring alkaline phosphatase level to estimate postoperative liver failure after hepatectomy. Hepato-Gastroenterology. 2004;51(59):1434–8.

64. Nanashima A, Tobinaga S, Abo T, Nonaka T, Takeshita H, Hidaka S, Sawai T, Nagayasu T. Reducing the incidence of post-hepatectomy hepatic complications by preoperatively applying parameters predictive of liver function. J Hepatobiliary Pancreat Sci. 2010;17(6):871–8.

65. Reissfelder C, Rahbari NN, Koch M, Kofler B, Sutedja N, Elbers H, Buchler MW, Weitz J. Postoperative course and clinical significance of biochemical blood tests following hepatic resection. Br J Surg. 2011;98(6):836–44.

66. Du ZG, Wei YG, Chen KF, Li B. An accurate predictor of liver failure and death after hepatectomy: a single institution's experience with 478 consecutive cases. World J Gastroenterol. 2014;20(1):274–81.

67. Pozin VM. Change in the electric activity of the heart in reversible local disorders of the coronary circulation in chronic experiments on dogs. Kardiologiia. 1966;6(4):29–35.

68. Yokoyama Y, Ebata T, Igami T, Sugawara G, Ando M, Nagino M. Predictive power of prothrombin time and serum total bilirubin for postoperative mortality after major hepatectomy with extrahepatic bile duct resection. Surgery. 2014;155(3):504–11.

69. Ercolani G, Grazi GL, Calliva R, Pierangeli F, Cescon M, Cavallari A, Mazziotti A. The lidocaine (MEGX) test as an index of hepatic function: its clinical usefulness in liver surgery. Surgery. 2000;127(4):464–71.

70. Delis SG, Bakoyiannis A, Dervenis C, Tassopoulos N. Perioperative risk assessment for hepatocellular carcinoma by using the MELD score. J Gastrointest Surg. 2009;13(12):2268–75.

71. Huang L, Li J, Yan JJ, Liu CF, Wu MC, Yan YQ. Prealbumin is predictive for postoperative liver insufficiency in patients undergoing liver resection. World J Gastroenterol. 2012;18(47):7021–5.

72. Huo TI, Lui WY, Wu JC, Huang YH, King KL, Loong CC, Lee PC, Chang FY, Lee SD. Deterioration of hepatic functional reserve in patients with hepatocellular carcinoma after resection: incidence, risk factors, and association with intrahepatic tumor recurrence. World J Surg. 2004;28(3):258–62.

73. Hyder O, Pulitano C, Firoozmand A, Dodson R, Wolfgang CL, Choti MA, Aldrighetti L, Pawlik TM. A risk model to predict 90-day mortality among patients undergoing hepatic resection. J Am Coll Surg. 2013;216(6):1049–56.

74. Makuuchi M, Sano K. The surgical approach to HCC: our progress and results in Japan. Liver Transpl. 2004;10(2 Suppl 1):S46–52.

75. Hemming AW, Scudamore CH, Shackleton CR, Pudek M, Erb SR. Indocyanine green clearance as a predictor of successful hepatic resection in cirrhotic patients. Am J Surg. 1992;163(5):515–8.

76. Fan ST, Lai EC, Lo CM, Ng IO, Wong J. Hospital mortality of major hepatectomy for hepatocellular carcinoma associated with cirrhosis. Arch Surg. 1995;130(2):198–203.

77. Chong CC, Wong GL, Chan AW, Wong VW, Fong AK, Cheung YS, Wong J, Lee KF, Chan SL, Lai PB, Chan HL. Liver stiffness measurement predicts high-grade post-hepatectomy liver failure: A prospective cohort study. J Gastroenterol Hepatol. 2017;32(2):506–14. doi:10.1111/jgh.13503. PubMed PMID: 27490702.

78. Cescon M, Colecchia A, Cucchetti A, Peri E, Montrone L, Ercolani G, Festi D, Pinna AD. Value of transient elastography measured with FibroScan in predicting the outcome of hepatic resection for hepatocellular carcinoma. Ann Surg. 2012;256(5):706–12. discussion 712–703

79. Sandrin L, Fourquet B, Hasquenoph JM, Yon S, Fournier C, Mal F, Christidis C, Ziol M, Poulet B, Kazemi F, Beaugrand M, Palau R. Transient elastography: a new noninvasive method for assessment of hepatic fibrosis. Ultrasound Med Biol. 2003;29(12):1705–13.

80. Jung KS, Kim SU, Choi GH, Park JY, Park YN, Kim DY, Ahn SH, Chon CY, Kim KS, Choi EH, Choi JS, Han KH. Prediction of recurrence after curative resection of hepatocellular carcinoma using liver stiffness measurement (FibroScan(R)). Ann Surg Oncol. 2012;19(13):4278–86.

81. Kim SU, Ahn SH, Park JY, Kim DY, Chon CY, Choi JS, Kim KS, Han KH. Prediction of postoperative hepatic insufficiency by liver stiffness measurement (FibroScan((R))) before curative resection of hepatocellular carcinoma: a pilot study. Hepatol Int. 2008;2(4):471–7.

82. Yoon JH, Choi JI, Jeong YY, Schenk A, Chen L, Laue H, Kim SY, Lee JM. Pre-treatment estimation of future remnant liver function using gadoxetic acid MRI in patients with HCC. J Hepatol. 2016;65(6):1155–62.
83. Wibmer A, Prusa AM, Nolz R, Gruenberger T, Schindl M, Ba-Ssalamah A. Liver failure after major liver resection: risk assessment by using preoperative Gadoxetic acid-enhanced 3-T MR imaging. Radiology. 2013;269(3):777–86.
84. Thian YL, Riddell AM, Koh DM. Liver-specific agents for contrast-enhanced MRI: role in oncological imaging. Cancer Imaging. 2013;13(4):567–79.
85. Tsuboyama T, Onishi H, Kim T, Akita H, Hori M, Tatsumi M, Nakamoto A, Nagano H, Matsuura N, Wakasa K, Tomoda K. Hepatocellular carcinoma: hepatocyte-selective enhancement at gadoxetic acid-enhanced MR imaging – correlation with expression of sinusoidal and canalicular transporters and bile accumulation. Radiology. 2010;255(3):824–33.
86. Wack KE, Ross MA, Zegarra V, Sysko LR, Watkins SC, Stolz DB. Sinusoidal ultrastructure evaluated during the revascularization of regenerating rat liver. Hepatology. 2001;33(2):363–78.
87. Ferenci P, Lockwood A, Mullen K, Tarter R, Weissenborn K, Blei AT. Hepatic encephalopathy--definition, nomenclature, diagnosis, and quantification: final report of the working party at the 11th World congresses of gastroenterology, Vienna, 1998. Hepatology. 2002;35(3):716–21.
88. Rahbari NN, Garden OJ, Padbury R, Brooke-Smith M, Crawford M, Adam R, Koch M, Makuuchi M, Dematteo RP, Christophi C, Banting S, Usatoff V, Nagino M, Maddern G, Hugh TJ, Vauthey JN, Greig P, Rees M, Yokoyama Y, Fan ST, Nimura Y, Figueras J, Capussotti L, Büchler MW, Weitz J. Posthepatectomy liver failure: a definition and grading by the International Study Group of Liver Surgery (ISGLS). Surgery. 2011;149(5):713–24. doi:10.1016/j.surg.2010.10.001. Epub 2011 Jan 14. PubMed PMID: 21236455.
89. Rahbari NN, Reissfelder C, Koch M, Elbers H, Striebel F, Buchler MW, Weitz J. The predictive value of postoperative clinical risk scores for outcome after hepatic resection: a validation analysis in 807 patients. Ann Surg Oncol. 2011;18(13):3640–9.
90. Skrzypczyk C, Truant S, Duhamel A, Langlois C, Boleslawski E, Koriche D, Hebbar M, Fourrier F, Mathurin P, Pruvot FR. Relevance of the ISGLS definition of posthepatectomy liver failure in early prediction of poor outcome after liver resection: study on 680 hepatectomies. Ann Surg. 2014;260(5):865–70. discussion 870
91. McCormack L, Petrowsky H, Jochum W, Furrer K, Clavien PA. Hepatic steatosis is a risk factor for postoperative complications after major hepatectomy: a matched case-control study. Ann Surg. 2007;245(6):923–30.
92. Kishi Y, Abdalla EK, Chun YS, Zorzi D, Madoff DC, Wallace MJ, Curley SA, Vauthey JN. Three hundred and one consecutive extended right hepatectomies: evaluation of outcome based on systematic liver volumetry. Ann Surg. 2009;250(4):540–8.
93. Roberts KJ, Bharathy KG, Lodge JP. Kinetics of liver function tests after a hepatectomy for colorectal liver metastases predict post-operative liver failure as defined by the international study group for liver surgery. HPB (Oxford). 2013;15(5):345–51.
94. Tsai S, Marques HP, de Jong MC, Mira P, Ribeiro V, Choti MA, Schulick RD, Barroso E, Pawlik TM. Two-stage strategy for patients with extensive bilateral colorectal liver metastases. HPB (Oxford). 2010;12(4):262–9.
95. Adam R, Laurent A, Azoulay D, Castaing D, Bismuth H. Two-stage hepatectomy: a planned strategy to treat irresectable liver tumors. Ann Surg. 2000;232(6):777–85.
96. Kauffmann R, Fong Y. Post-hepatectomy liver failure. Hepatobiliary Surg Nutr. 2014;3(5):238–46.
97. Pandanaboyana S, Bell R, Hidalgo E, Toogood G, Prasad KR, Bartlett A, Lodge JP. A systematic review and meta-analysis of portal vein ligation versus portal vein embolization for elective liver resection. Surgery. 2015;157(4):690–8.
98. Zhang GQ, Zhang ZW, Lau WY, Chen XP. Associating liver partition and portal vein ligation for staged hepatectomy (ALPPS): a new strategy to increase resectability in liver surgery. Int J Surg. 2014;12(5):437–41.

99. Spolverato G, Pawlik TM. Liver-directed therapies: surgical approaches, alone and in combi-
     nation with other interventions. Am Soc Clin Oncol Educ Book. 2014; 101–10. Available at
     http://meetinglibrary.asco.org/record/89021/edbook#overview (checked on 08/01/2017).
100. Yamanaka N, Okamoto E, Oriyama T, Fujimoto J, Furukawa K, Kawamura E, Tanaka T,
     Tomoda F. A prediction scoring system to select the surgical treatment of liver cancer. Further
     refinement based on 10 years of use. Ann Surg. 1994;219:342–6.
101. Kubota K, Makuuchi M, Kusaka K, Kobayashi T, Miki K, Hasegawa K, Harihara Y, Takayama
     T. Measurement of liver volume and hepatic functional reserve as a guide to decision-making
     in resectional surgery for hepatic tumors. Hepatology. 1997;26:1176–81
102. Vauthey JN, Chaoui A, Do KA, Bilimoria MM, Fenstermacher MJ, Charnsangavej C, Hicks
     M, Alsfasser G, Lauwers G, Hawkins IF, Caridi J. Standardized measurement of the future
     liver remnant prior to extended liver resection: methodology and clinical associations.
     Surgery. 2000;127:512–9.
103. Ribero D, Chun YS, Vauthey JN. Standardized liver volumetry for portal vein embolization.
     Semin Intervent Radiol. 2008;25:104–9.
104. Uchiyama K, Mori K, Tabuse K, Ueno M, Ozawa S, Nakase T, Kawai M, Tani M, Tanimura
     H, Yamaue H. Assessment of liver function for successful hepatectomy in patients with
     hepatocellular carcinoma with impaired hepatic function. J Hepatobiliary Pancreat Surg.
     2008;15:596–602.
105. Du ZG, Li B, Wei YG, Yin J, Feng X, Chen X. A new scoring system for assessment of
     liver function after successful hepatectomy in patients with hepatocellular carcinoma.
     Hepatobiliary Pancreat Dis Int. 2011;10:265–9.

Early Recovery After Surgery Pathways for Hepatic Surgery

8

Ryan W. Day and Thomas A. Aloia

Introduction

Enhanced recovery (ER) and fast-track protocols for perioperative surgical care have existed for at least 20 years [1]. ER was originally described in the context of colorectal surgery. Many of the same ER principles have been transferred to other operations and even entire surgical disciplines. Given the issues of multiple approaches, varying magnitudes of hepatectomy, frequent use of cytotoxic chemotherapy, anemia, and multivisceral resection, implementation of ER in liver surgery is a daunting task. While many elements are similar between different disciplines, there are some elements that are unique to liver surgery [2]. ER pathways encompass the preoperative, intraoperative, and postoperative time period. The foundation of an ER program is patient education and engagement. The four pillars of care that rest on this foundation and support the program are early feeding, early ambulation, goal-directed fluid therapy, and opiate-sparing analgesia (Fig. 8.1).

Several clinical trials and meta-analyses, which support individual elements of enhanced recovery pathways, as well as their composite effects, have been published [3, 4]. These studies have determined that patients who are managed with an enhanced recovery protocol have superior outcomes including shortened length of stay, improved functional outcomes, and decreased costs [5]. The goal of this chapter is to review the individual components of ER and evidence for the elements that form a modern clinical care pathway in liver surgery.

The authors have no conflicts of interest or disclosures.

R.W. Day, MD
Department of Surgery, Mayo Clinic Hospital in Arizona, Phoenix, AZ, USA

T.A. Aloia, MD (✉)
Department of Surgical Oncology, The University of Texas MD Anderson Cancer Center, Houston, TX, USA
e-mail: taaloia@mdanderson.org

© Springer International Publishing AG 2018
F.G. Rocha, P. Shen (eds.), *Optimizing Outcomes for Liver and Pancreas Surgery*, DOI 10.1007/978-3-319-62624-6_8

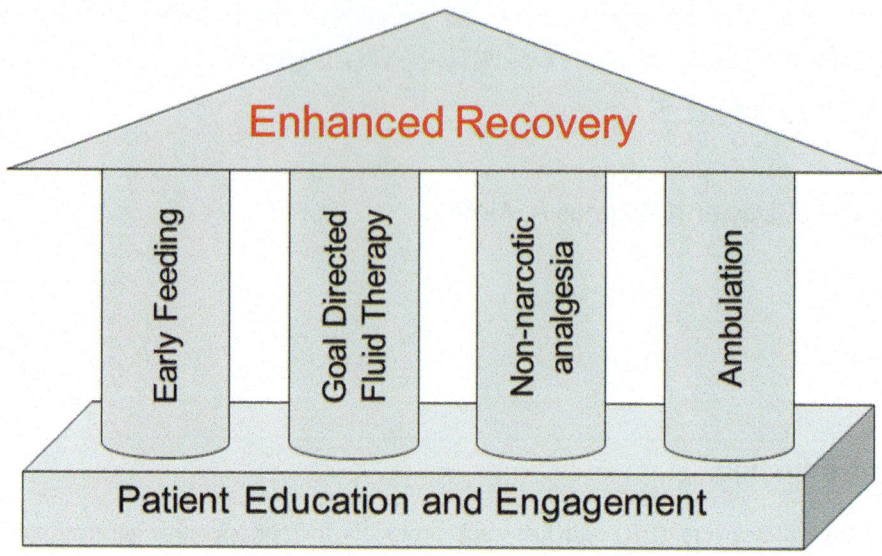

Fig. 8.1 The foundations of enhanced recovery programs are patient education and engagement. The fundamental pillars built on that foundation are early feeding, goal-directed fluid therapy, non-narcotic analgesia, and ambulation

For information regarding current best practices for ER in liver surgery, the Society of American Gastrointestinal and Endoscopic Surgeons SMART Enhanced Recovery Program maintains an up-to-date list of protocols [6]. Additionally, the authors have previously published our experience and ER protocol currently in use at the authors' institution (Fig. 8.2) [7].

Preoperative Care

Preoperative Evaluation and Education

Liver surgery encompasses a broad spectrum of procedures with varying magnitudes and impact on the patient's physiology. The preoperative evaluation of any patient planned for liver surgery should include a broad history and physical exam that reviews all comorbid conditions, paying particular attention to stigmata of liver disease, prior intra-abdominal procedures, and uncontrolled medical conditions.

Cirrhosis or undiagnosed liver disease needs to be fully explored prior to undertaking even minor liver operations. A thorough history and physical exam including a social history must be obtained on all patients. Many oncologic patients will also have prior exposure to intra-abdominal surgical procedures, radiation therapy, and/ or neoadjuvant cytotoxic chemotherapy. Depending on prior history and planned intervention, the evaluation should also include liver function tests, imaging, and even non-tumor liver pathology diagnosis with liver biopsy. In order to optimize

	Factors	Enhanced Recovery	Conventional
Pre-operative	Education	Open and MIS liver surgery patient education material provided, as well as, ER Specific Patient Education material provided includes information about ER principles, patient and care-giver expectations and pain management.	Open and MIS liver surgery patient education material provided.
	Fluid Management	Saline lock IV in pre-op holding	KVO IV
	Preoperative Fasting	Solids up to 6 hours prior to surgery. Clear liquids permissible up to 2hrs before surgery	Clear liquids after lunch day prior to surgery, NPO post midnight.
	Carb loading	Yes. 100g day prior to surgery and 50g day of surgery	None
	Bowel State	No mechanical bowel preparation required	Mechanical bowel preparation used selectively
	Preventive Analgesia	Celecoxib 400 mg PO, Pregabalin 150 mg PO (Age>65 75 mg PO), Tramadol 300 mg PO morning of surgery; Anxiolytics and Anti-nausea medication as needed	Anxiolytics and Anti-nausea medication as needed
Intra-operative	Perioperative Steroids	Dexamethasone 10mg intravenous on induction of anesthesia	No
	Opioid Sparing Anesthesia	Yes, PROMPT	No
	Total Intravenous Analgesia	Dexamethasone 10 mg IV at induction; IV Acetaminophen 1 gram q 6 hours.; Propofol as main anesthetic agent; IV Dexmedetomidine; IV ketamine; IV Lidocaine; Infusions will be titrated by anesthesiologists per patient as needed	Combined protocol with narcotics and inhalational agents
	Fluid Management	Goal directed: Monitor SV	Goal directed: unmonitored
	Regional Analgesia	MIS: Local anesthetic wound infiltration with long-acting liposomal bupivacaine (Exparel). Open: Epidural	MIS: Local anesthetic wound infiltration with short-acting lidocaine/bupivacaine. Open: Epidural
	Drains	Limit to only when absolutely indicated	Selectively used
Post-operative	Opioid Sparing Analgesia	Yes. Pregabalin 75 mg po BID, start pm POD0 x 48h; Acetaminophen 500 mg po x 1 POD0; celecoxib 200 mg PO BID, start POD1; Tramadol 50mg PO q6h, start POD1 x 48h; Hydromorphone 0.5 mg IV q 30 minutes prn breakthrough pain not relieved within 30 mins of oxycodone; No Patient Controlled Anesthetic	Epidural, PCA hydromorphone, hydrocodone, acetaminophen
	PRN Analgesia	Epidural patient: per pain service; Non-epidural patient: Mild pain (1-3): Acetaminophen 500 mg PO q6h; Moderate pain (4-6): Tramadol 50 mg PO q6h; Severe pain (7-10): Hydromorphone 0.5 mg q15 min x 2	hydromorphone, tramadol, hydrocodone
	Tubes	No NGT	Selective NGT
	Early Ambulation	Yes. Day of surgery: Sit on edge of bed; POD1 Out of bed to chair and ambulation at least 4 times daily	Yes. Day of surgery: Sit on edge of bed; POD1 Out of bed to chair and selective ambulation at least 4 times daily
	Fluid Management	Hepatobiliary fluid protocol, Minimize IVF rate, SL after 600cc PO and use Tranfusion guidelines	Hepatobiliary fluid protocol, Minimize IVF rate and use Tranfusion guidelines
	Early Oral Intake	Patients allowed clear liquids on day of surgery. Regular diet POD1	NPO x ice POD0, POD1 clears, POD2 regular
	Ready for discharge criteria	Formalized: Independently ambulatory, good pain control, tolerating diet, bowel function, no infections, comorbidities under control	Unwritten: Independtly ambulatory, good pain control, tolerating diet, bowel function, no infections, comorbidities under control

Fig. 8.2 MD Anderson enhanced recovery in liver surgery protocol (Reprinted from Day et al. [7])

postoperative outcomes, the magnitude of liver resection has to be considered in the context of any pre-existing conditions. In the case of large volume resections, preoperative planning including CT volumetry, MRI, and portal venous embolization with monitoring of kinetic growth rate may be necessary [8, 9].

Prior to undergoing surgery, optimization of chronic medical conditions is of critical importance. Hyperglycemia should prompt evaluation of glycemic control including fasting blood glucose and HgbA1c levels. Uncontrolled diabetes has been associated with adverse postoperative outcomes including wound infections, organ space infection, and even hepatic tumor recurrence [10, 11]. Chronic cardiopulmonary comorbidities may require preoperative evaluation, intervention, and even modification of intraoperative approach. Importantly, functional status should also be assessed prior to surgery. Several methods are currently used including the Easter Cooperative Oncology Group System (ECOG), Karnofsky scoring, and the 6-min walk test, to name a few [12, 13]. Patient surveys can also help with assessing patient's functional status before surgery [14]. The purpose of this workup is to identify correctable deficits that can be addressed preoperatively with physical conditioning, nutritional counseling, blood glucose control, and smoking cessation (e.g., STRONG for Surgery) [15].

Any complete preoperative evaluation of a patient undergoing liver surgery should include extensive, preoperative education. As the complexity of liver operations has increased, so have the branch points in perioperative care. Perioperative care requires the participation of the patient, and setting expectations for postoperative care helps to ensure active participation in the process. Multimodal pain control, early ambulation, and timely discharge from the hospital require the patient to be informed in order to both set expectations and allow for appropriate planning [16]. Often the preoperative education material will encompass a broad spectrum of topics that may be overwhelming for a nonmedical professional. It is, therefore, important to have all conversations in the patient's language of choice and to provide written information that reinforces the oral discussion. Patients should also be given adequate opportunity to ask questions of their surgeon prior to any intervention. All of these elements of education also serve to decrease patient anxiety prior to the planned surgical intervention [17].

Nutrition

As part of the preoperative evaluation, it is important to assess the patient's nutritional status. Particular attention should be directed toward recent weight loss, which may indicate underlying malnutrition. At the same time, obesity does not eliminate the possibility of malnutrition, as sarcopenic obesity is increasingly recognized as a risk factor for poor postoperative outcomes. Therefore, laboratory tests including albumin, prealbumin, ferritin, and others should be used to supplement the workup to help stratify patients into risk categories for perioperative malnutrition. Albumin lower than 3.5 g/dL and prealbumin less than 18 mg/dL both serve as accurate predictors of postoperative morbidity [18, 19]. Optimizing preoperative nutrition and addressing pre-existing malnutrition have been associated with improved outcomes [20].

Once chronic malnutrition has been stratified and addressed, planning specific to surgical intervention can occur. Traditional perioperative guidelines advised patients to undergo long periods of fasting prior to surgical intervention. In an effort to maintain euvolemia and glycemic balance, patients without gastroduodenal impairment can safely be advised to continue clear liquids until 2 h prior to anesthesia induction in accordance with recent American Anesthesiologist's Association (ASA) guidelines on fasting [21]. Controversy continues regarding the role of bowel prep in elective colorectal surgery, but in liver surgery, it is unnecessary and should be avoided [22].

As part of a preoperative nutritional regimen, carbohydrate loading should at least be considered. There is some evidence that preoperative carbohydrate loading helps to provide adequate energy stores for postoperative healing and maintains glycemic balance even in diabetic patients. Carbohydrate loading has been associated with decreased postoperative insulin resistance, patient discomfort, and improved healing [23–25]. A solution containing 100 g of carbohydrates should be administered the evening prior to surgery and an additional 50 g carbohydrate solution administered the morning of surgery. There are several commercial products available as well as more available and inexpensive supplements, such as apple juice. The role of preoperative education is critical to ensure compliance with preoperative carbohydrate loading.

Venous Thromboembolism Prophylaxis

Venous thromboembolism (VTE) presents an important preventable source of postoperative morbidity. The strategy utilized for prophylaxis of VTE should be individualized for each patient. The patient's prior medical history, body mass index, malignant indication, and planned operation must be considered when making decisions regarding anticoagulation strategies. Some patients will present on chronic anticoagulation for a prior episode of deep vein thrombosis (DVT) or VTE. The modified Caprini Risk Assessment model for VTE in surgical patients can be used to predict patient risk for surgical intervention [26]. Given the frequent presence of malignancy and the need for abdominal surgery, the vast majority of liver surgery patients will fall into the moderate- to high-risk Caprini categories.

Prior to the induction of anesthesia, all patients without contraindication should have mechanical thromboprophylaxis in the form of sequential compression devices and/or TED hose applied. The Americas Hepato-Pancreato-Biliary Association has also published guidelines for anticoagulation therapy in patients undergoing liver surgery [27]. Given the elevated risk of bleeding during and after liver surgery, both AHPBA and Chest guidelines indicate that chemical VTE prophylaxis should be held until hemostasis is confirmed. For most patients this will include withholding preoperative chemical prophylaxis and beginning chemical prophylaxis in the postoperative period when the risk of bleeding is judged to be low. Depending on the planned procedure, the need for vascular reconstruction may require intraoperative systemic anticoagulation. Communication and coordination with anesthesia colleagues are essential in these instances.

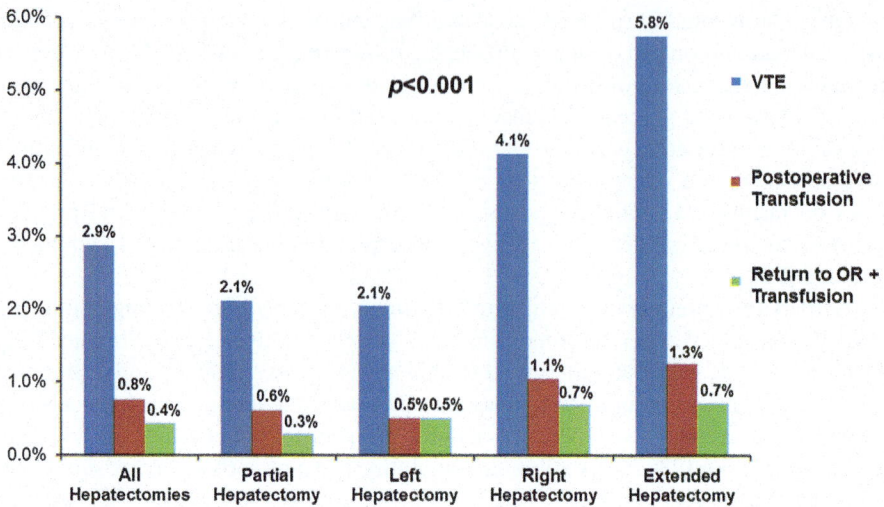

Fig. 8.3 Rates of post-hepatectomy venous thromboembolism, postoperative transfusion, and return to OR from the 2005–2009 NSQIP participant use file (Reprinted from Tzeng et al. [37])

After undergoing hepatectomy, patients will often have an elevated international normalized ratio (INR). Historically this was thought to be associated with a decreased risk of thromboembolism; however, recent studies have shown that the risk for thromboembolism after major liver surgery is significant and directly proportional to the amount of resected liver regardless of INR (Fig. 8.3). This has spurred searches for a more accurate objective measure of anticoagulation status. Thromboelastography may ultimately fill that role as a measure of assessing the various components of clotting capabilities. Patients who are operated on for hepatic malignancy are also at increased risk for thromboembolism after discharge from the hospital. It is, therefore, appropriate to anticoagulate these patients with low molecular weight heparin for up to 4 weeks after surgery [28].

Preemptive Pain Control

The incisions required for major hepatic surgery are typically quite extensive and associated with significant postoperative pain. Although minimally invasive strategies should be utilized when deemed safe by the surgeon, the penetrance of these strategies remains limited to specialized centers. A strategy for multimodal pain management should be developed prior to any intervention. Opiate-sparing analgesia strategies are a cornerstone of ER. Adequate preventative strategies result in less intraoperative and postoperative need for narcotics [29]. For complicated patients who have a history of chronic narcotic use or exposure, preoperative consultation with pain management specialists may have benefits including a coordinated plan for multimodal postoperative pain control.

Strategies to preemptively manage postsurgical pain begin with the administration of several nonnarcotic neuromodulators in the preoperative holding area. These medications generally include a combination of oral pregabalin, gabapentin, NSAIDs, and opiate-like narcotics such as tramadol. Discussion with anesthesiologists may allow for the coordination and the use of intraoperative neuraxial and regional blocks that can result in decreased postoperative pain, narcotic utilization, and postoperative nausea and vomiting.

Perioperative Care

Perioperative Antimicrobial Prophylaxis

In order to limit postoperative infections as a source of postoperative morbidity, appropriately antimicrobial prophylaxis should be administered perioperatively. For most patients, the administration of a cephalosporin like cefoxitin should provide adequate coverage and be administered less than 1 h prior to surgical incision and redosed every 4 h during the operation [30]. Additional antimicrobial coverage for gram-negative and anaerobic organisms is indicated when liver surgery is coordinated with other procedures that provide a potential source of contamination or if intra-abdominal contamination is encountered inadvertently.

Postoperatively all antibiotics should be stopped within 24 h of surgery, unless there is a documented source of established infection requiring further treatment. Postoperatively continuing antibiotics without treating a definitive site of established infection has not been associated with a decrease in infectious complications [31]. For preoperative skin preparation, chlorhexidine-alcohol 2% solution or betadine-alcohol should be used in preference to povidone-iodine alone [32].

Fluid Therapy

Intravenous fluid resuscitation is essential to performing surgery under general anesthesia. However the use of these fluids does have potentially deleterious physiologic effects. Particularly in liver surgery, attention has to be paid to the volume status of patients. The goal should be to maintain euvolemia or even slight dehydration with low central venous pressures (CVP) prior to and during parenchymal transection. The intraoperative management of CVP is essential to limiting blood loss and obviating the need for blood transfusion. While excessive bleeding is the most immediate consequence of over hydration, it is not the only one. Prolonged ileus due to excessive bowel edema, difficulty with ventilation due to pulmonary edema, and anasarca can also adversely impact patient outcomes.

Intravenous fluids should be titrated to physiologic goals. This requires a partnership with open communication between surgeon and anesthetist. Goal-directed fluid therapy has been shown to decrease morbidity, mortality, and costs [33]. While physiologic goals should be used for fluid hydration, there remains significant disagreement as to the best end point for resuscitation. Certain parameters have been long-standing pieces of management including blood pressure, heart, and urine output. Newer parameters include stroke volume, esophageal perfusion monitoring, lactate clearance, and cardiac index. These parameters will continue to be investigated, but it is clear that none of these variables can be used as a sole end point in a vacuum without considering the clinical context and other physiologic parameters.

Intraoperative Body Temperature Regulation

Similar to the goal of maintaining euvolemia, another goal should be to maintain normothermic body temperature. This can be somewhat challenging especially with unexpected large volume blood loss and/or long procedures. The hypothermic patient will be difficult to manage intraoperatively due to coagulopathy as well as postoperatively where hypothermia has been associated with wound infections, dehiscence, and prolonged length of stay.

There are several commercially available devices for keeping the ambient temperature around the patient warm. These include forced high-flow air heating devices and on-table warming blankets. The surgeon should also pay particular attention to the temperature of any fluids that are introduced into the abdominal cavity. These fluids should be prewarmed so as not to contribute to hypothermia.

Perioperative Blood Transfusion and Alternative Strategies for Management of Anemia

Blood transfusion is a generally well-tolerated intervention; however, it is not entirely benign. The risks of blood transfusion include transfusion reaction, transfusion-related lung injury, the risk of transmitting infectious disease, and transfusion-related immunomodulation. It is, therefore, worthwhile to take steps to prevent blood transfusion even if complications are rare.

Preoperative workup for patients should include assessment of symptoms related to anemia as well as biochemical analysis of anemia. If discovered in the preoperative workup, it is important to discern the etiology of the anemia and take steps to ensure preoperative optimization of the patient's anemia. If symptomatic, preoperative blood transfusion is indicated. Although iron infusion and erythropoietin treatment are theoretically possible, in practice the moderately anemic but asymptomatic patient with a liver tumor who needs to progress to operation simply assumes a higher risk of perioperative blood transfusion.

Intraoperatively, efforts should be undertaken to limit blood transfusion. The maintenance of low CVP during parenchymal transection has been associated with decreased blood loss and a lower need for transfusion. Additionally, the authors utilize the two-surgeon technique for parenchymal transection, which has been associated with less intraoperative blood loss [34]. Prompt correction of coagulopathy and maintenance of normothermia are also important steps to limiting perioperative transfusion.

Limitation of Narcotics

The limitation of intraoperative narcotics is largely a function of teamwork and communication between surgeon and anesthetist. The use of preemptive pain control, regional neuraxial blocks, and field blocks (e.g., TAP block) can all limit the need for intraoperative and postoperative narcotic use. While most patients will require some amount of narcotic medications, it is important to recognize that narcotics have several deleterious effects. Respiratory depression, potential narcotic dependence, constipation, and a prolonged period of time until recovery of bowel function are all concerns. The use of non-narcotic adjuvants including NSAIDs and acetaminophen is a vital component of any enhanced recovery pathway.

Use of Intra-abdominal Drains, Enteric Tubes, and Urinary Catheters

Historically, liver surgeons have frequently utilized surgical drains in the operative bed. While patients and procedures that are deemed high risk may still require drainage, every effort should be made to limit the placement of surgical drains. Biliary leak remains a concern after hepatectomy, but with adjunct intraoperative procedures in order to detect bile leaks, the rate can be dramatically decreased [35]. The air leak cholangiogram test and other similar procedures have been shown to reduce the rate of biliary leakage and can help alleviate the need for postoperative drainage.

In patients undergoing liver surgery alone, there is rarely an indication for nasogastric drainage. In fact, evidence from the colorectal surgery literature shows even patients undergoing major bowel resections do not require routine use of nasogastric tubes for enteric drainage. Refraining from placing nasogastric tubes has several positive effects on patient recovery including earlier advancement of diet, earlier ambulation, easier maintenance of normovolemia, and easier maintenance of electrolyte levels. If enteric drainage must be performed after surgery, it is important to remove the nasogastric tube as early as feasible in the postoperative course in order to facilitate prompt recovery.

The use of temporary indwelling urinary catheters is routine in liver surgery. The procedure length of many liver-focused interventions will require the placement of a urinary catheter. Additionally, the monitoring of urine output facilitates goal-directed fluid therapy both during the operation and in the immediate recovery period. As soon as patients are ambulatory postoperatively, any indwelling urinary drainage catheter should be removed. This can usually be accomplished on postoperative day 1 or 2. If the need for hourly urinary output monitoring mandates a catheter cannot be removed at this point, the surgical team should continually reassess the need for urinary drainage in order to remove the catheter as soon as possible. Older males may have issues with urinary retention that can be avoided or reversed with preemptive administration of tamsulosin.

Postoperative Care

Postoperative Nausea and Vomiting Prophylaxis

Many anesthetic techniques and drugs have been associated with clinically significant levels of nausea and vomiting. These side effects can prolong the period of time between operation and initiation of a diet. In turn, this can increase the time period where patients require intravenous fluids and can increase hospital length of stay. Furthermore, patients who are still under some effects of anesthetics are at higher risk for aspiration events, while they remain sedated.

To limit postoperative nausea and vomiting, chemoprophylaxis should be administered in the operating room, prior to extubation. Corticosteroids like dexamethasone administered prior to incision can help decrease postoperative nausea and vomiting while limiting the patient's inflammatory response to surgery. There are a myriad of other antiemetic options available as well.

Postoperative Pain Control

Similar to preoperative and intraoperative management, postoperative pain management should focus on a multimodal, narcotic-sparing analgesia strategies. A significant number of patients undergoing open liver surgery can be managed with nonnarcotic agents reserving low-dose narcotics for significant breakthrough pain. Acetaminophen, nonsteroidal anti-inflammatory medications, regional neuraxial blocks, and/or field blocks should be utilized to minimize narcotic requirements. Non-pharmacologic treatments such as ice packs, massage, and acupuncture are additional adjuncts that can limit narcotic exposure.

General Postoperative Management

The goals for early postoperative management are centered around early normalization of the patient's diet and activity. Having a formal order set and pathway for postoperative management, which patients routinely progress along, makes it easy to identify patients who deviate from the expected recovery. The individuals who do deviate from the normal postoperative course should be promptly identified and thoroughly investigated for surgical complications. If a surgical complication is identified, every effort should be made to manage the complication in an effective and timely manner and limit the potential harm from subsequent complications.

Postoperative Diet Management

After most routine liver surgeries, there is no reason to limit a patient's diet postoperatively. Those individuals who have no contraindication to early feeding should be allowed to take in clear liquids on the same day as the surgery and regular diet by the next morning. The authors avoid the use of full liquid diets, as up to 30% of patients are lactose intolerant. The role of intravenous fluids should be limited to situations where the patient is unable to sustain euvolemia with oral liquids. In the early postoperative period, intravenous fluids can be discontinued with as little as 600 cc of oral intake. Postoperative nausea and vomiting as well as the routine use of nasogastric tubes for enteric drainage will obviously interfere with the ability to rapidly normalize a patient's diet.

Postoperative Mobilization

Mobilization in the early postoperative period is another key to realizing the benefits of ER. Almost all patients can begin mobilization immediately after surgery. A surprising number of lay people and even medical professionals continue to perpetuate the idea that the early postoperative period should not include ambulation or activity. The practice of early ambulation will reduce ileus, improve pulmonary function, and decrease the risk of postoperative thromboembolic events. Limiting extraneous drains, IV tubing, and urinary catheters can help facilitate early mobilization by empowering patients and limiting the time and effort needed to begin ambulating. For patients who have baseline difficulty with ambulation and mobility, physical and occupational therapists should be engaged early in the hospitalization.

Outcomes of ER Protocols

The outcomes of ER protocols in liver surgery have been described in the surgical literature. Decreased morbidity, cost, and hospital length of stay have all been demonstrated in numerous randomized controlled trials [3, 4]. Recent reports have also focused on improved functional outcomes as characterized by the patient-reported outcomes [7]. These studies have shown that management with a clinical care pathway leads to a quicker return to baseline of life interference and can also facilitate early return to intended oncologic therapies (RIOT) for patients undergoing oncologic resection (Fig. 8.4) [36].

Combined, the literature indicates that perioperative management with a clinical care pathway has the ability to improve not only objective outcome measures but patient's quality of life as well. Each outcome measure can also have broad positive downstream effects with some examples including less time exposed to hospital-acquired pathogens and less time outside the labor force spent in recovering from surgery.

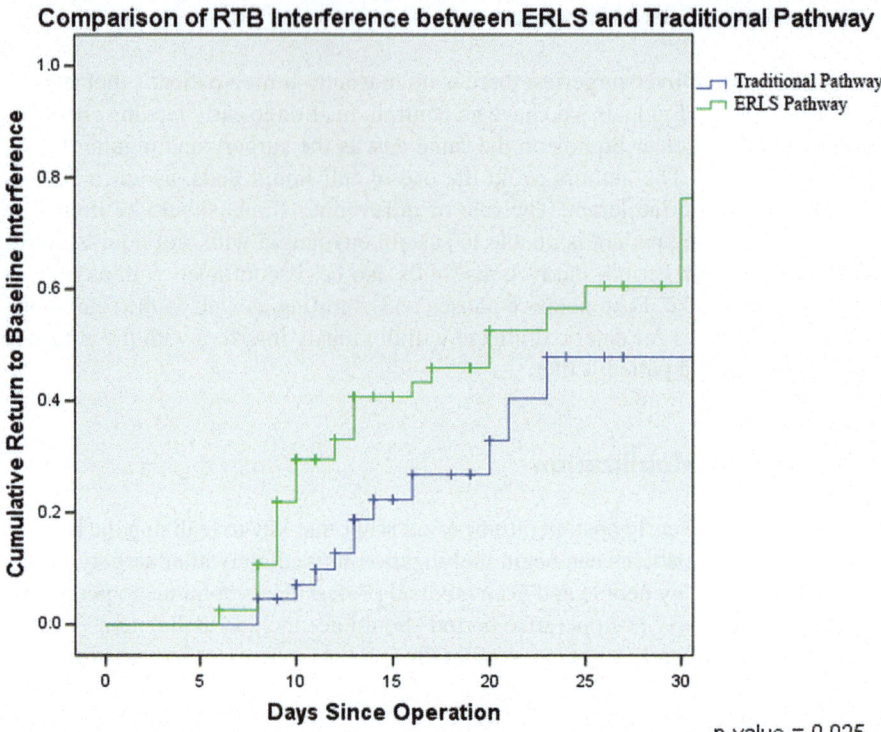

Fig. 8.4 Time to return of baseline interference measured by the MDASI-GI survey after hepatectomy managed on enhanced recovery versus traditional pathways (Reprinted from Day et al. [7])

References

1. Kehlet H, Wilmore DW. Fast-track surgery. Br J Surg. 2005;92(1):3–4. doi:10.1002/bjs.4841.
2. Melloul E, Hubner M, Scott M, Snowden C, Prentis J, Dejong CH, Garden OJ, Farges O, Kokudo N, Vauthey JN, Clavien PA, Demartines N. Guidelines for perioperative care for liver surgery: enhanced recovery after surgery (ERAS) society recommendations. World J Surg. 2016;40(10):2425–40. doi:10.1007/s00268-016-3700-1.
3. Song W, Wang K, Zhang RJ, Dai QX, Zou SB. The enhanced recovery after surgery (ERAS) program in liver surgery: a meta-analysis of randomized controlled trials. Spring. 2016;5:207. doi:10.1186/s40064-016-1793-5.
4. Hughes MJ, McNally S, Wigmore SJ. Enhanced recovery following liver surgery: a systematic review and meta-analysis. HPB (Oxford). 2014;16(8):699–706. doi:10.1111/hpb.12245.
5. Stottmeier S, Harling H, Wille-Jorgensen P, Balleby L, Kehlet H. Pathogenesis of morbidity after fast-track laparoscopic colonic cancer surgery. Color Dis. 2011;13(5):500–5. doi:10.1111/j.1463-1318.2010.02274.x.
6. SAGES SMART Enhanced Recovery Program. 2017. https://www.sages.org/smart-enhanced-recovery-program/. Accessed 28 Mar 2017.
7. Day RW, Cleeland CS, Wang XS, Fielder S, Calhoun J, Conrad C, Vauthey JN, Gottumukkala V, Aloia TA. Patient-reported outcomes Accurately measure the value of an enhanced recovery program in liver surgery. J am Coll Surg. 2015;221(6):1023–1030. e1021–1022. doi:10.1016/j.jamcollsurg.2015.09.011.

8. Shindoh J, Truty MJ, Aloia TA, Curley SA, Zimmitti G, Huang SY, Mahvash A, Gupta S, Wallace MJ, Vauthey JN. Kinetic growth rate after portal vein embolization predicts posthepatectomy outcomes: toward zero liver-related mortality in patients with colorectal liver metastases and small future liver remnant. J Am Coll Surg. 2013;216(2):201–9. doi:10.1016/j.jamcollsurg.2012.10.018.

9. Lim MC, Tan CH, Cai J, Zheng J, Kow AW. CT volumetry of the liver: where does it stand in clinical practice? Clin Radiol. 2014;69(9):887–95. doi:10.1016/j.crad.2013.12.021.

10. Fukuda H. Patient-related risk factors for surgical site infection following eight types of gastrointestinal surgery. J Hosp Infect. 2016;93(4):347–54. doi:10.1016/j.jhin.2016.04.005.

11. Kaneda K, Uenishi T, Takemura S, Shinkawa H, Urata Y, Sakae M, Yamamoto T, Kubo S. The influence of postoperative glycemic control on recurrence after curative resection in diabetics with hepatitis C virus-related hepatocellular carcinoma. J Surg Oncol. 2012;105(6):606–11. doi:10.1002/jso.22137.

12. Karnofsky DA. Cancer chemotherapeutic agents. CA Cancer J Clin. 1964;14:67–72.

13. Hsieh CB, Tsai CS, Chen TW, Chu HC, Yu JC, Chen DR. Correlation between SF-36 and six-minute walk distance in liver donors. Transplant Proc. 2010;42(9):3597–9. doi:10.1016/j.transproceed.2010.06.033.

14. Cleeland CS, Mendoza TR, Wang XS, Chou C, Harle MT, Morrissey M, Engstrom MC. Assessing symptom distress in cancer patients: the M.D. Anderson symptom inventory. Cancer. 2000;89(7):1634–46.

15. Certain. 2016. Strong for surgery. http://www.becertain.org/strong_for_surgery. Accessed 30 Sept 2016.

16. Takamoto T, Hashimoto T, Inoue K, Nagashima D, Maruyama Y, Mitsuka Y, Aramaki O, Makuuchi M. Applicability of enhanced recovery program for advanced liver surgery. World J Surg. 2014;38(10):2676–82. doi:10.1007/s00268-014-2613-0.

17. Granziera E, Guglieri I, Del Bianco P, Capovilla E, Dona B, Ciccarese AA, Kilmartin D, Manfredi V, De Salvo GL. A multidisciplinary approach to improve preoperative understanding and reduce anxiety: a randomised study. Eur J Anaesthesiol. 2013;30(12):734–42. doi:10.1097/EJA.0b013e3283652c0c.

18. Djaladat H, Bruins HM, Miranda G, Cai J, Skinner EC, Daneshmand S. The association of preoperative serum albumin level and American Society of Anesthesiologists (ASA) score on early complications and survival of patients undergoing radical cystectomy for urothelial bladder cancer. BJU Int. 2014;113(6):887–93. doi:10.1111/bju.12240.

19. Lucas DJ, Haider A, Haut E, Dodson R, Wolfgang CL, Ahuja N, Sweeney J, Pawlik TM. Assessing readmission after general, vascular, and thoracic surgery using ACS-NSQIP. Ann Surg. 2013;258(3):430–9. doi:10.1097/SLA.0b013e3182a18fcc.

20. Lin MY, Liu WY, Tolan AM, Aboulian A, Petrie BA, Stabile BE. Preoperative serum albumin but not prealbumin is an excellent predictor of postoperative complications and mortality in patients with gastrointestinal cancer. Am Surg. 2011;77(10):1286–9.

21. Brady M, Kinn S, Stuart P. Preoperative fasting for adults to prevent perioperative complications. Cochrane Database Syst Rev. 2003;4:CD004423. doi:10.1002/14651858.CD004423.

22. Zmora O, Mahajna A, Bar-Zakai B, Rosin D, Hershko D, Shabtai M, Krausz MM, Ayalon A. Colon and rectal surgery without mechanical bowel preparation: a randomized prospective trial. Ann Surg. 2003;237(3):363–7. doi:10.1097/01.SLA.0000055222.90581.59.

23. Nygren J, Thorell A, Ljungqvist O. Preoperative oral carbohydrate nutrition: an update. Curr Opin Clin Nutr Metab Care. 2001;4(4):255–9.

24. Hausel J, Nygren J, Lagerkranser M, Hellstrom PM, Hammarqvist F, Almstrom C, Lindh A, Thorell A, Ljungqvist O. A carbohydrate-rich drink reduces preoperative discomfort in elective surgery patients. Anesth Analg. 2001;93(5):1344–50.

25. Svanfeldt M, Thorell A, Hausel J, Soop M, Rooyackers O, Nygren J, Ljungqvist O. Randomized clinical trial of the effect of preoperative oral carbohydrate treatment on postoperative whole-body protein and glucose kinetics. Br J Surg. 2007;94(11):1342–50. doi:10.1002/bjs.5919.

26. Caprini JA. Individual risk assessment is the best strategy for thromboembolic prophylaxis. Dis Mon. 2010;56(10):552–9. doi:10.1016/j.disamonth.2010.06.007.

27. Aloia TA, Geerts WH, Clary BM, Day RW, Hemming AW, D'Albuquerque LC, Vollmer CM Jr, Vauthey JN, Toogood GJ. Venous thromboembolism prophylaxis in liver surgery. J Gastrointest Surg. 2016;20(1):221–9. doi:10.1007/s11605-015-2902-4.
28. Merkow RP, Bilimoria KY, McCarter MD, Cohen ME, Barnett CC, Raval MV, Caprini JA, Gordon HS, Ko CY, Bentrem DJ. Post-discharge venous thromboembolism after cancer surgery: extending the case for extended prophylaxis. Ann Surg. 2011;254(1):131–7. doi:10.1097/SLA.0b013e31821b98da.
29. Cillo JE Jr, Dattilo DJ. Pre-emptive analgesia with pregabalin and celecoxib decreases postsurgical pain following maxillomandibular advancement surgery: a randomized controlled clinical trial. J Oral Maxillofac Surg. 2014;72(10):1909–14. doi:10.1016/j.joms.2014.05.014.
30. Bratzler DW, Houck PM, Surgical Infection Prevention Guidelines Writers W, American Academy of Orthopaedic S, American Association of Critical Care N, American Association of Nurse A, American College of S, American College of Osteopathic S, American Geriatrics S, American Society of A, American Society of C, Rectal S, American Society of Health-System P, American Society of PeriAnesthesia N, Ascension H, Association of periOperative Registered N, Association for Professionals in Infection C, Epidemiology, Infectious Diseases Society of A, Medical L, Premier, Society for Healthcare Epidemiology of A, Society of Thoracic S, Surgical Infection S. Antimicrobial prophylaxis for surgery: an advisory statement from the National Surgical Infection Prevention Project. Clin Infect Dis. 2004;38(12):1706–15. doi:10.1086/421095.
31. Togo Y, Tanaka S, Kanematsu A, Ogawa O, Miyazato M, Saito H, Arai Y, Hoshi A, Terachi T, Fukui K, Kinoshita H, Matsuda T, Yamashita M, Kakehi Y, Tsuchihashi K, Sasaki M, Ishitoya S, Onishi H, Takahashi A, Ogura K, Mishina M, Okuno H, Oida T, Horii Y, Hamada A, Okasyo K, Okumura K, Iwamura H, Nishimura K, Manabe Y, Hashimura T, Horikoshi M, Mishima T, Okada T, Sumiyoshi T, Kawakita M, Kanamaru S, Ito N, Aoki D, Kawaguchi R, Yamada Y, Kokura K, Nagai J, Kondoh N, Kajio K, Yoshimoto T, Yamamoto S. Antimicrobial prophylaxis to prevent perioperative infection in urological surgery: a multicenter study. J Infect Chemother. 2013;19(6):1093–101. doi:10.1007/s10156-013-0631-8.
32. Darouiche RO, Wall MJ Jr, Itani KM, Otterson MF, Webb AL, Carrick MM, Miller HJ, Awad SS, Crosby CT, Mosier MC, Alsharif A, Berger DH. Chlorhexidine-alcohol versus Povidone-iodine for surgical-site antisepsis. N Engl J Med. 2010;362(1):18–26. doi:10.1056/NEJMoa0810988.
33. Correa-Gallego C, Tan KS, Arslan-Carlon V, Gonen M, Denis SC, Langdon-Embry L, Grant F, Kingham TP, DeMatteo RP, Allen PJ, D'Angelica MI, Jarnagin WR, Fischer M. Goal-directed fluid therapy using stroke volume variation for resuscitation after low central venous pressure-assisted liver resection: a randomized clinical trial. J Am Coll Surg. 2015;221(2):591–601. doi:10.1016/j.jamcollsurg.2015.03.050.
34. Day RW, Brudvik KW, Vauthey JN, Conrad C, Gottumukkala V, Chun YS, Katz MH, Fleming JB, Lee JE, Aloia TA. Advances in hepatectomy technique: toward zero transfusions in the modern era of liver surgery. Surgery. 2016;159(3):793–801. doi:10.1016/j.surg.2015.10.006.
35. Zimmitti G, Vauthey JN, Shindoh J, Tzeng CW, Roses RE, Ribero D, Capussotti L, Giuliante F, Nuzzo G, Aloia TA. Systematic use of an intraoperative air leak test at the time of major liver resection reduces the rate of postoperative biliary complications. J Am Coll Surg. 2013;217(6):1028–37. doi:10.1016/j.jamcollsurg.2013.07.392.
36. Aloia TA, Zimmitti G, Conrad C, Gottumukalla V, Kopetz S, Vauthey JN. Return to intended oncologic treatment (RIOT): a novel metric for evaluating the quality of oncosurgical therapy for malignancy. J Surg Oncol. 2014;110(2):107–14. doi:10.1002/jso.23626.
37. Tzeng C-WD, Katz MHG, Fleming JB, Pisters PWT, Lee JE, Abdalla EK, Curley SA, Vauthey J-N, Aloia TA. Risk of venous thromboembolism outweighs post-hepatectomy bleeding complications: analysis of 5651 National Surgical Quality Improvement Program patients. HPB. 2012;14(8):506–51.

Evolving Role of Drains, Tubes and Stents in Pancreatic Surgery

9

Camilo Correa-Gallego and Peter J. Allen

Introduction

As recently as 30 years ago, major pancreatic resections were associated with morbidity and mortality rates that were considered prohibitive by many. Over the last several decades, through better training, technical advances, and the development of intensive perioperative care and interventional endoscopy and radiology, these procedures have become significantly safer. Pancreaticoduodenectomy is now associated with postoperative mortality as low as 1% in many high-volume centers.

Part of the evolution of pancreatic resection involved the routine implementation of every possible safety measure to prevent complications or to assist in diagnosing and managing them. These included routine stenting of the common bile duct to relieve jaundice preoperatively, routine construction of the pancreaticojejunal anastomosis over a stent, routine drainage of the surgical bed, and routine placement of gastric decompression and jejunostomy feeding tubes. Many of these have been slowly abandoned at most centers; however, intense debate still surrounds some of these techniques.

While there are high-quality randomized data on some of these issues, practice patterns haven't adapted accordingly and in most cases are dictated by practical issues, dogma, or personal bias. Here we review the most relevant data regarding the use of stents and drains in pancreatic surgery and present our current practice and recommendations.

C. Correa-Gallego, MD (✉)
Memorial Sloan Kettering Cancer Center, New York, NY, USA
e-mail: correagj@mskcc.org

P.J. Allen, MD
Department of Surgery, Memorial Sloan Kettering Cancer Center, New York, NY, USA

© Springer International Publishing AG 2018
F.G. Rocha, P. Shen (eds.), *Optimizing Outcomes for Liver and Pancreas Surgery*, DOI 10.1007/978-3-319-62624-6_9

Preoperative Biliary Drainage

The most common presenting sign for patients with malignancy of the periampullary region is obstructive jaundice. While a significant proportion of these patients will be asymptomatic, the deleterious systemic consequences of uncontrolled hyperbilirubinemia may still occur. Furthermore, symptoms such as pruritus can be debilitating and have a significant impact on the quality of life. Thus, some have advocated preoperative drainage of the biliary system in patients with resectable periampullary malignancies, given widespread availability of endoscopic retrograde cholangiopancreatography and its perceived safety profile. On the other hand, the purported benefits of routine preoperative drainage in this patient population (namely, resolution of symptoms in symptomatic patients while awaiting surgery, restoration of the enterohepatic cycle, and a potential decrease in postoperative morbidity) have proven to be largely theoretical, and now there are high-quality phase III data that demonstrate the deleterious effects of routine stenting.

A seminal study originating from the Netherlands in 2010 evaluated this issue in the only modern randomized controlled trial to date evaluating preoperative endoscopic biliary decompression for these patients [1]. In their multicenter study, they randomized 202 patients with newly diagnosed pancreatic head cancer and bilirubin levels between 2.3 and 14.6 mg/dL to preoperative biliary drainage for 4–6 weeks vs. immediate surgery which was to be performed within a week of enrollment. The primary endpoint was the development of serious complications within 120 days after randomization. Serious complications were defined as complications related to the drainage procedure or the surgical intervention that required additional medical, endoscopic, or surgical management, and that resulted in prolongation of the hospital stay, readmission to the hospital, or death [1]. The reported overall rate of serious complications in this study favored the immediate surgery group (39 vs. 74%; RR 0.54–95% [CI], 0.41–0.71; $P < 0.001$), complications related to surgery were equivalent (37 vs. 47%; $P = 0.14$), and there was no difference in mortality rates or length of hospital stay. The observed drainage-related complications included a 15% rate of stent occlusion, 30% need for exchange, and 26% incidence of cholangitis. Figure 9.1 shows the cumulative incidence of complications, and Table 9.1 details the specific complications in these patients. Based on these results, the authors concluded that the morbidity associated with the drainage procedure itself had an additive effect on the postoperative morbidity of patients undergoing pancreatic head resection for cancer and recommended against its routine use in this population.

A Cochrane systematic review of all available randomized studies (including the abovementioned study by van der Gaag et al.) evaluating preoperative biliary drainage was published in 2012 [2]. In this study, Fang et al. assessed the impact of this intervention on survival, serious morbidity (defined as Clavien-Dindo grade 3 or 4), and quality of life. Furthermore, they sought to assess differences in total length of hospital stay and cost. They identified six randomized trials of which four used percutaneous transhepatic biliary drainage and the remaining two used endoscopic sphincterotomy and stenting. The pooled analysis of 520 patients (of which 51% underwent preoperative biliary drainage) showed no difference in mortality, but

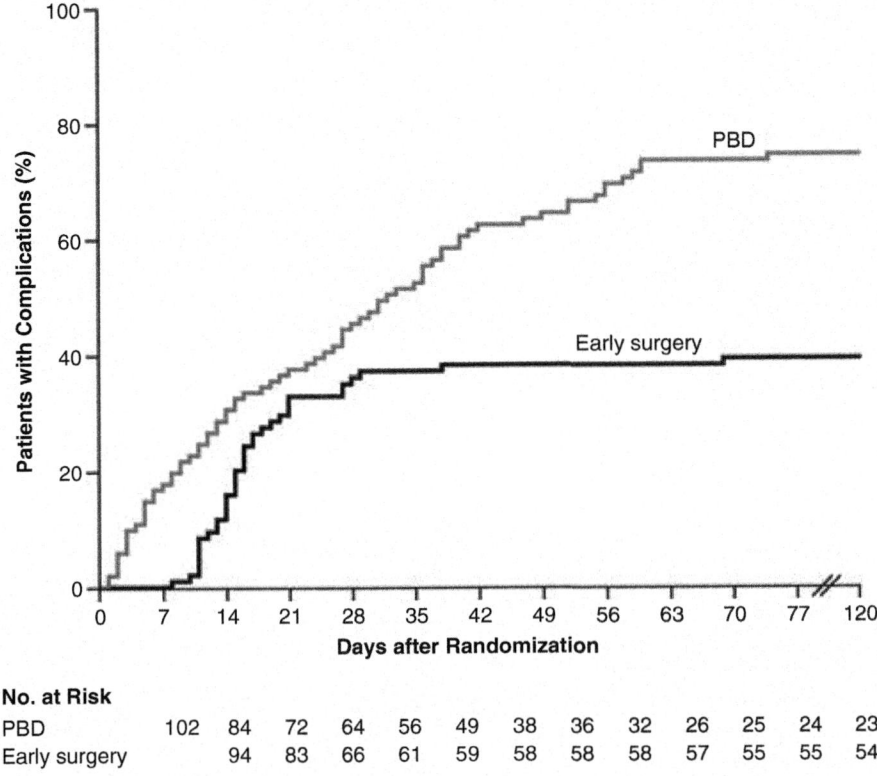

Fig. 9.1 Proportion of patients with complications

importantly, it showed a significantly higher incidence of serious morbidity in the preoperative drainage group with a rate ratio (RaR) of 1.66 (95% CI 1.28–2.16; $P = 0.002$). There was no difference in length of hospital stay and not enough data reported for analysis of cost or quality of life. Based on the available level 1 data, the authors concluded that there was no evidence to support or refute routine preoperative biliary drainage in patients with obstructive jaundice. However, this review also underscored the fact that preoperative biliary drainage may be associated with an increased rate of adverse events and thus questioned the safety of this practice [2].

This Cochrane review included old studies that evaluated patients undergoing percutaneous drainage, a technique used less frequently today for periampullary malignancies. Furthermore, several of these trials included patients with hilar and other types of biliary obstruction. However, the concept of preoperative decompression, as well as its purported benefits and observed results, may be reasonably extrapolated to patients with periampullary lesions.

Table 9.1 Serious complications within 120 days after randomization[a]

Complication	Early surgery (N = 94) no. (%)	Preoperative biliary drainage (N = 102) no. (%)
Related to preoperative biliary drainage		
Any	2 (2)	47 (46)
Pancreatitis	0	7 (7)
Cholangitis[b]	2 (2)	27 (26)
Perforation	0	2 (2)
Hemorrhage after ERCP[c]	0	2 (2)
Related to stent		
Occlusion	1 (1)	15 (15)
Need for exchange	2 (2)	31 (30)
Related to surgery		
Any	35 (37)	48 (47)
Pancreaticojejunostomy leakage[d]	11 (12)	8 (8)
Grade A	1 (1)	0
Grade B	4 (4)	4 (4)
Grade C	6 (6)	4 (4)
Hemorrhage after pancreatectomy[c]	4 (4)	2 (2)
Delayed gastric emptying	9 (10)	18 (18)
Biliary leakage	3 (3)	1 (1)
Gastrojejunostomy or duodenojejunostomy leakage	2 (2)	4 (4)
Intra-abdominal abscess	3 (3)	2 (2)
Wound infection	7 (7)	13 (13)
Portal vein thrombosis	1 (1)	0
Pneumonia	5 (5)	9 (9)
Cholangitis	3 (3)	3 (3)
Myocardial infarction	0	4 (4)
Need for repeated laparotomy[e]	13 (14)	12 (12)

[a]The numbers refer to patients who had one or more complications. ERCP denotes endoscopic retrograde cholangiopancreatography
[b]In two patients, cholecystitis occurred in connection with cholangitis, prompting antibiotic treatment, without the need for cholecystectomy
[c]Hemorrhage was defined as bleeding that required the transfusion of at least four units of packed red cells during a 24-h period or bleeding that led to repeat laparotomy or another intervention
[d]Grade A refers to transient biochemical leakage that does not require treatment, grade B refers to leakage that is managed with prolonged or percutaneous drainage, and grade C refers to leakage requiring repeat laparotomy
[e]This category refers to complications of either preoperative biliary drainage or another surgical procedure

Author's Practice

In our practice, preoperative biliary drainage is rarely necessary in asymptomatic patients with resectable periampullary lesions that have no evidence of systemic dysfunction related to the hyperbilirubinemia. Since the level 1 data noted above had an upper limit of 14 mg/dl as a cutoff, some will consider stenting in patients with a bilirubin higher than 14. When attempting resection in a patient with a very high bilirubin (>15 mg/dl), we will typically admit the patient the night before resection for preoperative hydration, as postoperative renal failure is one of the primary postoperative complications in this group of patients. Portal dissection in the absence of a preoperative stent is typically more straightforward with less inflammation and a better ability to grossly assess tumor margin. Unfortunately, many patients who do not require stenting will have this done prior to referral to a surgeon. We continue to emphasize to our community of gastroenterologists that patients should be referred for surgical evaluation prior to the placement of a biliary stent.

There are several instances where we do feel that preoperative drainage is necessary. When preoperative systemic therapy is to be given, preoperative drainage with a self-expanding metal stent is appropriate. A metal, rather than a plastic, stent should be utilized as these patients will typically receive months of treatment before resection. We will also typically stent any patient in which a major vascular reconstruction is anticipated. Intraoperative ischemia, and postoperative vascular thrombosis, can often be tolerated in a non-jaundiced liver but may result in liver necrosis in the setting of deep jaundice. Finally, any patient in which prolonged preoperative evaluation is felt to be necessary should also be considered for decompression.

Pancreatic Duct Drainage

Stenting of the Pancreatic Duct (PD) for Distal Pancreatectomy

Several small studies have reported the use of PD stents to decrease postoperative pancreatic leak and fistula from the cut surface of the distal pancreas. This practice is based on the assertion that the pressure gradient between the main pancreatic duct and the duodenum is decreased by disruption and/or stenting of the sphincter of Oddi. Theoretically, this intervention has the potential to decrease the incidence of clinically relevant postoperative pancreatic fistula (POPF). One of the earlier studies published in 2008 reported on ten patients who underwent preoperative endoscopic placement of a 3 cm, 7 Fr transampullary pediatric feeding tube [3]. There were no POPF, as defined by the ISGPF guidelines [4]. However, 20% of patients developed acute pancreatitis as a result of the preoperative endoscopic retrograde cholangiopancreatography (ERCP). This paper was later retracted due to prior publication, and there is no follow-up study on a large patient population published to date.

A second study from the Methodist Hospital in Houston reported on the use of intraoperative transampullary duct stenting (TAPDS) in 16 patients undergoing distal pancreatectomy [5]. In this cohort, Fischer et al. report significantly lower POPF rates and shorter length of stay after resection in patients undergoing TAPDS compared to 42 historical controls. The technique described in the manuscript involves identification of the pancreatic duct after transection of the gland, direct antegrade insertion of a soft pediatric feeding tube in the lumen of the duct, and confirmation of transampullary placement by palpation of the duodenum. The theoretical advantage of this approach is that it obviates the need for preoperative ERCP and the risk of post-procedural pancreatitis.

Lastly, Rieder et al. published a single-surgeon prospective study comparing a prospective cohort of 25 patients who underwent PD with preoperative endoscopic sphincterotomy and stent placement to a historical cohort of 23 patients without stent [6]. Similarly to the study of Abe et al., no POPFs were identified in the intervention group, while the historical cohort had an incidence of 22% (5/23 patients) that was statistically significant ($P = 0.02$). The groups were comparable with respect to their baseline characteristics and postoperative outcomes (other than POPF). This study should be interpreted with caution as it has several limitations. Namely, certain factors known to influence the incidence of POPF such as glad texture and duct size were not reported; the operative time was significantly longer in the controls which raises questions about surgeon's expertise or case complexity; furthermore, even though there was a significant difference in the incidence of POPF, this did not translate in a decrease in the overall morbidity, which can be at least partially explained by the addition of the morbidity related to the endoscopic sphincterotomy and stent placement [7].

A meta-analysis of five prospective studies (including the ones mentioned above) was published in abstract form in 2013. A pooled analysis of 223 patients did not show a significant difference in the rate of POPF between those with and without a PD stent. The authors concluded that pancreatic duct stents for the prevention of pancreatic duct leaks following distal pancreatectomy cannot be routinely recommended [8].

Operative Stenting of the Pancreatic Duct for Pancreaticoduodenectomy

The theoretical benefits of this technique include more precise placement of the fine stitches required to build this anastomosis and protection from leakage early in the healing stages as the pancreatic enzymes are diverted away from the interface between the pancreatic duct and the jejunal mucosa. Some groups routinely place a transanastomotic stent that is exteriorized through a Hoffmeister-type enterotomy and through the abdominal wall, while others place a short stent to drain directly into the jejunal loop used for the reconstruction.

A randomized trial published in 2006 and originating from Johns Hopkins enrolled 238 patients and randomized them to receive a stent (S) or no stent (NS) during the creation of the pancreaticojejunostomy [9]. In this trial, a 6 cm stent was placed in the pancreatic duct and left to drain in the jejunal loop where it was secured with an absorbable suture as shown in Fig. 9.2. Furthermore, they stratified patients according to pancreatic texture (soft vs. hard) as this has been shown to correlate with the risk of POPF. Their study, however, showed no difference in the incidence of POPF between the S and NS groups on either stratum. For patients with hard pancreas, the POPF rates were 2 and 5% ($P = 0.4$) for patients with and without stents, respectively. The corresponding rates for patients with soft pancreas were 21 and 11% ($P = 0.1$).

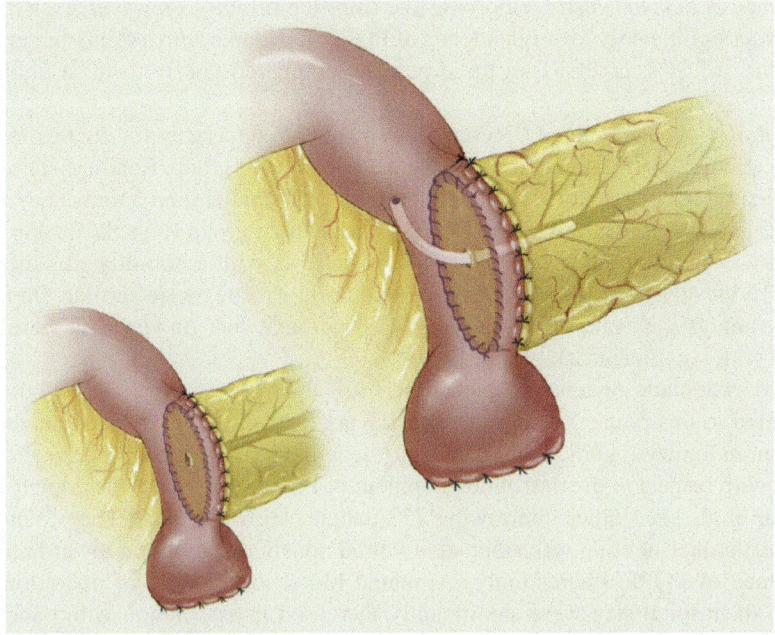

Fig. 9.2 Schematic of the placement of the pancreatic duct stent. In both illustrations, an end-to-side pancreaticojejunostomy is depicted. On the *left panel*, no stent is shown. On the *right panel*, a 6-cm-long stent is depicted, with 3 cm residing in the jejunal lumen and 3 cm residing in the pancreatic duct. The stent is secured in place with one nonabsorbable suture

Furthermore, they did not detect any difference in the severity of the POPF or the frequency with which their occurrence altered the management of the patients. Based on these data, the authors concluded that internal pancreatic duct stenting does not decrease the incidence or severity of postoperative pancreatic fistula [9].

Poon et al. published a similar trial and included 120 patients who were randomized 1:1 to have either an external stent inserted across the anastomosis to drain the pancreatic duct or no stent. They found a significantly lower pancreatic fistula rate in patients with a stent (7 vs. 20%, $P = 0.03$). Overall morbidity and mortality rates were equivalent. They performed a multivariate analysis and reported that the lack of pancreaticojejunostomy stenting and pancreatic duct diameter <3 mm were significantly associated with the development of POPF [10].

In a multicentric study conducted in France, 158 patients were randomized to either have an external transanastomotic stent placed ($n = 77$) or no stent ($n = 81$). As part of the inclusion criteria for this trial, patients had to have a soft pancreas and a small duct (diameter <3 mm). These criteria provided an enriched population of high-risk pancreata [11]. They found that the group that had a PD stent placed had a significantly lower overall PF compared to those without a stent (26 vs. 42%; $P = 0.034$). Furthermore, these findings were also associated with a decreased incidence of delayed gastric emptying and overall morbidity. However, even though there was significantly lower incidence of POPF in patients with a stent, the reported incidence of 26% of POPF in these patients compared poorly to most published series.

Motoi et al. randomized 93 consecutive patients undergoing a duct-to-mucosa pancreaticojejunostomy into a stented and a non-stented group. Randomization was stratified by the pancreatic duct diameter greater or smaller than 3 mm. They found a lower rate of clinically relevant POPF in the stented group (6 vs. 22%; $P = 0.04$) which was limited only to the subgroup of patients with a non-dilated pancreatic duct (10 vs. 40%; $P = 0.03$). Morbidity and mortality rates were similar. On multivariate analysis, elevated BMI, non-dilated pancreatic duct, and no stent were associated with significant risk of POPF.

Two systematic reviews have been performed and summarize most of the data presented to this point. Xiong et al. in 2012 pooled data from five randomized and 11 nonrandomized studies and found no benefit with the use of pancreatic duct stents with respect to the risk of development of POPF [12]. In the meta-analysis by Markar et al., six studies comprising 732 patients were included. They found that pancreatic duct stenting was associated with a nonsignificant trend toward reduced incidence of POPF. Interestingly, estimated blood loss, length of operation, and length of hospital stay were significantly increased in association with pancreatic stent placement. They concluded that there were insufficient data to confidently reject the null hypothesis that stenting has no beneficial effect [13].

Lastly, a recent multi-institutional study retrospectively evaluated a nonrandomized cohort of patients who underwent pancreaticoduodenectomy with or without stent placement at the surgeon's discretion over a 14-year period [14]. Their outcomes were stratified based on a previously validated pancreatic fistula risk score (FRS) which includes well-known and reproducible risk factors for the development of POPF, namely, soft or normal pancreatic parenchyma, non-pancreatic adenocarcinoma histology, small pancreatic duct diameter, and elevated intraoperative blood loss [15]. Approximately 18% of patients in this cohort had a transanastomotic pancreatic duct stent placed. These patients had higher median FRS (6 vs. 3; $P < 0.001$). Furthermore, they found that the incidence of clinically relevant POPF was no different in patients with low FRS. However, in the subgroup of high-risk patients (FRS 7–10), the use of a transanastomotic stent was associated with lower POPF rates (14 vs. 36%; $P = 0.03$), lower severe complication rate, and shorter hospital stay. The authors concluded that pancreatic stents may offer benefit in the group of patients at inherent high risk for anastomotic complications. While these results are enticing, this study is limited by its retrospective nature that spans over a decade during which definitions of POPF have evolved and management strategies couldn't have been adjusted for. Furthermore, the subgroup of interest (FRS 7–10) includes only 72 patients, which should raise question about adequate power to draw strong conclusions.

Author's Practice

The data presented regarding the utility of PD stenting (either internal or external) in reducing the incidence of POPF is heterogeneous and difficult to interpret. Most studies are small in nature, span different eras, and use different definitions of POPF and techniques for PD stenting. Furthermore, in some of the studies that report a benefit from pancreatic duct stenting, the fistula rates reported are exceedingly high either in the control group, the intervention group, or both. Based on the presented data, as argued in the studies by McMillan et al. [14] and Motoi et al. [16], it may be reasonable to use PD stenting in patients at high risk of POPF such as those with a small duct diameter and/or soft gland. On the other hand, for patients undergoing distal pancreatectomy, the data available don't justify the morbidity associated with an endoscopic sphincterotomy and preoperative placement of a trans-sphincteric stent. It is not our practice to place PD stents during the construction of pancreaticojejunal anastomoses or preoperatively prior to distal pancreatectomy.

Operative Drainage of the Surgical Bed

To Drain or Not to Drain?

Routine use of surgical drains after pancreatic resection is a topic of intense debate in the surgical community. Historically, most abdominal operations called for routine drain placement; however, this practice has slowly been abandoned through the years. For pancreatic resection, this practice has evolved much more slowly, given the potentially catastrophic consequences of an uncontrolled postoperative pancreatic leak. The gradual evolution to the abandonment of routine drainage was recently disrupted by the publication of a multicenter randomized controlled trial of "drain vs. no drain" which showed significantly increased morbidity and mortality in patients undergoing pancreaticoduodenectomy without drain placement [17]. This trial and other randomized studies will be reviewed here. We also included a discussion on the management of surgical drains when they are used, specifically as it pertains duration of drainage and the measurement of amylase levels.

There are now three randomized controlled trials evaluating the use of routine operative drainage after pancreatic resection. The first study published in 2001 by Conlon et al. [18] randomized 179 patients undergoing pancreatic resection (139 pancreaticoduodenectomy and 40 distal pancreatectomy) to have no drains placed ($n = 91$) or to have closed-suction drainage placed ($n = 88$).There was no difference in the incidence or type of postoperative complications between the groups. The composite endpoint of intra-abdominal fluid collection, intra-abdominal abscess, enterocutaneous fistula, and pancreatic fistula occurred more commonly in patients in the drain group (19 pts. vs. 8 pts.; $P < 0.02$), with 11/19 (12.5%) experiencing a pancreatic fistula in the drain group compared to none in the no-drain group. The authors concluded that routine placement of drains after pancreatic resection failed to reduce the incidence or severity of fistula-related morbidity, the need for additional interventional radiology-guided procedures, or the mortality rate in these procedures. A little over a decade after the publication of this randomized controlled trial, the same group published a retrospective analysis of their practice over a 5-year time period [19]. This study of 1122 patients revealed an interesting trend within our institution where of the six high-volume pancreatic surgeons, one-third were "routine drainers," one-third were "selective drainers," and one-third were "routine non-drainers." Overall, 49% of patients had undergone operative drainage, thus allowing for valuable comparisons to be made. Patients without operative drains experienced lower-grade $\geq$ 3 morbidity rates (26 vs. 33%; $P = 0.01$), shorter hospital stays (7 vs. 8 days; $P < 0.01$), fewer readmissions (20 vs. 27%; $P = 0.01$), and lower rates of clinically relevant (grade $\geq$ 3) POPF (16 vs. 20%; $P = 0.05$). Similar reoperation rates (both <1%) need for interventional radiology procedures (15% vs. 19%; $P = 0.1$), and mortality rates (2 vs. 1%; $P = 0.3$) were seen in both groups. Based on these findings, the authors concluded that the routine use of surgical drains after pancreatic resection could be safely abandoned. This study also highlighted the difficulties of changing surgical dogma. Even at the institution where the first RCT showing no benefit of routine drainage was performed, a third of pancreatic surgeons continue to routinely place intraperitoneal drains. Figure 9.3 shows the trends over time of the different surgeons in this cohort and the incidence of grade $\geq$ 3 POPF.

In 2014 Van Buren et al. published the results of a multicenter RCT that was halted before complete accrual (for patients undergoing pancreaticoduodenectomy) due to disproportionately high mortality in patients who were randomized to no drain [17]. Their publication reports the results of 137 patients randomized up to that point. In this study, the group randomized to no drain had a higher incidence of gastroparesis, fluid collection, intra-abdominal abscess (10 vs. 25%; $P = 0.027$), severe diarrhea, interventional radiology-guided procedures, and a longer duration of hospitalization. At the point of analysis, the mortality rates were 12 and 3% in

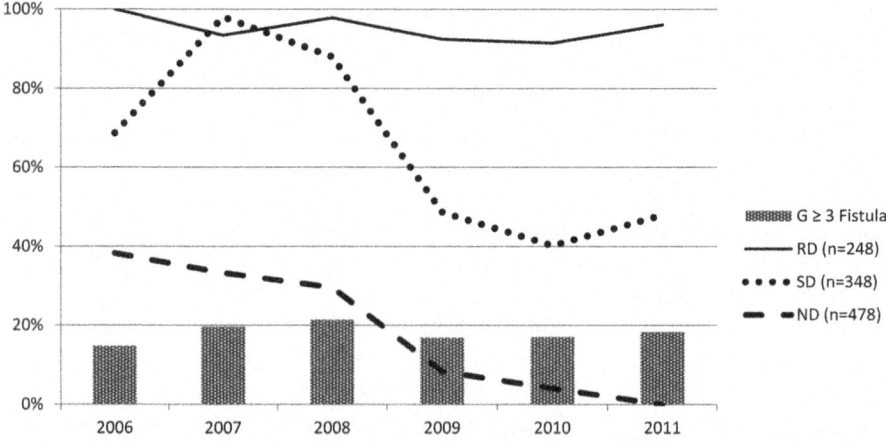

Fig. 9.3 Trends over years. *Lines:* prophylactic drainage trends over years per surgeon type. *Bars:* incidence of G $\geq$ 3 fistula overall. *RD* routine drainers, *SD* selective drainers, *ND* routine non-drainers

patients randomized to no drain and drain, respectively. Given these findings, the study was stopped, and the overall conclusion from the trial was that pancreatic resection without operative drainage was not safe.

The third and most recent RCT on prophylactic drainage after pancreatic surgery was published in 2016 from Dr. Buchler's group in Germany [20]. This non-inferiority trial randomized 395 patients undergoing pancreaticoduodenectomy between 2007 and 2015 to intra-abdominal drainage in the standard fashion versus no drainage. The primary outcome measure was re-intervention rate (re-laparotomy or interventional radiology-guided procedures). They found that re-intervention rates were not inferior in the no-drain group (drain 21%, no drain 17%; $P < 0.001$). Clinically relevant POPF was lower in the no-drain group (6 vs. 12%; $P = 0.03$) as were fistula-associated complications (13 vs. 26%; $P < 0.001$). It is important to mention, given the concerns raised by the Van Buren trial, that in-hospital mortality was the same in both groups (drain 3.0%, no drain 3.1%; $P = 0.936$) and consistent with the reported literature.

Management of Surgically Placed Drains

Beyond the decision to use prophylactic intra-abdominal drains, there are different recommendations regarding the management of these drains once placed, specifically as it pertains the duration of drainage and measurement of amylase levels. We reviewed two relevant studies addressing these questions.

Bassi et al. reported a randomized controlled trial comparing early versus late removal of surgically placed intra-abdominal drains after pancreatic resection [21]. They randomized 114 patients who had undergone pancreatic resection with intra-peritoneal drain placement and who had a low risk for pancreatic fistula as established by their institutional criteria (amylase value in drains ≤5000 U/L on postoperative day 1) to have their drains removed on postoperative day 3 (early) versus postoperative day 5 (late). They found a lower incidence of POPF (2 vs. 26%; $P < 0.001$) for patients in the early group. Other abdominal complications and pulmonary complications were also lower in the patients who underwent early drain removal. These patients also experienced shorter hospital stays and fewer readmissions. On multivariate analysis, timing of drain removal and unintentional preoperative weight loss were independent risk factors for the development of POPF. The authors concluded that operative drains should be removed on postoperative day 3 in patients who had low-drain amylase levels on postoperative day 1 given the higher incidence of postoperative complications with prolonged drainage.

Recently, the group from the Massachusetts General Hospital published their experience with routine measurement of daily amylase values in operative drains to predict the development of POPF and guide drain management [22]. In this study, they prospectively analyzed two independent cohorts of patients undergoing pancreaticoduodenectomy. In the first cohort ($n = 126$), daily amylase levels were obtained from the surgically placed drains, and POD 1 amylase was found to have the highest correlation with the development of POPF with a concordance index of

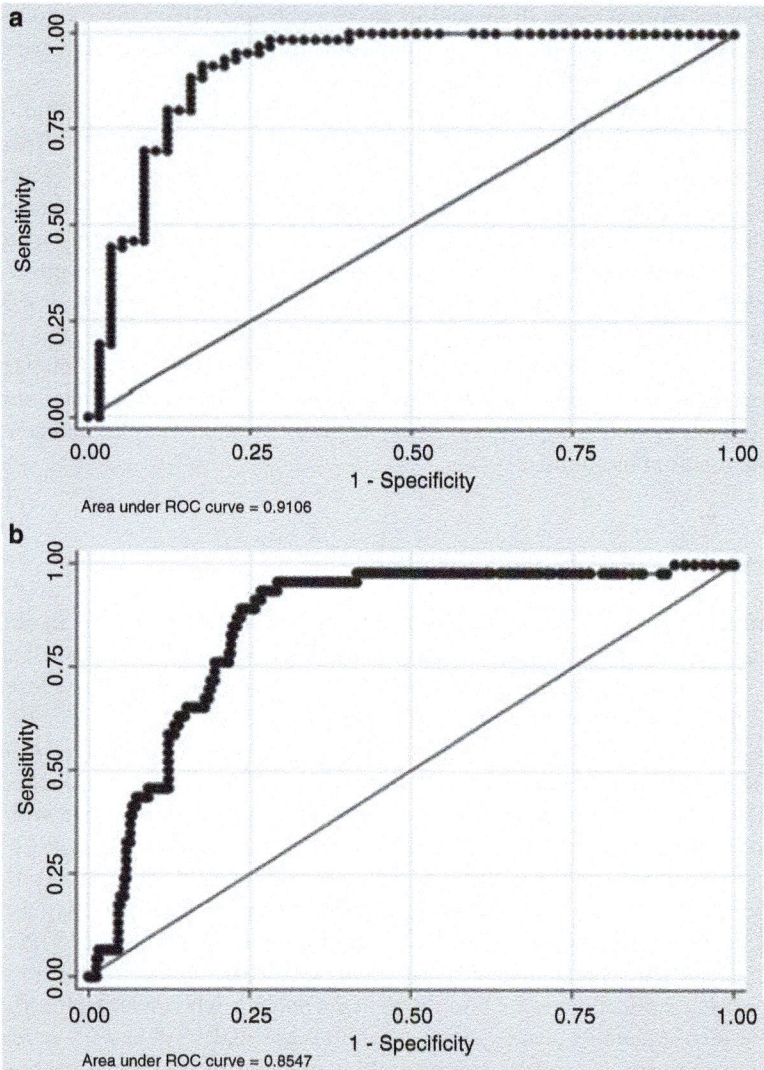

Fig. 9.4 (a) ROC curve of POD 1 drain amylase level as a predictor of PF in the training cohort of patients undergoing PD (*n* = 126), with an AUC of 0.911. Values along the *diagonal straight line* reflect no predictive ability. (b) ROC curve of POD 1 drain amylase level as a predictor of PF in the validation cohort of patients undergoing PD (*n* = 369), with an AUC of 0.855. Values along the *diagonal straight line* reflect no predictive ability

0.91 (Fig. 9.4a). A drain amylase of 612 U/L had a sensitivity of 93% and specificity of 79%. In the independent validation cohort, the observed concordance index was 0.85 (Fig. 9.4b). Postoperative day 1 drain amylase ≤600 U/L was found on 62% of patients (229/369) in this cohort. These patients had a significantly lower incidence of POPF compared to patients with amylase >600 (1 vs. 31%; $P < 0.001$; OR = 52).

On a multivariate model, amylase level on postoperative day 1 was a stronger predictor of POPF than gland texture and duct diameter. The authors concluded that surgically placed drains should be removed on postoperative day 1 in patients whose amylase level is ≤600 U/L.

Author's Practice
Surgical drains are very infrequently used in our practice, and their use is even further decreasing with time. Although we do not feel that it is inappropriate to drain, we do feel that surgeons should not feel obligated to place drains. While it is hard to argue that drains cause pancreatic leaks and POPF, the evidence suggests that they fail to improve early detection and effectively control leaks without additional drainage when they do occur. As discussed above, interventional radiology-guided procedures are not less frequent (and perhaps even more frequent) in patients with surgically placed drains, as are readmissions, mostly due to drain-related complications. It also is plausible that closed-suction drains generate enough negative pressure and disrupt tissue apposition to a degree that prevents adequate healing of the pancreaticojejunal anastomosis. We feel that the lack of abdominal drains allows patients to feel more mobile and may accelerate their recovery.

The only recent evidence to support ongoing routine drainage is the Van Buren study noted above. It is hard to reconcile these results with the randomized trial from our institution and from Heidelberg. If the increased mortality was secondary to the lack of a drain in a patient with a POPF, then it suggests that these patients were not rescued from a potentially reversible event. More than 1000 patients have undergone pancreatic resection without a drain at our center, and the operative mortality in that group is just under 2%. In the study from Heidelberg, the postoperative mortality rate was 3% in the no-drain group. Many of the participating centers in the Van Buren study were not high-volume centers, and it is unclear if the surgical expertise or interventional/endoscopic support was present to appropriately manage these patients. It is important to underscore that in the absence of drains, special attention needs to be paid to changes in vital signs, laboratory values, and physical examination so that immediate imaging and intervention can be obtained in those in whom a leak is suspected. This heightened index of suspicion and a low threshold for cross-sectional imaging are paramount for prompt recognition of pancreatic leaks which allows for timely intervention before potentially catastrophic consequences ensue.

Gastric Decompression and Jejunal Feeding Tubes

Gastric decompression with either nasogastric (NG) or orogastric (OG) tubes is commonplace in patients undergoing general anesthetic for major surgery. Historically, after major gastrointestinal procedures, postoperative NG decompression was considered a routine measure to avoid the potential consequences associated with prolonged ileus and delayed gastric emptying. This practice has been slowly abandoned with time as studies have shown no association between duration of NG decompression and surgical outcomes. However, patients undergoing major pancreatic resections are still too often subject to prolonged NG drainage due to the belief that doing so may decrease the incidence, severity, or ultimate impact of common complications such as delayed gastric emptying or POPF.

While there is little high power data evaluating this practice in pancreatic resections, here we review two recent studies that address the issue and reached similar conclusions [23, 24]. In a prospective study from Baylor College of Medicine, Fisher et al. evaluated 100 consecutive patients undergoing pancreatic resection (64 pancreaticoduodenectomy and 36 distal pancreatectomy). All patients had NG placed at the time of surgery, but only the first 50 patients kept it postoperatively. The groups were adequately balanced, and they found no difference in outcomes including delayed gastric emptying, anastomotic leak, wound complications, or respiratory complications. The rate of postoperative placement or replacement of NG tubes was similar between the groups (4 vs. 8%; $P = 0.7$). The authors conclude that it is safe to selectively use postoperative NG decompression only in patients with a clear indication [23]. In a similar study from UT Southwestern, Roland et al. reported their outcomes after 231 consecutive pancreatectomies. Two-thirds of their patients had routine NG placement in the OR, while in the latter third of their cohort, OG tubes were placed for surgery but removed prior to extubation. Reinsertion was required in 19% of patients in either arm, and their outcomes (including minor or major morbidity and length of stay) were similar, underscoring the author's conclusion fact that the routine use of NG tubes can be safely avoided after pancreatic resection.

Author's Practice
Routine postoperative NG decompression is not used in our practice unless there is a clear indication for it (e.g., previous GI obstruction, diabetic gastroparesis, etc.). Nearly every patient will have the NG tube removed at the time of extubation or on the morning of postoperative day 1.

Jejunostomy Feeding Tubes

Routine placement of surgical jejunostomy tubes (JT) at the time of pancreatic resection was historically justified by the high incidence of POPF and the inability to provide enteral nutrition while avoiding stimulation of pancreatic enzyme release and activation. In that setting, a JT placed intraoperatively constituted a lifeline that allowed for nutritional support even in the ambulatory setting while avoiding the need for parenteral nutrition and its potential complications. Lower incidence of POPF and ready access to bedside or radiology-guided nasojejunal (NJ) tube placement, or endoscopically placed JT in modern-day practices, make the routine placement of JTs unnecessary and potentially hazardous.

Nussbaum et al. recently reported outcomes of 126 patients who had operatively placed JT at the time of pancreaticoduodenectomy at a major hepatobiliary center [25]. In this cohort, 14% of patients developed a complication directly related to the feeding tube (i.e., pericatheter infection, pneumatosis intestinalis, severe feeding tube intolerance, and catheter malfunction); 50% of these patients (7% of total cohort) required a reoperation. A second study by Zhu et al. compared the effectiveness of JT and NJ tubes [26]. This study showed better outcomes in patients who had NJ tubes. Specifically, these patients had a lower incidence of intestinal obstruction and catheter-related complications. Feeding tube removal time and length of hospital stay were significantly shorter in patients with NJ tubes. The authors concluded that the use of NJ feeding tubes is safer than JTs.

Author's Practice
We do not routinely use NJ or JT feeding tubes. In the case of inability of oral intake by POD 7–10 due to persistent DGE or concern for uncontrolled POPF, a NJ is usually placed as a bridge to resumption of oral intake. In patients with prolonged DGE, an endoscopically placed JT can be placed to allow for enteral feeding, while the DGE resolves.

Conclusions

The latest generation of surgeons has seen a phenomenal evolution of the practice of pancreatic resection, which has gone from highly morbid and rarely performed to safe and widely available at high-volume centers. In addition, there has been a concomitant shift in the application of the use of biliary and pancreatic stents and drains. However, major pancreatic resection still carries measurable morbidity and mortality, and the systematic, judicious analysis of individual center's outcomes is germane to continued improvement. It is important that care be directed by the highest-quality data available, and in areas where there isn't high-quality data, every effort must be made to generate that data. Furthermore, surgeons should strive to limit our bias and openly interpret and apply scientific evidence as it becomes available.

References

1. van der Gaag NA, Rauws EA, van Eijck CH, Bruno MJ, van der Harst E, Kubben FJ, et al. Preoperative biliary drainage for cancer of the head of the pancreas. N Engl J Med. 2010;362(2):129–37.
2. Fang Y, Gurusamy KS, Wang Q, Davidson BR, Lin H, Xie X, et al. Pre-operative biliary drainage for obstructive jaundice. Cochrane Database Syst Rev. 2012;9:CD005444.
3. Abe N, Sugiyama M, Suzuki Y, Yamaguchi T, Mori T, Atomi Y. Preoperative endoscopic pancreatic stenting: a novel prophylactic measure against pancreatic fistula after distal pancreatectomy. J Hepato-Biliary-Pancreat Surg. 2008;15(4):373–6.
4. Bassi C, Dervenis C, Butturini G, Fingerhut A, Yeo C, Izbicki J, et al. Postoperative pancreatic fistula: an international study group (ISGPF) definition. Surgery. 2005;138(1):8–13.
5. Fischer CP, Bass B, Fahy B, Aloia T. Transampullary pancreatic duct stenting decreases pancreatic fistula rate following left pancreatectomy. Hepato-Gastroenterology. 2008;55(81):244–8.

6. Rieder B, Krampulz D, Adolf J, Pfeiffer A. Endoscopic pancreatic sphincterotomy and stenting for preoperative prophylaxis of pancreatic fistula after distal pancreatectomy. Gastrointest Endosc. 2010;72(3):536–42.
7. Dumonceau JM. Distal pancreatectomy: another indication for prophylactic pancreatic stenting? Gastrointest Endosc. 2010;72(3):543–5.
8. Alkaade S, Abu Dayyeh BK, Baron TH. Meta-analysis of preoperative placement of pancreatic stents to prevent postoperative leaks after distal pancreatectomy. Gastrointest Endosc. 2013;77(5):AB382.
9. Winter JM, Cameron JL, Campbell KA, Chang DC, Riall TS, Schulick RD, et al. Does pancreatic duct stenting decrease the rate of pancreatic fistula following pancreaticoduodenectomy? Results of a prospective randomized trial. J Gastrointest Surg. 2006;10(9):1280–90.
10. Poon RT, Fan ST, Lo CM, Ng KK, Yuen WK, Yeung C, et al. External drainage of pancreatic duct with a stent to reduce leakage rate of pancreaticojejunostomy after pancreaticoduodenectomy: a prospective randomized trial. Ann Surg. 2007;246(3):425–33. discussion 33–5
11. Pessaux P, Sauvanet A, Mariette C, Paye F, Muscari F, Cunha AS, et al. External pancreatic duct stent decreases pancreatic fistula rate after pancreaticoduodenectomy: prospective multicenter randomized trial. Ann Surg. 2011;253(5):879–85.
12. Xiong JJ, Altaf K, Mukherjee R, Huang W, Hu WM, Li A, et al. Systematic review and meta-analysis of outcomes after intraoperative pancreatic duct stent placement during pancreaticoduodenectomy. Pancreas. 2012;41(8):1413–4.
13. Markar SR, Vyas S, Karthikesalingam A, Imber C, Malago M. The impact of pancreatic duct drainage following Pancreaticojejunostomy on clinical outcome. J Gastrointest Surg. 2012;16(8):1610–7.
14. McMillan MT, Ecker BL, Behrman SW, Callery MP, Christein JD, Drebin JA, et al. Externalized stents for pancreatoduodenectomy provide value only in high-risk scenarios. J Gastrointest Surg. 2016;20(12):2052–62.
15. Callery MP, Pratt WB, Kent TS, Chaikof EL, Vollmer CM Jr. A prospectively validated clinical risk score accurately predicts pancreatic fistula after pancreatoduodenectomy. J Am Coll Surg. 2013;216(1):1–14.
16. Motoi F, Egawa S, Rikiyama T, Katayose Y, Unno M. Randomized clinical trial of external stent drainage of the pancreatic duct to reduce postoperative pancreatic fistula after pancreaticojejunostomy. Br J Surg. 2012;99(4):524–31.
17. Van Buren G 2nd, Bloomston M, Hughes SJ, Winter J, Behrman SW, Zyromski NJ, et al. A randomized prospective multicenter trial of pancreaticoduodenectomy with and without routine intraperitoneal drainage. Ann Surg. 2014;259(4):605–12.
18. Conlon KC, Labow D, Leung D, Smith A, Jarnagin W, Coit DG, et al. Prospective randomized clinical trial of the value of intraperitoneal drainage after pancreatic resection. Ann Surg. 2001;234(4):487–93. discussion 93–4
19. Correa-Gallego C, Brennan MF, D'Angelica M, Fong Y, Dematteo RP, Kingham TP, et al. Operative drainage following pancreatic resection: analysis of 1122 patients resected over 5 years at a single institution. Ann Surg. 2013;258(6):1051–8.
20. Witzigmann H, Diener MK, Kienkotter S, Rossion I, Bruckner T, Barbel W, et al. No need for routine drainage after pancreatic head resection: the dual-center, randomized, controlled PANDRA trial (ISRCTN04937707). Ann Surg. 2016;264(3):528–37.
21. Bassi C, Molinari E, Malleo G, Crippa S, Butturini G, Salvia R, et al. Early versus late drain removal after standard pancreatic resections: results of a prospective randomized trial. Ann Surg. 2010;252(2):207–14.
22. Ven Fong Z, Correa-Gallego C, Ferrone CR, Veillette GR, Warshaw AL, Lillemoe KD, et al. Early drain removal--the middle ground between the drain versus no drain debate in patients undergoing pancreaticoduodenectomy: a prospective validation study. Ann Surg. 2015;262(2):378–83.
23. Fisher WE, Hodges SE, Cruz G, Artinyan A, Silberfein EJ, Ahern CH, et al. Routine nasogastric suction may be unnecessary after a pancreatic resection. HPB. 2011;13(11):792–6.

24. Roland CL, Mansour JC, Schwarz RE. Routine nasogastric decompression is unnecessary after pancreatic resections. Arch Surg. 2012;147(3):287–9.
25. Nussbaum DP, Zani S, Penne K, Speicher PJ, Stinnett SS, Clary BM, et al. Feeding jejunostomy tube placement in patients undergoing pancreaticoduodenectomy: an ongoing dilemma. J Gastrointest Surg. 2014;18(10):1752–9.
26. Zhu X, Wu Y, Qiu Y, Jiang C, Ding Y. Comparative analysis of the efficacy and complications of nasojejunal and jejunostomy on patients undergoing pancreaticoduodenectomy. JPEN J Parenter Enteral Nutr. 2014;38(8):996–1002.

Strategies for Prevention and Treatment of Pancreatic Fistula

10

Priya M. Puri and Charles M. Vollmer Jr.

Introduction

Historically, pancreatic surgery was generally avoided due to its technical difficulties and high mortality and morbidity rates. However, in recent decades, mortality rates after pancreatectomy have decreased to less than 5% [1, 2]. This can be attributed to the development of high-volume, specialized pancreatic centers, as well as innovations in surgical techniques and perioperative management [3, 4]. Despite this progress, however, the incidence of postoperative morbidity remains high and can range from 30–60% [1]. Delayed gastric emptying, post-pancreatectomy hemorrhage, and pancreatic fistula are the three major procedure-specific complications associated with pancreatic surgery [5–7]. Postoperative pancreatic fistula (POPF) is considered the most common of these and the most significant determinant of postoperative morbidity and mortality associated with major pancreatic resections. [2, 8, 9]. POPF leads to increased length of hospital stay and resource utilization and thus has a significant economic impact on healthcare systems [10–12].

Definition of Pancreatic Fistula

A general definition of pancreatic fistula is an abnormal communication between the pancreatic ductal epithelium and another surface containing pancreas-derived, degradative enzyme-rich fluid [5]. Reported POPF incidence ranges from 2% to 33% [13–18]. The significant variability in this incidence can be attributed, in part, to the broad spectrum of its historical definitions [19]. This dilemma was addressed in 2005, when the International Study Group of Pancreatic Fistula (ISGPF) – an international panel of

P.M. Puri • C.M. Vollmer Jr. (✉)
Department of Surgery, University of Pennsylvania Perelman School of Medicine,
Philadelphia, PA, USA
e-mail: Charles.Vollmer@uphs.upenn.edu

© Springer International Publishing AG 2018
F.G. Rocha, P. Shen (eds.), *Optimizing Outcomes for Liver and Pancreas Surgery*, DOI 10.1007/978-3-319-62624-6_10

high-volume pancreatic surgical experts – convened to establish a universal definition of POPF by consensus [5]. According to the ISGPF, a broad definition of POPF is "output via an operatively placed drain (or a subsequently placed, percutaneous drain) of any measurable volume of drain fluid on or after postoperative day 3, with an amylase content greater than 3 times the upper normal serum value."[5] The ISGPF defined POPF based on a tiered clinical grading system, dividing pancreatic fistulas into grades A, B, and C. Grade A fistulas are biochemical leaks and cause little, if any, deviation from the normal clinical course. These asymptomatic leaks are the most common fistula in most series and are characterized by a threshold of elevated (>3× the upper limit of normal serum amylase concentration) drain amylase only. Grades B and C fistulas, on the other hand, deviate from the expected clinical course. They are often a major source of morbidity and are thus categorized as clinically relevant fistulas (CR-POPF). Among CR-POPF, grade C fistulas are more severe (but less common) than grade B and are characterized by at least one of three qualifiers: an operative intervention under general anesthesia, some element of organ failure, or fistula-attributed death. Table 10.1 depicts the ISGPF clinical grading system, based on the following nine criteria: clinical conditions, specific treatment, ultrasound (US) or computed tomography (CT) findings, persistent drainage, death related to POPF, signs of infections, sepsis, and readmission [5]. Because the ISGPF grading system is defined according to the clinical impact on the patient's hospital course, it cannot be used as a predictive measure and can only be accurately ascribed once the patient's clinical course has been fully developed [3]. However, the new standardized definition has allowed for the systematic investigation of risk factors [8]. While the original proposal has been one of the most widely cited contributions to modern pancreatic surgery, it has recently been revisited and further refined [20].

Risk Factors for Pancreatic Fistula

Numerous risk factors have historically been cited for the development of pancreatic fistula, including endogenous, perioperative, and operative contributions [1]. The relevance of each of these risk factors varies depending on the type of major

Table 10.1 ISGPF parameters for POPF grading

Parameter	Grade A	Grade B	Grade C
Clinical state	Well	Often well	Ill appearing/bad
Specific treatment[a]	No	Yes/no	Yes
US/CT	Negative	Negative/positive	Positive
Drainage beyond 3 weeks[b]	No	Usually yes	Yes
Reoperation	No	No	Yes
POPF-related death	No	No	Possibly yes
Signs of infections	No	Yes	Yes
Sepsis	No	No	Yes
Readmission	No	Yes/no	Yes/no

Adapted from Bassi et al. [5]
[a]Partial (peripheral) or total parenteral nutrition, antibiotics, enteral nutrition, somatostatin analog, and/or minimal invasive drainage
[b]With or without a drain in situ

pancreatic resection [14]. However, the ISGPF consensus definition does not differentiate between fistulas origination from various types of pancreatic resections – despite their fundamental biological differences [1, 14]. Although POPF occurs less frequently after pancreatoduodenectomy (22–26%), compared with distal pancreatectomy (30%), it is associated with a greater average complication burden [14, 21]. Much of the fistula literature is focused on POPF after pancreatoduodenectomy (PD). Thus, a majority of this section will be focused on risk factors for POPF after PD. A brief section later in this chapter will be dedicated to POPF after distal pancreatectomy (DP), where risk factor elucidation has been more elusive.

Risk factors for the development of POPF after PD fall into three general categories including endogenous influences such as age, cardiovascular comorbidities, diabetes mellitus, gender, disease pathology, pancreatic duct diameter, and pancreatic remnant texture; perioperative factors, including neoadjuvant therapy and the use of prophylactic somatostatin analogs; and operative drivers such as anastomotic technique, intraoperative blood loss, operative time, drain placement, and the use of transanastomotic stents [1].

Endogenous Factors

Age
Increasing age is known to contribute to the severity of other endogenous risk factors that correlate with increased incidence of CR-POPF, such as fatty infiltration [22]. Thus, advanced age can be seen as an important secondary risk factor contributing to the development of CR-POPF [1].

Cardiovascular Comorbidities
There is evidence that patients with coronary artery disease have a significantly higher risk for developing POPF. Contrarily, hypertension is thought to be a protective factor against it. Despite these trends, larger cohort studies are necessary to provide better insight into coronary artery disease as a risk factor and hypertension as a protective factor for the development of POPF.

Diabetes Mellitus
The literature surrounding diabetes as a contributor to fistula development offers contradictory results, with some studies suggesting diabetes as a risk factor, while others suggesting it as a protective factor. Though there is no general consensus, logical connections can be drawn between the presence of diabetes and how it may reduce the risk of fistula development [1]. Diabetic patients have less fat and more fibrosis in their pancreas compared to nondiabetic patients. It is known that fibrotic glands hold suture more effectively, and thus the pancreatic fibrosis induced by diabetes may explain the reduced fistula risk in such patients [23]. A post-ISGPF study supported this conclusion, reporting that diabetic patients were more likely to have a firm pancreatic gland and a decreased incidence of CR-POPF [24].

Gender

Though male gender is often reported to be correlated with elevated fistula rates, there is a lack of substantial evidence of its role as a prominent risk factor for fistula development [1].

Disease Pathology

Disease pathology is recognized as an important contributor to fistula development and, depending on the histology, can either escalate or diminish the risk of fistula [1]. Several studies have shown that patients with chronic pancreatitis and pancreatic adenocarcinoma had lower fistula rates than did patients with ampullary cancer, bile duct cancer, duodenal neoplasms, or cystic neoplasms [18, 25–28]. A possible explanation for this finding is that patients with pancreatitis and pancreatic adenocarcinoma generally have firm glands and dilated ducts, two factors that are favorable for anastomotic connection, thereby reducing the risk of fistula development. Most other pathologies tend to have soft glands and small ducts, which are known to increase fistula risk [8].

Pancreatic Duct Diameter

Much of the literature demonstrates that a small or narrow pancreatic duct diameter ($\leq$ 3 mm) is perhaps the most significant risk factor for fistula development [1, 18, 29]. Small diameter ducts are associated with greater pancreatic juice output volume, have a greater probability of constriction, and can accommodate a limited number of sutures – all increasing the risk of fistula development [30, 31]. Furthermore, it has been reported that each 1 mm increment decrease in duct size is associated with a discrete increase in CR-POPF risk [8]. Additionally, small duct size is also strongly correlated to other fistula risk factors, such as fatty pancreas and soft glands [23]. The coexistence of a diminutive duct and soft gland can significantly elevate the risk of pancreatic fistula.

Pancreatic Remnant Texture

Soft pancreatic gland texture is perhaps the most widely recognized risk factor of POPF [23, 32]. This can be explained by several factors including the belief that soft glands are a) unable to hold suture as effectively as firm glands, b) often associated with small main ducts, and c) more likely to retain robust exocrine function than are firm glands [8]. One study indicates that soft pancreas, total pancreatic fat, and BMI are significantly associated with each other, and all can be linked to the development of CR-POPF [23]. Moreover, several investigations have demonstrated soft pancreatic parenchyma as a major risk factor for CR-POPF, indicating that it can differentiate between biochemical and clinically relevant fistulas [33]. Because soft pancreatic parenchyma is an extremely strong predictor of CR-POPF, it is a central component of more advanced fistula risk metrics [8, 34].

Perioperative Influences

Neoadjuvant Therapy

Several studies have concluded that patients who have undergone neoadjuvant therapy – chemo +/– radiation – have reduced occurrence of pancreatic fistula [35–37]. A possible biological explanation for this trend is that preoperative radiation damages acinar cells, thereby decreasing exocrine secretion and reducing the volume of pancreatic juice that comes into contact with the anastomosis or, alternatively, by creating fibrosis [35, 38]. That being said, because of the severe side effects of radiation, neoadjuvant therapy should not be administered to patients without a malignant condition just because it is protective factor against pancreatic fistula [39]. Furthermore, although neoadjuvant therapy is associated with a lower overall fistula occurrence, further, better-designed studies are necessary to elucidate its impact on CR-POPF, especially since its use is highly correlated to the presence of protective factors like pancreatic cancer.

Operative Factors

Intraoperative Blood Loss

Elevated intraoperative blood loss is a well-established risk factor for fistula. Furthermore, studies have shown that *excessive* intraoperative blood loss is a significant risk factor for CR-POPF. In fact, blood loss is considered a risk factor for values as low as 400 ml. Blood loss can be categorized into tiers, with each sequential tier representing escalating risk [8, 18].This categorization system has been validated [40].

Operative Time

PD is a complex procedure, with an inherently long operative time, ranging from 4–6 h for uncomplicated cases. A multivariate analysis in one study revealed operating time of ≥285 min to be a significant predictor for pancreatic fistula [27]. Other studies have shown operative time to be significant in univariate analyses only [32, 41]. A possible explanation for this is that operative time is highly correlated with intraoperative blood loss [1].

Putting It All Together for PD

Assessing the true impact of each of these risk factors was difficult before the advent of the universal, consensus-driven definition for pancreatic fistula established by the ISGPF in 2005, which differentiates between biochemical fistula and CR-POPF. Since then, several attempts have been made to comprehensively assess CR-POPF risk – to determine which factors contribute most to fistula risk and how to infer an individual patient's aggregate risk [1]. Ultimately, this culminated in the development of the Fistula Risk Score (FRS). The FRS is an externally validated system for the prediction of CR-POPF after PD, resulting from an extensive multivariate analysis of 54 endogenous, perioperative, and operative risk variables [8, 40]. Following a regression analysis, four significant risk factors emerged: soft gland texture, high-risk pathology (anything other than pancreatic adenocarcinoma or pancreatitis), small pancreatic duct diameter (<5 mm), and elevated intraoperative blood loss (>400 ml). These factors were then weighted and assigned quantitative values, as shown in Table 10.2.

Table 10.2 The Fistula Risk Score for the prediction of CR-POPF after pancreatoduodenectomy

Risk factor	Parameter	Quantitative value
Gland texture	Firm	0
	Soft	2
Pathology	Pancreatic adenocarcinoma or pancreatitis	0
	Ampullary, duodenal, cystic, islet cell, etc.	1
Pancreatic duct diameter (mm)	≥5	0
	4	1
	3	2
	2	3
	≤1	4
Intraoperative blood loss (ml)	≤400	0
	401–700	1
	701–1000	2
	>1000	3
		Total score 0–10

Adapted from Callery et al. [8]

The values assigned to these four risk factors can then be aggregated to create a simple scoring system on a scale from 0 to 10, spanning over four discrete zones, with 0 indicating negligible risk, 1–2 low risk, 3–6 moderate risk, and 7–10 high risk [40]. The FRS system allows for the simple assessment of individual patients' CR-POPF risk after PD at an important point of time – intraoperatively, when the anastomosis is created and decisions regarding mitigation strategies begin.

Risk Factors for Distal Pancreatectomy

Though there are numerous identified risk factors for POPF development following DP, the aggregate risk has not been fully explored, and an analogous risk score system like the FRS has not been developed for POPF risk following DP [42]. Reasons for this may be a dearth of studies with high patient accrual that specifically assess pancreatic fistula risk factors for DP (an operation performed with one-third of the frequency of PD) and the fact that few studies have assessed every major known risk factor [1]. Nonetheless, it is important to note the various risk factors associated with fistula development following DP. These drivers can be divided into endogenous factors and operative variables. Younger age is reported to be a risk factor for fistula following DP, with one study showing that patients younger than 65 were around three times more likely to develop a CR-POPF [43]. A possible explanation for this is that exocrine function decreases with aging, resulting in a lower risk for fistula [43, 44]. Obesity and elevated BMI are also common risk factors associated with fistula development after DP, which is probable because BMI is also strongly correlated with other known risk factors such as total pancreatic fat and soft pancreatic parenchyma [23, 33, 42]. Fistula risk associated with DP might also be dependent on disease pathology, with pancreatic disease pathologies, such as pancreatic adenocarcinoma and chronic pancreatitis, associated with lower risk than non-pancreatic disease pathologies, such as gastric adenocarcinoma and renal carcinoma [45]. A large-volume pancreatic remnant is another reported risk factor for CR-POPF development [46].

One operative risk for fistula development following DP is the method of closure. However, this risk factor is still highly debated, with several studies citing non-stapler closure as a risk factor, while others suggesting the opposite, and others yet finding no significant differences between stapled and non-stapled closure [1]. A less controversial operative risk factor is ligation of the main pancreatic duct. Quite obviously, failure to ligate the main pancreatic duct is known to be associated with increased risk of fistula [43, 47, 48]. However, while often described in the literature as "risk factors," these might more rightly be conceived as mitigation strategies (chosen at the behest of the surgeon) rather than innate causes of CR-POPF. Duration of operation is another risk factor for fistula development following DP, with an increased operative time of >210 min as a strong predictor for fistula development in one study [49]. Lastly, site of transection is another consideration. Transection at the body has been found to be associated with higher pancreatic fistula rates in comparison to transection at the neck of the pancreas [49].

Mitigation Strategies: "Prevention as Management"

Postoperative care following PD is challenged with the difficulties of managing pancreatic fistula, which is considered to be the most difficult and resolute complication in pancreatic surgery [29]. We believe the best management strategy is to never develop a fistula in the first place. The FRS has become a valuable yet simple tool for the assessment of individual CR-POPF risk after PD and allows surgeons to make risk-adjusted decisions regarding its management. The primary and ultimate goal is "prevention as management" – to utilize this established tool in order to obviate the occurrence, and minimize the impact, of pancreatic fistula. Putative prevention and mitigation strategies include technical factors (i.e., the type of reconstruction and/or the anastomotic technique), as well as technological factors such as the use of prophylactic somatostatin analogs, tissue sealants, autologous tissue patches, transanastomotic stents, and the selective utilization of intraperitoneal drains.

Type of Reconstruction

The two primary types of reconstructive techniques following PD are pancreaticojejunostomy (PJ) and pancreaticogastrostomy (PG), with PJ being the traditional and most widely used method. This technique unites the remnant pancreatic tissue with the jejunum, thereby reestablishing enteric flow of pancreatic juice [29]. PG, on the other hand, was first introduced in clinical practice by Waugh and Clagett in 1946. There are several potential advantages of PG when compared to the classical PJ: the proximity of the stomach to the pancreas enables tension-free anastomosis; the thick gastric wall and the exceptional blood supply to the stomach improve anastomotic healing; and lastly, the gastric acid of the stomach can inactivate pancreatic enzymes and can thereby prevent disruption of the anastomosis [50]. Numerous studies have attempted to draw comparisons between fistula rates following PG versus those following PJ, the most notable of which was by Yeo et al. who conducted a randomized trial comparing PG and PJ in 145 consecutive patients undergoing PD. Results from this study showed no significant difference in pancreatic fistula incidence between PG and PJ reconstruction (12.3% for PG and 11.1% for PJ) [41].This is supported by other prospective studies that have also found comparable fistula rates between the two anastomotic techniques [51, 52]. In contrast, other notable randomized studies reported results indicating that PG is beneficial for mitigating the occurrence of CR-POPF [53, 54]. Despite this, meta-analyses still conclude that there is inadequate evidence to prove PG advantage over PJ for fistula mitigation [55]. However, the importance of risk-based evaluation of mitigation strategies is essential. A recent study specifically characterizing high-risk pancreatic anastomoses during pancreato-duodenectomy found that PG anastomosis was associated with a higher rate of CR-POPF [56]. In this study, PG – a generally less commonly utilized reconstruction technique [57] – was chosen at a significantly higher rate in high FRS risk (FRS 7–10) patients than in lower-risk (FRS 0–6) patients [56]. Because of this, it is suggested that in high-risk scenarios, surgeons should adhere to the reconstruction techniques that they practice routinely [58].

Anastomotic Technique

The type of PJ anastomosis technique is another important factor to consider in regard to fistula mitigation, i.e., duct-to-mucosa PJ versus invagination PJ. The duct-to-mucosa anastomosis involves sewing the pancreatic duct directly to the bowel mucosa, while the invagination anastomosis joins the pancreatic parenchyma and external capsule into the bowel [29]. Though the duct-to-mucosa PJ technique was originally considered to be associated with lower fistula rates compared to the invagination PJ technique, a more recent randomized trial found lower fistula rates with the invagination PJ technique [26, 59–63]. These findings held true after multivariate analysis and even the rates of grade B CR-POPF were lower for patients in the invagination cohort (5 vs. 14%, $p = 0.03$) [59]. Despite these findings, additional studies are needed to establish the most efficacious anastomotic technique after PD. Neither approach has been found to be superior when judged by the FRS in a risk-adjusted analysis [56].

Additionally, Roux-en-Y reconstruction (RYR) has recently been compared to conventional loop reconstruction (CLR). RYR uses separate jejunal limbs, separating the pancreatic anastomosis from the biliary anastomosis [61, 64]. Although it is logical to reason that RYR may limit the activation of pancreatic enzymes by biliary secretion and thereby reduce POPF risk, no significant differences have been found in fistula rates with RYR compared to CLR [65, 66]. Given its relative infrequent application worldwide, the Roux approach has not yet been subject to analysis by the FRS.

Lastly, mitigation strategies involving the absence of a pancreaticoenteric anastomosis include duct occlusion and total pancreatectomy. Duct occlusion, however, is used infrequently and has not been proven especially effective [67]. A total pancreatectomy – the complete removal of the pancreas – is only considered in extremely high-risk situations, as it is associated with absolute endocrine and exocrine insufficiency [68]. This is often employed as a "salvage" alternative to manage a severe fistula once it has manifest but is usually fraught with high mortality. Thus, when evaluating reconstruction type, it is essential to assess each patient's individual risk.

The Use of Prophylactic Somatostatin Analogs

In addition to the aforementioned operative factors, numerous technological mitigation strategies also exist. These include the use of prophylactic somatostatin analogs, tissue sealants, autologous tissue patches, transanastomotic stents, and intraperitoneal drains. Some surgeons advocate the perioperative administration of prophylactic octreotide in the hope of preventing or decreasing the severity of fistula. The predicted effect of somatostatin analogs is to reduce the volume of fistula output, thereby potentially mitigating the natural course [69]. Their use, however, is controversial. While several randomized trials are in favor of the use of prophylactic somatostatin analogs, others oppose it [29]. Furthermore, a systematic review and meta-analysis of these showed no conclusive evidence of a significant advantage with this practice. This can be explained not only by the small sample sizes of the studies but also by the fact that the studies were published between 1990 and 2009 and therefore lacked a consistent definition of POPF [70]. Though the ambiguous results are largely due to the historically liberal definition of fistula, [19] they persist even in a Cochrane Review conducted in the current era using the rigorous ISGPF definition [71]. In fact, an analysis of a large clinical series subjected to the FRS revealed octreotide to confer harm, perhaps paradoxically, as risk for CR-POPF escalated [72]. Alternatively, a recent randomized trial has proposed that the somatostatin analog pasireotide may provide clinical value; however, it requires multicenter validation yet, is costly (around $3000/case), and is not readily available to most clinicians. Because there is no solid evidence for the advantages of somatostatin analogs yet, we suggest they should not be a primary preventative measure in mitigating POPF [3].

Tissue Sealants and Patches

Currently, the literature surrounding the benefits of using tissue sealants in the prevention of POPF is conflicting. Overall, there is no conclusive evidence from randomized trials that application of fibrin glue sealant to the surface of a pancreatic anastomosis reduces the incidence of POPF after PD [73, 74]. In regard to the potential mitigation effects of autologous tissue patches, some retrospective studies conclude that this strategy is associated with a lower incidence of POPF after both PD and DP. However, further, more robustly designed, randomized trials are necessary to validate these introductory results [75, 76].

Transanastomotic Stents

Some surgeons recommend the placement of transanastomotic stents (either internal or external) as a potential mitigation strategy against POPF. Several rationales exist for this, including diversion of proteolytic enzymes from the anastomotic site, decompression of the pancreatic remnant, and facilitation of precise suturing of the anastomosis [77]. However, much of the literature on transanastomotic stent placement is controversial. Two randomized controlled trials found no benefit to fistula mitigation from the use of internal stents [78, 79]. Furthermore, one retrospective study using risk adjustment with the FRS found that the use of stents, primarily internal stents, may have led to short-term and long-term adverse outcomes in patients, particularly those with elevated POPF risk [80].

While the majority of data suggest that internal stents have little, or negative effect on fistula occurrence, external stents appear to be beneficial in reducing CR-POPF incidence. This may be because external stents are less likely to migrate than internal stents, which are shorter and not fixed in place [1]. Secondly, external stents may be more effective at diverting pancreatic secretion away from the anastomotic site [81]. Third, they may facilitate more precise suture placement. Meta-analyses of several randomized control trials suggest a lower incidence of POPF with the use of external stents. However, many of these studies failed to account for other POPF risk factors, and a more recent, retrospective study used the FRS for risk adjustment to compare CR-POPF occurrence between patients who received an external stent versus those who received no stent [77]. Results from this study revealed that among patients who received an external stent, only those in the high CR-POPF risk zone (FRS 7–10) demonstrated significantly reduced rates of CR-POPF [77]. In fact, the indiscriminate use of external stents in lesser risk scenarios conferred worse outcomes. This study sheds light upon the benefits of risk stratification and its importance in evaluating the efficacy of fistula mitigation strategies.

Intraperitoneal Drain Placement

Routine placement of intraperitoneal drains is another fistula mitigation strategy that, though having been a conventional approach during PD, is now increasingly questioned in regard to its value. Drains are used in an attempt to evacuate blood, bile, chyle, or pancreatic juice that may accumulate after surgery [1]. However, the perceived clinical benefit of routine drain placement has been a challenged because of its perceived lack of value in other gastrointestinal surgeries [82–85] as well as concerns about infection, trauma to visceral tissues, and erosion at the anastomotic site [86]. Several retrospective studies attempting to understand this have produced mixed results [86, 87]. One randomized control trial found drains to be unnecessary and potentially harmful, increasing the risk of POPF development [88]. It is important to note that this study, and many of the previous ones, was conducted in the pre-ISGPF era. They therefore lacked a precise definition of POPF, conflating biochemical fistulas and clinically relevant fistulas. A recent, randomized controlled trial attempted to address this. The objective of this study was to test the hypothesis that PD without the use of routine intraperitoneal drainage does not increase the frequency or severity of complications. It was found that the elimination of drains in PD increases the frequency and severity of complications. Notably, this study was terminated early by the Data Safety Monitoring Board due to an extremely high mortality rate in patients undergoing PD without intraperitoneal drainage [89].

A follow-up analysis of this particular randomized control trial aimed to understand the frequency and severity of CR-POPFs after PD, specifically, in the context of fistula risk using the FRS. It was found that patients with moderate (FRS 3–6) and high risk (FRS 7–10) had significantly fewer CR-POPFs when intraperitoneal drains were used. Furthermore, CR-POPFs among this moderate- and high-risk patient group were more severe – with longer hospital stays, higher rates of grade C CR-POPF, and a 21% higher mortality rate when drains were not used. In the roughly 30% of patients with negligible and low risk (FRS 0–2), drain placement offered no benefits and in fact resulted in higher CR-POPF incidence, though the difference was not statistically significant in an underpowered sample size [90]. Based on this study, it is suggested that patients undergoing PD can be individually stratified by FRS, as there is a benefit to selective drainage based on risk of CR-POPF. Those with moderate and high CR-POPF risk should have routine intraperitoneal drain placement, while those with negligible and low risk can be safely obviated. Table 10.3 shows specific risk factor combinations for patients with negligible and low CR-POPF risk, for which drain placement can be avoided.

Furthermore, the optimal timing of drain removal must also be considered in order to mitigate CR-POPF risk. While traditionally intraperitoneal drains had been removed around postoperative day (POD) 7 or later, [4, 91, 92] more recent studies have demonstrated a potential benefit to early drain removal [93, 94]. In fact, a randomized study in 2010 found a significant reduction (nearly 25%) in POPF incidence when drains were removed on POD 3 compared to POD 5 [94]. Though this study proved the benefits of early drain removal, it did so in isolation only. An important risk-adjusted analysis of a randomized study in 2015 sought to determine

Table 10.3 Risk factor combinations for patients with negligible and low CR-POPF risk

Gland texture	Pathology	Pancreatic duct diameter (mm)	Intraoperative blood loss (ml)	FRS
Firm	PDAC or pancreatitis	≥5	≤400	0
Firm	PDAC or pancreatitis	≥5	401–700	1
Firm	PDAC or pancreatitis	≥5	701–1000	2
Firm	PDAC or pancreatitis	4	≤400	1
Firm	PDAC or pancreatitis	4	401–700	2
Firm	PDAC or pancreatitis	3	≤400	2
Firm	Other	≥5	≤400	1
Firm	Other	≥5	401–700	2
Firm	Other	4	≤400	2
Soft	PDAC or pancreatitis	≥5	≤400	2

Adapted from McMillan et al. [90]

the risk-adjusted optimal timing for drain removal based on drain and serum amylase values from POD 1, which are known to be accurate postoperative predictors of
CR-POPF. This study found that CR-POPF rates were significantly lower in moderate and high FRS patients with POD 1 drain fluid amylase (DFA) of ≤5000 U/L
when drain removal occurred on POD 3 versus POD ≥5. These patients also had
shorter hospital stays and experienced fewer complications [95]. Thus, patients who
receive intraperitoneal drains, namely, moderate- and high-risk patients, should be
evaluated postoperatively for drain amylase volume in order to determine whether
or not early drain removal is beneficial as a fistula mitigation strategy. Based on this,
the drain management protocol shown in Fig. 10.1 was established. This clinical
care protocol demonstrates that routine intraperitoneal drain placement is recommended for moderate and high FRS risk patients, specifically. Furthermore, based
on the POD 1 DFA, drains should be removed either early (on POD 3) if DFA
≤5000 U/L or based on the surgeon's discretion if DFA >5000 U/L. Another multicenter study prospectively evaluated and confirmed the advantage of this drain management protocol for PD by showing that significant decreases in CR-POPF were
achieved [96].

Strategies for Risk Mitigation in High-Risk Cases

With the establishment of FRS, a high-risk (FRS 7–10) cohort can be identified by
the aggregate of weighted FRS variables. This clinical scenario, though relatively
rare (≈10% of all cases), has been found to have the highest rates of CR-POPF and
develop considerably worse outcomes than when these variables were considered in
isolation [56]. This reinforces the importance of utilizing the FRS in risk assessment, especially for this uncommon but clinically challenging situation. Table 10.4
presents 20 high Fistula Risk Score scenarios. A multinational, retrospective study
including 5323 PDs performed by 62 surgeons at 17 institutions provides insight as
to the efficacy of fistula mitigation strategies within this cohort specifically [56].

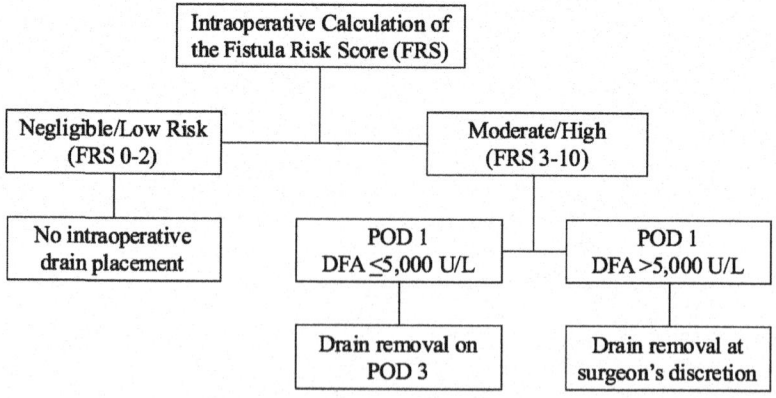

Fig. 10.1 Drain management protocol (Adapted from McMillan et al. [90])

Table 10.4 Twenty high-risk FRS scenarios

Gland texture	Pathology	Pancreatic duct diameter (mm)	Intraoperative blood loss (ml)	FRS
Soft	PDAC or pancreatitis	≤1	401–700	7
Soft	PDAC or pancreatitis	≤1	701–1000	8
Soft	PDAC or pancreatitis	≤1	>1000	9
Soft	PDAC or pancreatitis	2	701–1000	7
Soft	PDAC or pancreatitis	2	>1000	8
Soft	PDAC or pancreatitis	3	>1000	7
Soft	Other	≤1	≤ 400	7
Soft	Other	≤1	401–700	8
Soft	Other	≤1	701–1000	9
Soft	Other	≤1	>1000	10
Soft	Other	2	401–700	7
Soft	Other	2	701–1000	8
Soft	Other	2	>1000	9
Soft	Other	3	701–1000	7
Soft	Other	3	>1000	8
Soft	Other	4	>1000	7
Firm	PDAC or pancreatitis	≤1	>1000	7
Firm	Other	≤1	701–1000	7
Firm	Other	≤1	>1000	8
Firm	Other	2	>1000	7

Adapted from Ecker et al. [56]
Abbreviations: *PDAC* pancreatic ductal adenocarcinoma, *EBL* estimated blood loss, *FRS* Fistula Risk Score

This study found that the use and type of transanastomotic stents had the greatest impact on CR-POPF incidence in this study. The results were in line with previous randomized control trials, finding a reduction in CR-POPF rate with external stenting when compared to no stenting and an increase in CR-POPF with the use of internal stents when compared to no stenting. Furthermore, another mitigation strategy – prophylactic octreotide administration – was found to be independently associated with *increased* CR-POPF and postoperative complication burden. The importance of risk adjustment is once again emphasized, as previous non-risk-adjusted settings showed no concrete evidence in support of or against the use of somatostatin analogs. Finally, the use of PG reconstruction was found to be inferior to PJ anastomoses in this particular setting. An "optimal" approach to this scenario including the use of a PJ anastomosis, external stent, and intraperitoneal drain, as well as exclusion of octreotide, performed significantly better than other combinations and dropped the CR-POPF rate to just 13%, from an otherwise expected rate of roughly 30% in these especially challenging cases. Prospective randomized studies with appropriate risk adjustment are needed to further confirm optimal management strategies in high-risk scenarios.

Table 10.5 Mitigation strategies based on FRS zone

FRS zone	Negligible risk	Low risk	Moderate risk	High risk
% Frequency	8.13	22.6	58.8	10.5
% CR-POPF	0.7	5.2	14.3	31.6
Drains	0	0	+	+
Somatostatin analog	0	0	0	0
Internal stent	0	0	0	−
External stent	0	0	−	+
PG vs. PJ	0	0	PJ	PJ

Overview of Pancreatic Fistula Risk

The primary goal in addressing pancreatic fistula should be "prevention as management" by utilizing various mitigation strategies appropriately, and with discrimination, in order to reduce the occurrence of CR-POPF after pancreatic resection. However, based on the contemporary literature, it is necessary to implement a risk adjustment approach when evaluating CR-POPF risk and developing fistula mitigation strategies. It is essential to understand a patient's overall CR-POPF risk, taking into consideration the composite risk, rather than individual factors in isolation. Table 10.5 depicts the distribution of cases and the frequency of CR-POPF within each FRS risk zone, as well as the effect of mitigation strategies based on FRS zone – with 0 indicating no effect, + indicating a beneficial effect, and – indicating a harmful effect. The FRS has proven to be a well-established, validated, and simple method to assess composite risk for pancreatoduodenectomy. However, such a tool is not yet available for distal pancreatectomy, as risk modeling for this operation has thus far been unfruitful.

Management and Treatment of Pancreatic Fistula

If mitigation strategies fail, several management approaches exist for the treatment of CR-POPF once one occurs. These management and treatment strategies include conservative therapy and interventional techniques and differ depending on the severity of the fistula. Fistula severity can be assigned based on a complication-specific adaptation of the six-point Modified Accordion Severity Grading System, as shown in Table 10.6, which is specifically for POPF [97–99]. Accordion grades 1–3 correspond to grade B CR-POPF, and nonoperative management, while accordion grades 4–6 correspond to grade C CR-POPF, sometimes requiring reoperation.

It is important to note that the vast majority of CR-POPFs can be managed conservatively. Frequently, the only thing necessary is prolonged drainage from the initially placed operative drain. This can most often be achieved by a slow "backing out" process of the drain over a matter of 2–4 weeks. For this sort of patient, who is clinically stable with a relatively low-output leak, a strict nil per os (NPO) policy is

Table 10.6 Modified Accordion Severity Grading System for postoperative pancreatic fistula

Fistula Accordion Severity Grade	Description	Severity weight
1	Discharge from hospital with original operatively placed drain, with no other interventions required	0.110
2	The use of therapeutic (not prophylactic) somatostatin analogs, antibiotics, or total parenteral nutrition or total enteral nutrition, via pre-existing nasogastric or jejunostomy tubes, is required for the treatment of POPF	0.260
3	Any operative procedure short of general anesthesia is required for POPF management: complex wound management, percutaneous drain placement or aspiration of an amylase-rich collection postoperatively, angiographic procedure for control of a pseudoaneurysm secondary to POPF, or endoscopic procedure	0.370
4	Reoperation under general anesthesia is required for an anastomotic leak from the pancreaticojejunostomy or pancreaticogastrostomy Alternatively, single organ failure secondary to POPF (e.g., renal failure, pulmonary failure, neurologic failure, etc.) has developed	0.600
5	Reoperation under general anesthesia for an anastomotic leak is required, *and* single organ failure secondary to POPF (e.g., renal failure, pulmonary failure, neurologic failure, etc.) has developed Alternatively, multisystem (≥ 2) organ failure secondary to POPF has developed	0.790
6	Death attributable to POPF has occurred	1.000

Adapted from McMillan et al. [97]

not required, and diet advancement is preferred to achieve better overall nutrition. Although practiced elsewhere, we have not found great utility in multiple drain interrogation procedures, although certain fistulas may progress to a heightened clinical scenario if they are poorly drained, and they may require an "upsizing" or repositioning of the original drain, if not additional drainage. Most fistulas will heal and seal on their own as the patient's general nutrition and stamina normalize. Antibiotics are usually invoked with this sort of approach, as most CR-POPFS demonstrate bacterial infection.

One of the central components of conservative therapy for significant POPFs is nutritional support. Most patients with POPF are in a hypercatabolic state, resulting in high basal energy expenditure [3]. Additionally, patients with high-output fistulas (>200 mL of exocrine secretion per day) may also have fluid, electrolyte imbalances, and nutritional depletion [100]. There are two common types of nutritional support: total parenteral nutrition (TPN) and enteral nutrition (EN). TPN blocks all food-induced pancreatic secretions, thereby eliminating the release of gastrointestinal hormones. However, long-term TPN may have negative consequences, namely, caused by the absence of food in the gastrointestinal tract, lack of bile salts and proteolytic enzymes, motility dysfunction, and changes in the serum levels of hormones [101]. These changes may lead to wound infection, sepsis, hyperglycemia, gastrointestinal mucosa atrophy, gut barrier dysfunction, pancreas atrophy, and decrease in enzyme secretion or synthesis [102, 103]. On the other hand, EN largely avoids these consequences by stimulating the release of certain gastrointestinal peptides, which form a negative feedback control system and can inhibit pancreatic secretion [103]. Furthermore, a randomized controlled trial evaluating the clinical implications of TPN versus EN in patients with CR-POPF demonstrated the benefits of EN. This study found that EN support increased by more than twofold the probability of fistula closure, shortened the time to closure, and was associated with faster recovery, lower rates of nutrition-related complications, and lower cost than TPN [104]. According to the European Society for Clinical Nutritional and Metabolism (ESPEN), patients with a CR-POPF should receive EN of up to 20–25 kcal/kg body weight/day [105].

Another component of conservative therapy for CR-POPF, traditionally, has been the administration of somatostatin analogs in a *therapeutic* manner. Like their efficacy as a mitigation strategy, however, there is no solid evidence that somatostatin analogs result in a higher closure rate for POPF compared with other treatments. Thus, the administration of somatostatin analogs should not be used as a standard treatment, particularly given their added cost [3].

Interventional techniques, specifically interventional radiology, also play a significant role in the management of post-pancreatectomy complications [106]. One such technique is the image-guided percutaneous drainage of peripancreatic fluid collections/abscesses, which can be done for patients with a CR-POPF who are hemodynamically stable and have an acceptable coagulation panel and if there is a safe access route for a needle. After the administration of prophylactic broad-spectrum antibiotics, the fluid collection is punctured using real-time imaging guidance, and the fluid is aspirated. A drainage catheter is placed into the fluid collection and it is emptied, after which post-drainage imaging is retrieved to ensure complete or near-complete fluid emptying [3]. Studies have shown that over 85% of patients were successfully managed with percutaneous drainage and did not need a reoperation [106, 107]. Nonetheless, disadvantages to percutaneous drainage do exist and include the need of daily care and regular flushing of the catheter, frequent monitoring, and re-intervention to determine appropriate time for catheter removal, possible localized skin irritation and infections, prolonged duration of treatment, delay of oral refeeding, and longer hospital stay [108]. Special nursing needs are also required for patients after their discharge.

Endoscopic ultrasound (EUS)-guided transmural drainage is being increasingly used for the management of POPF, after both PD and DP [109, 110]. Anatomically, this is more realistically used for DP where the stomach's normal topography is not affected by any reconstruction process, as opposed to the situation with PD. Several retrospective studies comparing endoscopic and percutaneous drainage concluded the two techniques have a nearly equal treatment success rate [108, 111–113]. However, these studies contained multiple limitations, and it is important to note the objective advantages of EUS-guided drainage, namely, offered by the high-resolution imaging of the fluid collection, pancreas, and surrounding vasculature [3]. However, specialty expertise of this approach may not be universally available.

The majority of CR-POPF can be managed nonoperatively. Some, however, do require surgical intervention and thus qualify as ISGPF grade C fistulas. For example, failure or contraindication of radiologic endovascular procedures requires emergency relaparotomy to control ongoing bleeding in the case of hemorrhage from a pseudoaneurysm. Unfortunately, this is associated with high morbidity and significantly increased risk of mortality [7]. Though other indications of relaparotomy are not uniform across different studies, there are general guidelines dictating the need for an operative intervention. These include the following: deteriorating general conditions despite maximal supporting care, infected intra-abdominal collections that are inaccessible to percutaneous or endoscopic drainage, suspected peritonitis due to visceral perforation, and drainage limb necrosis [114, 115].

Furthermore, there are multiple surgical options for pancreatic stump management at relaparotomy. These include debridement and drainage of the peripancreatic region (with or without bridge stenting of the main pancreatic duct), attempted repair of the leakage site, construction of a new pancreaticoenteric anastomosis (not advised), resection of the pancreaticoenteric anastomosis with remnant ligation or closure, and completion pancreatectomy (which is often associated with subsequent mortality) [3]. The surgical option is usually determined by intraoperative findings, as well as the patient's clinical stability. Resource utilization, cost of care, and probability of death escalate significantly with each grade of CR-POPF, as well as with baseline risk of CR-POPF development [11, 116–118].

References

1. McMillan MT, Vollmer CM. Predictive factors for pancreatic fistula following pancreatectomy. Langenbecks Arch Surg. 2014;339(7):811–24.
2. Vollmer CM Jr, Sanchez N, Gondek S, et al. A root-cause analysis of mortality following major pancreatectomy. J Gastrointest Surg. 2012;16(1):89–102. discussion 102–3
3. Malleo G, Pulvirenti A, Marchegiani G, Butturini G, Salvia R, Bassi C. Diagnosis and management of postoperative pancreatic fistula. Langenbecks Arch Surg. 2014;399(7):801–10.
4. Yeo CJ, et al. Six hundred fifty consecutive pancreaticoduodenectomies in the 1990s: pathology, complications, and outcomes. Ann Surg. 1997;226(3):248–57. discussion 257–60
5. Bassi C, et al. Postoperative pancreatic fistula: an international study group (ISGPF) definition. Surgery. 2005;138(1):8–13.
6. Wente MN, Bassi C, Dervenis C, Fingerhut A, Gouma DJ, Izbicki JR, et al. Delayed gastric emptying (DGE) after pancreatic surgery: a suggested definition by the International Study Group of Pancreatic Surgery (ISGPS). Surgery. 2007 Nov;142(5):761–8.
7. Wente MN, Veit JA, Bassi C, Dervenis C, Fingerhut A, Gouma DJ, et al. Postpancreatectomy hemorrhage (PPH): an International Study Group of Pancreatic Surgery (ISGPS) definition. Surgery. 2007 July;142(1):20–5.
8. Callery MP, et al. A prospectively validated clinical risk score accurately predicts pancreatic fistula after pancreatoduodenectomy. J Am Coll Surg. 2013;216(1):1–14.
9. Allen PJ, Gonen M, Brennan MF, et al. Pasireotide for postoperative pancreatic fistula. N Engl J Med. 2014;370(21):2014–22.
10. Enestvedt CK, Diggs BS, Cassera MA, et al. Complications nearly double the cost of care after pancreaticoduodenectomy. Am J Surg. 2012;204:332–8.
11. Pratt WB, Maithel SK, Vanounou T, Huang ZA, Callery MP, Vollmer CM. Clinical and economic validation of the International Study Group of Pancreatic Fistula (ISGPF) classification scheme. Ann Surg. 2007;245(3):443–51.
12. Vollmer CM. The economics of pancreas surgery. Surg Clin North Am. 2013;93:711–28.

13. Buchler MW, et al. Pancreatic fistula after pancreatic head resection. Br J Surg. 2000;87(7):883–9.
14. Pratt W, et al. Postoperative pancreatic fistulas are not equivalent after proximal, distal, and central pancreatectomy. J Gastrointest Surg. 2006;10(9):1264–78. discussion 1278–9
15. Lermite E, et al. Risk factors of pancreatic fistula and delayed gastric emptying after pancreaticoduodenectomy with pancreaticogastrostomy. J Am Coll Surg. 2007;204(4):588–96.
16. Shrikhande SV, Barreto G, Shukla PJ. Pancreatic fistula after pancreaticoduodenectomy: the impact of a standardized technique of pancreaticojejunostomy. Langenbecks Arch Surg. 2008;393(1):87–91.
17. Balzano G, et al. Fast-track recovery programme after pancreatico-duodenectomy reduces delayed gastric emptying. Br J Surg. 2008;95(11):1387–93.
18. Pratt WB, Callery MP, Vollmer CM Jr. Risk prediction for development of pancreatic fistula using the ISGPF classification scheme. World J Surg. 2008;32(3):419–28.
19. Bassi C, et al. Pancreatic fistula rate after pancreatic resection. The importance of definitions. Dig Surg. 2004;21(1):54–9.
20. Bassi C, et al. The 2016 update of the International Study Group (ISGPS) definition and grading of postoperative pancreatic fistula: 11 years after. Surgery. 2016;161(3):584–91.
21. Harnoss JC, Ulrich AB, Harnoss JM, et al. Use and results of consensus definitions in pancreatic surgery: a systematic review. Surgery. 2014;155:47–57.
22. Rosso E, et al. The role of "fatty pancreas" and of BMI in the occurrence of pancreatic fistula after pancreaticoduodenectomy. J Gastrointest Surg. 2009;13(10):1845–51.
23. Mathur A, et al. Fatty pancreas: a factor in postoperative pancreatic fistula. Ann Surg. 2007;246(6):1058–64.
24. Addeo P, et al. Pancreatic fistula after a pancreaticoduodenectomy for ductal adenocarcinoma and its association with morbidity: a multicentre study of the French Surgical Association. HPB (Oxford). 2014;16(1):46–55.
25. Veillette G, et al. Implications and management of pancreatic fistulas following pancreaticoduodenectomy: the Massachusetts General Hospital experience. Arch Surg. 2008;143(5):476–81.
26. Bartoli FG, et al. Pancreatic fistula and relative mortality in malignant disease after pancreaticoduodenectomy. Review and statistical meta-analysis regarding 15 years of literature. Anticancer Res. 1991;11(5):1831–48.
27. de Castro SM, et al. Incidence and management of pancreatic leakage after pancreatoduodenectomy. Br J Surg. 2005;92(9):1117–23.
28. Aranha GV, et al. Current management of pancreatic fistula after pancreaticoduodenectomy. Surgery. 2006;140(4):561–8. discussion 568–9
29. Callery MP, Pratt WB, Vollmer CM Jr. Prevention and management of pancreatic fistula. J Gastrointest Surg. 2009;13(1):163–73.
30. Hamanaka Y, et al. Pancreatic juice output after pancreatoduodenectomy in relation to pancreatic consistency, duct size, and leakage. Surgery. 1996;119(3):281–7.
31. Sato N, et al. Risk analysis of pancreatic fistula after pancreatic head resection. Arch Surg. 1998;133(10):1094–8.
32. Lin JW, et al. Risk factors and outcomes in postpancreaticoduodenectomy pancreaticocutaneous fistula. J Gastrointest Surg. 2004;8(8):951–9.
33. Gaujoux S, et al. Fatty pancreas and increased body mass index are risk factors of pancreatic fistula after pancreaticoduodenectomy. Surgery. 2010;148(1):15–23.
34. Wellner UF, et al. A simple scoring system based on clinical factors related to pancreatic texture predicts postoperative pancreatic fistula preoperatively. HPB (Oxford). 2010;12(10):696–702.
35. Ishikawa O, et al. Concomitant benefit of preoperative irradiation in preventing pancreas fistula formation after pancreatoduodenectomy. Arch Surg. 1991;126(7):885–9.
36. Lowy AM, et al. Prospective, randomized trial of octreotide to prevent pancreatic fistula after pancreaticoduodenectomy for malignant disease. Ann Surg. 1997;226(5):632–41.

37. Cheng TY, et al. Effect of neoadjuvant chemoradiation on operative mortality and morbidity for pancreaticoduodenectomy. Ann Surg Oncol. 2006;13(1):66–74.
38. Ahmadu-Suka F, et al. Exocrine pancreatic function following intraoperative irradiation of the canine pancreas. Cancer. 1988;62(6):1091–5.
39. Hishikawa Y, et al. Radiotherapy of pancreatic fistula. Radiat Med. 1986;4(1):27–8.
40. Miller BC, et al. A multi-institutional external validation of the fistula risk score for pancreatoduodenectomy. J Gastrointest Surg. 2014;18(1):172–9. discussion 179–80
41. Yeo CJ, et al. A prospective randomized trial of pancreaticogastrostomy versus pancreaticojejunostomy after pancreaticoduodenectomy. Ann Surg. 1995;222(4):580–8. discussion 588–92
42. Weber SM, et al. Laparoscopic left pancreatectomy: complication risk score correlates with morbidity and risk for pancreatic fistula. Ann Surg Oncol. 2009;16(10):2825–33.
43. Yoshioka R, et al. Risk factors for clinical pancreatic fistula after distal pancreatectomy: analysis of consecutive 100 patients. World J Surg. 2010;34(1):121–5.
44. Watanabe H, et al. Aging is associated with decreased pancreatic acinar cell regeneration and phosphatidylinositol 3-kinase/Akt activation. Gastroenterology. 2005;128(5):1391–404.
45. Ridolfini MP, et al. Risk factors associated with pancreatic fistula after distal pancreatectomy, which technique of pancreatic stump closure is more beneficial? World J Gastroenterol. 2007;13(38):5096–100.
46. Sugimoto M, et al. Risk factor analysis and prevention of postoperative pancreatic fistula after distal pancreatectomy with stapler use. J Hepatobiliary Pancreat Sci. 2013;20(5):538–44.
47. Bilimoria MM, et al. Panreatic leak after left pancreatectomy is reduced following main pancreatic duct ligation. Br J Surg. 2003;90(2):190–6.
48. Pannegeon V, et al. Pancreatic fistula after distal pancreatectomy: predictive risk factors and value of conservative treatment. Arch Surg. 2006;141(11):1071–6. discussion 1076
49. Ban D, et al. Stapler and nonstapler closure of the pancreatic remnant after distal pancreatectomy: multicenter retrospective analysis of 388 patients. World J Surg. 2012;36(8):1866–73.
50. Mason GR. Pancreatogastrostomy as reconstruction for pancreatoduodenectomy: review. World J Surg. 1999;23:221–6.
51. Duffas JP, et al. A controlled randomized multicenter trial of pancreatogastrostomy or pancreatojejunostomy after pancreatoduodenectomy. Am J Surg. 2005;189(6):720–9.
52. Bassi C, et al. Reconstruction by pancreaticojejunostomy versus pancreaticogastrostomy following pancreatectomy: results of a comparative study. Ann Surg. 2005;242(6):767–71. discussion 771–3
53. Fernandez-Cruz L, et al. Pancreatogastrostomy with gastric partition after pylorus-preserving pancreatoduodenectomy versus conventional pancreatojejunostomy: a prospective randomized study. Ann Surg. 2008;248(6):930–8.
54. Topal B, et al. Pancreaticojejunostomy versus pancreaticogastrostomy reconstruction after pancreaticoduodenectomy for pancreatic or periampullary tumours: a multicentre randomised trial. Lancet Oncol. 2013;14(7):655–62.
55. He T, et al. Pancreaticojejunostomy versus pancreaticogastrostomy after pancreaticoduodenectomy: a systematic review and meta-analysis. Dig Surg. 2013;30(1):56–69.
56. Ecker BL, et al. The characterization and optimal management of high-risk pancreatic anastomosis during pancreatoduodenectomy. Ann Surg. (Manuscript in submission).
57. McMillan MT, Sprys M, Malleo G, Bassi C, Vollmer CM. Defining the practice of pancreatoduodenectomy around the world. HPB. 2015;17(12):1145–54.
58. Shrikhande SV, Sivasanker M, Vollmer CM, et al. Pancreatic anastomosis after pancreatoduodenectomy: a position paper by the International Study Group of Pancreatic Surgery (ISGPS). Surgery. (Manuscript in submission).
59. Berger AC, et al. Does type of pancreaticojejunostomy after pancreaticoduodenectomy decrease rate of pancreatic fistula? A randomized, prospective, dual-institution trial. J Am Coll Surg. 2009;208(5):738–47. discussion 247–9
60. Poon RT, Lo SH, Fong D, Fan ST, Wong J. Prevention of pancreatic anastomotic leakage after pancreaticoduodenectomy. Am J Surg. 2002;183:42–52.

61. Sikora SS, Posner MC. Management of the pancreatic stump following pancreaticoduode-nectomy. Br J Surg. 1995;82:1590–7.
62. Matsumoto Y, Fujii H, Miura K, Inoue S, Sekikawa T, Aoyama H, Oshnishi N, Sakai K, Suda K. Successful pancreatojejunal anastomosis for pancreatoduodenectomy. Surg Gynecol Obstet. 1992;175:555–62.
63. Stojadinovic A, Brooks A, Hoos A, Jacques DP, Conlon KC, Brennan MF. An evidence-based approach to the surgical management of resectable pancreatic adenocarcinoma. J Am Coll Surg. 2003;196:954–64.
64. Kingsnorth AN. Safety and function of isolated Roux loop pancreaticojejunostomy after Whipple's pancreaticoduodenectomy. Ann R Coll Surg Engl. 1994;76:175–9.
65. Grobmyer SR, et al. Roux-en-Y reconstruction after pancreaticoduodenectomy. Arch Surg. 2008;143(12):1184–8.
66. Funovics JM, et al. Progress in reconstruction after resection of the head of the pancreas. Surg Gynecol Obstet. 1987;164(6):545–8.
67. Tran K, et al. Occlusion of the pancreatic duct versus pancreaticojejunostomy: a prospective randomized trial. Ann Surg. 2002;236(4):422–8. discussion 428
68. Muller MW, et al. Is there still a role for total pancreatectomy? Ann Surg. 2007;246(6):966–74. discussion 974–5
69. Henegouwen MI, Gulik TM, Akkermans LMA, Jansen JB, Gouma DJ. The effect of octreo-tide on gastric emptying at a dosage used to prevent complications after pancreatic surgery: a randomised, placebo controlled study in volunteers. Gut. 1997;41:758–62.
70. Gans SL, van Westreenen HL, Kiewiet JJS, et al. Systematic review and meta-analysis of somatostatin analogues for the treatment of pancreatic fistula. Br J Surg. 2012;99:754–60.
71. Koti RS, Gurusamy KS, Fusai G, Davidson BR. Meta-analysis of randomized controlled tri-als on the effectiveness of somatostatin analogues for pancreatic surgery: a Cochrane review. HPB (Oxford). 2010;12(3):155–65.
72. McMillan M, et al. Prophylactic octreotide for pancreatoduodenectomy: more harm than good? HPB (Oxford). 2014;16(10):954–62.
73. Lillemoe KD, et al. Does fibrin glue sealant decrease the rate of pancreatic fistula after pancreaticoduodenectomy? Results of a prospective randomized trial. J Gastrointest Surg. 2004;8(7):766–72. discussion 772–4
74. Suc B, et al. Temporary fibrin glue occlusion of the main pancreatic duct in the prevention of intra-abdominal complications after pancreatic resection: prospective randomized trial. Ann Surg. 2003;237(1):57–65.
75. Iannitti DA, et al. Use of the round ligament of the liver to decrease pancreatic fistulas: a novel technique. J Am Coll Surg. 2006;203(6):857–64.
76. Hassenpflug M, et al. Decrease in clinically relevant pancreatic fistula by coverage of the pancreatic remnant after distal pancreatectomy. Surgery. 2012;152(3):164–71.
77. McMillan MT, et al. Externalized stents for pancreatoduodenectomy provide value only in high-risk scenarios. J Gastrointest Surg. 2016;20(12):2052–62.
78. Winter JM, et al. Does pancreatic duct stenting decrease the rate of pancreatic fistula fol-lowing pancreaticoduodenectomy? Results of a prospective randomized trial. J Gastrointest Surg. 2006;10(9):1280–90. discussion 1290
79. Smyrniotis V, et al. Does internal stenting of the pancreaticojejunostomy improve out-comes after pancreatoduodenectomy? A prospective study. Langenbecks Arch Surg. 2010;395(3):195–200.
80. Sachs TE, et al. The pancreaticojejunal anastomotic stent: friend or foe? Surgery. 2013;153(5):651–2.
81. Pessaux P, et al. External pancreatic duct stent decreases pancreatic fistula rate after pancreat-icoduodenectomy: prospective multicenter randomized trial. Ann Surg. 2011;253(5):879–85.
82. Gurusamy KS, et al. Routine abdominal drainage for uncomplicated laparoscopic cholecys-tectomy. Cochrane Database Syst Rev. 2007;4:CD006004.
83. Karliczek A, et al. Drainage or nondrainage in elective colorectal anastomosis: a systematic review and meta-analysis. Color Dis. 2006;8(4):259–65.

84. de Rougemont O, et al. Abdominal drains in liver transplantation: useful tool or useless dogma? A matched case-control study. Liver Transpl. 2009;15(1):96–101.
85. Aldameh A, McCall JL, Koea JB. Is routine placement of surgical drains necessary after elective hepatectomy? Results from a single institution. J Gastrointest Surg. 2005;9(5):667–71.
86. Fisher WE, Hodges SE, Silberfein EJ, Artinyan A, Ahern CH, Jo E, et al. Pancreatic resection without routine intraperitoneal drainage. HPB (Oxford). 2011;13(7):503–10.
87. Correa-Gallego C, et al. Operative drainage following pancreatic resection: analysis of 1122 patients resected over 5 years at a single institution. Ann Surg. 2013;258(6):1051–8.
88. Conlon KC, et al. Prospective randomized clinical trial of the value of intraperitoneal drainage after pancreatic resection. Ann Surg. 2001;234(4):487–93. discussion 493–4
89. Van Buren G 2nd, et al. A randomized prospective multicenter trial of pancreaticoduodenectomy with and without routine intraperitoneal drainage. Ann Surg. 2014;259(4):605–12.
90. McMillan, M., et al., The value of drains as a fistula mitigation strategy for pancreatoduodenectomy: something for everyone? Results of a randomized prospective multi-institutional study. J Gastroinest Surg. 2014;19(1):21–30.
91. Bottger TC, Junginger T. Factors influencing morbidity and mortality after pancreaticoduodenectomy: critical analysis of 221 resections. World J Surg. 1999;23:164–72.
92. Tran KTC, Smeenk HG, van Eijck CHJ, et al. Pylorus preserving pancreaticoduodenectomy versus standard whipple procedure: a prospective, randomized, multicenter analysis of 170 patients with pancreatic and periampullary tumors. Ann Surg. 2004;240:738–45.
93. Kawai M, Tani M, Terasawa H, et al. Early removal of prophylactic drains reduces the risk of intra-abdominal infections in patients with pancreatic head resection: prospective study for 104 consecutive patients. Ann Surg. 2006;244:1e7.
94. Bassi C, Molinari E, Malleo G, et al. Early versus late drain removal after standard pancreatic resections: results of a prospective randomized trial. Ann Surg. 2010;252:207e214.
95. McMillan MT, et al. Drain management after pancreatoduodenectomy: reappraisal of a prospective randomized trial using risk stratification. J Am Coll Surg. 2015;221(4):798–809.
96. McMillan MT, et al. Multicenter, prospective trial of selective drain management for pancreatoduodenectomy using risk stratification. Ann Surg. (Manuscript in submission).
97. McMillan MT, Christein JD, Callery MP, et al. Comparing the burden of pancreatic fistulas after pancreatoduodenectomy and distal pancreatectomy. Surgery. 2016;159(4):1013–22.
98. Strasberg SM, Linehan DC, Hawkins WG. The accordion severity grading system of surgical complications. Ann Surg. 2009;250(2):177–86.
99. Miller BC, Christein JD, Behrman SW, et al. Assessing the impact of a fistula after a pancreaticoduodenectomy using the post-operative morbidity index. HPB. 2013;15(10):781–8.
100. Bassi C, Malleo G. Pancreas: postoperative pancreatic fistula: use of enteral nutrition. Nat Rev Gastroenterol Hepatol. 2011;8:427–8.
101. Fong YM, Marano MA, Barber A, et al. Total parenteral nutrition and bowel rest modify the metabolic response to endotoxin in humans. Ann Surg. 1989;210:449–56.
102. Spiller RC, Trotman IF, Higgins BE, et al. The ileal brake-inhibition of jejunal motility after ileal fat perfusion in man. Gut. 1984;25:365–74.
103. O'Keefe SJD. Physiological response of the human pancreas to enteral and parenteral feeding. Curr Opin Cin Nutr Metab Care. 2006;9:622–8.
104. Klek S, Sierzega M, Turczynowski L, et al. Enteral and parenteral nutrition in the conservative treatment of pancreatic fistula: a randomized clinical trial. Gastroenterol. 2011;141:157–63.
105. Meier R, Ockenga J, Pertkiewicz M, et al. ESPEN guidelines on enteral nutrition: pancreas. Clin Nutr. 2006;25:275–84.
106. Sanjay P, Kellner M, Tait IS. The role of interventional radiology in the management of surgical complications after pancreatoduodenectomy. HPB. 2012;14:812–7.
107. Munoz-Bongrand N, Sauvanet A, Denys A, Sibert A, Vilgrain V, Belghiti J. Conservative management of pancreatic fistula after pancreaticoduodenectomy with pancreaticogastrostomy. J Am Coll Surg. 2004;199:198–203.
108. Kwon YM, Gerdes H, Schattner MA, et al. Management of peripancreatic fluid collections following partial pancreatectomy: a comparison of percutaneous versus EUS-guided drainage. Surg Endosc. 2013;27:2422–7.

109. Reddymasu SC, Pakseresht K, Moloney B, et al. Incidence of pancreatic fistula after distal pancreatectomy and efficacy of endoscopic therapy for its management: results from a tertiary care center. Case Rep Gastroenterol. 2013;7:332–9.
110. Bartoli E, Rebibo L, Robert B, et al. Efficacy of the double-pigtail stent as a conservative treatment for grade B pancreatic fistula after pancreatoduodenectomy with pancreatogastric anastomosis. Surg Endosc. 2013;28:1528–34.
111. Tilara A, Gerdes H, Allen P, et al. Endoscopic ultrasound-guided transmural drainage of postoperative pancreatic collections. J Am Coll Surg. 2014;218:33–40.
112. Azeem N, Baron TH, Topazian MD, et al. Outcomes of endoscopic and percutaneous drainage of pancreatic fluid collections arising after pancreatic tail resection. J Am Coll Surg. 2012;215:177–85.
113. Onodera M, Kawakami H, Kuwatani M, et al. Endoscopic ultrasound-guided transmural drainage for pancreatic fistula or pancreatic duct dilation after pancreatic surgery. Surg Endosc. 2011;26:1710–7.
114. Fuks D, Plessen G, Huet E, et al. Life-threatening postoperative pancreatic fistula (grade C) after pancreaticoduodenectomy: incidence, prognosis, and risk factors. Am J Surg. 2009;197:702–9.
115. Balzano G, Pecorelli N, Plemonti L, et al. Relaparotomy for a pancreatic fistula after a pancreaticoduodenectomy: a comparison of different surgical strategies. HPB. 2014;16:40–5.
116. Abbott DE, et al. Pancreas fistula risk prediction: implications for hospital costs and payments. HPB. 2016;19(2):140–6.
117. McMillan MT, Vollmer CM, Asbun HJ, et al. The characterization and prediction of ISGPF grade C fistulas following Pancreatoduodenectomy. J Gastrointest Surg. 2016;20:262.
118. McMillan MT, Allegrini V, Asbun HJ, et al. Incorporation of procedure-specific risk into the ACS-NSQIP surgical risk calculator improves the prediction of morbidity and mortality after Pancreatoduodenectomy. Ann Surg. 2016;265(5):978–86.

Minimally Invasive Pancreas Resections

11

Jan Grendar and Paul D. Hansen

Introduction

With improvements in technology of laparoscopic surgery and with increased avail- ability and utilization of this technique, there was enthusiasm to compare the lapa- roscopic and open approach in many types of procedures. Advantages of laparoscopy were identified in randomized trials in procedures performed for benign indications, such as cholecystectomy [1, 2], appendectomy [3, 4], or Roux-en-Y gastric bypass [5]. The biggest advantages are improved postoperative pain control, faster recov- ery, shorter time to oral intake, shorter length of stay, better quality of life, decreased blood loss, and lower incidence of incisional hernia. Comparison of cancer-specific outcomes in randomized trials after distal gastrectomy [6] or resections for colon and rectal adenocarcinoma [7, 8] showed non-inferiority of the laparoscopic approach in terms of lymph node harvest, margin negativity, recurrence, and overall survival.

Laparoscopic pancreatic procedures were attempted later than other technically easier operations as open pancreatectomies have been associated with significant risk. Perioperative mortality was historically in the 20–40% range [9, 10], an unac- ceptable number for modern surgery. Despite this risk and technical complexity, surgeons continued to remove cancers in the pancreas since curative resection was and until now is the only chance for long-term survival or cure [11]. With gradual improvements in outcomes [12, 13], it was possible to consider pancreatic resection to be a standard procedure performed by high-volume surgeons in high-volume specialized centers [14]. Gradually, minimally invasive pancreatic resections were also incorporated in practice in specialized centers, first laparoscopically [15, 16]

J. Grendar
Liver and Pancreas Surgery, Portland Providence Cancer Institute, Portland, OR, USA

P.D. Hansen (✉)
The Oregon Clinic, Providence Portland Cancer Center, Portland, OR, USA
e-mail: phansen@orclinic.com

© Springer International Publishing AG 2018
F.G. Rocha, P. Shen (eds.), *Optimizing Outcomes for Liver and Pancreas Surgery*, DOI 10.1007/978-3-319-62624-6_11

and more recently using the robotic platform [17, 18]. At the present time, minimally invasive approaches are employed for all types of pancreatic lesions including complex and multivisceral resections at an increasing rate [19]. Minimal invasiveness is not a synonym for minimal extent of disease or minimal complexity anymore. After sufficient experience with minimally invasive procedures was obtained, comparison studies assessed proposed advantages of this approach. Rationale and limitations of each type of minimally invasive pancreatic resection will be discussed in this chapter. Significance of this topic is also evident through an IHPBA initiative at the 2016 World Congress in Sao Paulo, Brazil, where a state-of-the-art conference on minimally invasive pancreatic resection was held.

Before proceeding with the detailed description of literature regarding each type of procedure, it is important to mention a fundamental issue with minimally invasive pancreatic resections – their incorporation into practice. Sufficient literature [14, 20–23] exists regarding the relationship between hospital and surgeon volume of complex pancreatic procedures and patient outcomes as well as learning curves after subspecialty training in HPB surgery [24]. Similarly there is an additional learning curve even for HPB surgeons experienced in open pancreatic resections [25–29]. Therefore, centers where minimally invasive pancreatic resections are not routinely performed but wish to incorporate these into their practice need to do so with appropriate initial training and supervision. Also, after incorporation of MIS technique, appropriate maintenance of high volume of this technique is required to preserve outcomes. Regional or nationwide programs of implementation [30] should be developed. This is especially true for minimally invasive pancreaticoduodenectomy as an example of a technically complex resection. Occasional laparoscopic resections to maintain competitiveness of that particular center have to be discouraged.

One of the limitations of current MIS pancreatectomy outcomes and comparison literature is its retrospective character that comes from a series of high-volume, minimally invasive HPB surgeons in high-volume centers. This is associated with questionable generalizability to all centers across North America. Also, outcomes in studies mentioned in this chapter further strengthen the point of appropriate incorporation of MIS technique into practice and maintenance of high volume of this technique after incorporation.

Current State of the Literature

Enucleation

Standard resections of the pancreas – pancreaticoduodenectomy and distal pancreatectomy – are complex procedures associated with significant perioperative risk [12, 13]. These procedures are required for malignant diagnoses in order to obtain satisfactory local treatment with negative margin as well as for appropriate lymph node harvest. For benign diseases or those with very low malignant potential and with well-defined and encapsulated lesions, parenchyma-sparing local resection and enucleation without lymphadenectomy has been suggested to be an effective treatment. This was first described as a standard procedure for insulinoma [31]. The debate regarding enucleation for small nonfunctioning NETs is less definitive due to association with increased risk of recurrence as well as lymph node positivity that can be seen even in small tumors [32] where enucleation would miss proper sampling of these nodes.

The rationale for decreasing the extent of resection is the reduction of perioperative risk due to avoidance of the need for anastomoses and minimization of surgical trauma as well as preservation of pancreatic function and its associated lower rate of postresection exocrine and endocrine dysfunction. Indeed, a review of 61 [33] and 119 patients undergoing enucleation [34] did not identify any patients with new onset diabetes requiring therapy with insulin supplementation. In a comparison of enucleation versus standard resection [35] though, there was similar risk in terms of perioperative morbidity and mortality with higher overall risk of postoperative pancreatic fistula (POPF) and clinically relevant postoperative pancreatic fistula (CR-POPF). This suggests that enucleation still represents a technically challenging procedure associated with significant risk. The lower volume of removed pancreatic tissue does not translate into a less significant procedure. Therefore, it is not surprising that only 9–22.5% of enucleations described in the literature were performed using minimally invasive approach [35–37].

A review of the literature describing minimally invasive pancreatic enucleation identifies mostly retrospective studies and prospectively collected cohorts. There are no randomized comparisons of minimally invasive and open enucleations or comparisons between different types of minimally invasive techniques.

Multiple case series of patients undergoing minimally invasive enucleation have been published. Given that the selection criteria for the MIS approach were highly variable, it is not unexpected that the perioperative results were also inconsistent. Older studies were summarized in 2009 in a systematic review by Briggs et al. [36]. At that time, 11 retrospective reviews included 101 patients (5–24 patients per study) who underwent laparoscopic pancreatic enucleations. Mean operative time was 132 min with a conversion rate of 23%. Overall pooled perioperative morbidity was 47% with an overall POPF rate of 30%. Mean length of stay was 7.8 days. Although more recent studies [32, 38, 39] describe similar mean operative time of 123–130 min, there has been a lower rate of conversion to an open procedure in 8.5–26% of patients and mean EBL of 64–220 ml. Overall morbidity was reduced to 10–17% with CR-POPF rates of 5–10%. Mean length of postoperative stay remained at 6–8.4 days. These results are in accordance with the expected improvement in outcomes. However, since we should expect a similar improvement in outcomes after open enucleations over time, a comparison of these results to historical open cohorts would be inappropriate. The most recent direct comparison of laparoscopic and open enucleations from Song et al. [39] showed shorter OR time and shorter length of postoperative stay after laparoscopic procedures, but when controlled for location of the lesion (head and uncinate process vs. neck, body, and tail of the pancreas), there were no significant differences between the two types of surgical approach in any of the outcomes.

There are no studies that have compared long-term outcomes such as recurrence rates, disease-free and overall survival, or patients' quality of life between laparoscopic and open enucleation.

The most significant difference between open and minimally invasive pancreatic enucleation is the lack of tactile feedback and inability to palpate the pancreas in order to precisely localize a deep lesion that is not readily visible upon inspection of the gland. Therefore, adjuncts such as intraoperative ultrasound play a major role when an MIS technique is selected [40]. Other surgical principles (described later) such as decision-making, drain management, and perioperative management are similar.

In summary, minimally invasive pancreatic enucleations are technically challenging but feasible and safe procedures when performed in specialized centers. Short-term perioperative outcomes are comparable to open enucleation.

Distal Pancreatectomy

Distal pancreatectomy is considered to be technically less challenging and is associated with lower perioperative risk compared to pancreaticoduodenectomy. This is due to the lack of the construction of multiple anastomoses. Therefore, it is widely accepted as the most common pancreatic resection performed minimally invasively [41, 42]. It was first described in a series of 12 patients with islet cell tumors by Gagner et al. [16] in the mid-1990s. Subsequently with the advance of robotic surgery, a robot-assisted distal pancreatectomy was described in the early 2000s [17, 43].

Since that time, many studies described experience with laparoscopic and robotic distal pancreatectomies. In population-based studies utilizing the National Inpatient Sample (NIS) database [44, 45], MIS technique was used in less than 5% of distal pancreatectomies prior to 2011. Comparison between outcomes after these relatively few laparoscopic procedures with open distal pancreatectomies showed either equivalency [44] or better outcomes in the laparoscopic distal pancreatectomy group in terms of lower overall complication rates, decreased mortality, and length of stay [45]. It is likely that selection bias can be responsible for some of these differences, although the laparoscopic population was significantly older and had more comorbidities than the open surgery cohort [45]. However, more recent studies suggest, the MIS technique is increasing in frequency. This has resulted in significant heterogeneity in the relative frequency of MIS approach as well as in rates of conversion from MIS to open procedures that span 3–33% in some series [46–49]. With increasing experience, these rates are expected to drop.

There are no randomized controlled trials comparing laparoscopic and open distal pancreatectomy. Many retrospective reviews of institutional experiences with minimally invasive techniques describe a wide range of outcomes in a combination of patient populations (benign diagnoses, premalignant, or malignant). The majority of comparisons were unmatched, while some studies utilized a matched design. The most commonly compared outcomes between MIS and open distal pancreatectomy were operative outcomes and perioperative risks.

Several unmatched comparisons demonstrated that the laparoscopic approach required significantly longer OR times than open operations [49–51], a difference that persisted in matched comparisons [49, 52]. Khaled et al. [53], however, did not identify any significant difference in OR time in their matched analysis. Two other studies [52, 54] found an association between an increased need for transfusion in the open approach. Multiple unmatched studies showed decreased intraoperative estimated blood loss (EBL) with laparoscopic techniques [48, 49, 51, 55, 56] that persisted in three matched comparisons [49, 52, 53]. Laparoscopic procedures were also associated with higher rates of successful splenic preservation [52, 53].

Multiple studies retrospectively reviewed and compared postoperative complications. The majority did not identify a statistically significant difference inoverall postoperative morbidity [51, 53–55]. Several studies found an association between laparoscopy and decreased rates of overall postoperative morbidity [47–49], including matched analyses in which there was no difference between the two approaches in overall complication rates. In another matched analysis [52], lower overall morbidity in laparoscopic group reached statistical significance (24 vs. 33%, p < 0.001). Variable results have been described for postoperative pancreatic fistula rates, where some studies found no difference in matched analysis [49, 51], whereas other showed less Grade B postoperative pancreatic fistulas (POPF) in the laparoscopic group [52]. Postoperative mortality was not different between methods [51].

A comparison between the two techniques in postoperative recovery showed less need for painkillers [55] and less time to normal diet [50] in the laparoscopic group. There was also a consistent association between decreased length of hospital stay and laparoscopic surgery [47–56] that persisted in matched comparisons [49, 52, 53].

When performing resections for a malignant diagnosis, it is important to not only assure perioperative and surgical safety but also oncologic appropriateness of the technique. Three systematic reviews and meta-analyses [57–59] including a recent Cochrane review focused on assessment of margin clearance, lymph node harvest, and recurrence at maximum follow-up and did not identify significant differences between laparoscopic and open approach in this pooled data.

Another important question is the additional cost associated with laparoscopy. Although it was found to be associated with increased cost upfront, the reduced subsequent postoperative cost resulted in an overall cost that was not significantly different from open surgery in some studies [51, 60], while overall cost was decreased in another retrospective review [61].

Several recent studies showed robotic distal pancreatectomy to be a safe option in terms of perioperative outcomes [18, 62–66]. Comparisons between laparoscopic and robotic technique suggest robotic resection to be superior in the ability to preserve spleen [64, 67], associated with decreased rate of conversion to open resection as well as increased lymph node harvest and reduced margin negativity in one study [62], while another non-matched comparison [66] failed to identify any difference in rate of conversion, length of postoperative stay, postoperative pancreatic fistula rate, lymph node harvest, or margin negativity between the techniques.

In summary, minimally invasive distal pancreatectomy is a safe procedure. Since the majority of postoperative complications are a consequence of postoperative pancreatic fistulas and POPF rates are not different between MIS and open procedures, we should not expect major differences in overall or severe complications between the techniques. Complications are therefore most likely the consequence of operating on the pancreas itself and depend on the characteristics of the gland and disease process or method of transection rather than the amount of tissue trauma to the surrounding tissues. The most important finding in this regard is that MIS distal pancreatectomy is not associated with worse rates of POPF, morbidity, and mortality as well as cancer-specific outcomes. The amount of tissue trauma is expected to influence speed of recovery. There is literature to support this rationale with less pain, decreased time to normal diet, and decreased length of stay in the hospital for MIS patients. These findings are consistent across studies. Shorter hospital stay is in return associated with decreased postoperative costs that balance the upfront increased OR cost of MIS techniques resulting in a comparable overall cost to open surgery. The robotic approach does not seem to offset the added cost with additional benefit compared to laparoscopy. These results support wider incorporation of laparoscopic techniques to the armamentarium of HPB surgeons. The ongoing Dutch prospective, randomized "LEOPARD" trial will hopefully supply the ultimate answer regarding future of laparoscopic distal pancreatectomy.

In our institution, there is a long and rich history of minimally invasive surgery. Over time and with increasing experience, selection criteria for laparoscopic versus open procedures have broadened across all institutions performing laparoscopic distal pancreatectomy so that virtually every patient is considered for laparoscopy. The only consideration for upfront open procedure is significant vascular involvement. Tumor size, the need for multivisceral resection, or other complex features are not an automatic contraindication to this approach. The procedure is continued laparoscopically as long as it is safe and feasible. The biggest limitation to a totally laparoscopic distal pancreatectomy is insufficient tactile feedback due to the occasional need for palpation to proceed in a safe manner. In these cases, we do not consider a hand port or a conversion to open procedure to be a failure. Without attachment to a particular technique, we strive to perform the safest procedure associated with the least postoperative risk and the fastest recovery of the patient for return to as normal function as possible. We believe that our experience and current literature satisfactorily describe laparoscopic distal pancreatectomy to be the better procedure for vast majority of patients, while the few challenging cases are indeed better served with conversion to an open distal pancreatectomy.

Pancreaticoduodenectomy

The first laparoscopic pancreaticoduodenectomy (LPD) was described in 1994 [15] on a patient with chronic pancreatitis. LPD is technically more challenging than distal pancreatectomy. Multiple steps requiring unique set of skills including three anastomoses decrease the enthusiasm of surgeons to incorporate this technique into their practice. Another potential issue is the relatively frequent need for major vascular resection and reconstruction. LPD is therefore viewed as more of a challenge for individual surgeons or departments.

Soon after the description of LPD, several centers around the world adopted this method and continued to refine it. With increasing experience, the criteria used to identify patients suitable for LPD were broadened [68–72]. Similar to other laparoscopic procedures, LPD was compared to open PD in several domains – intraoperative events, general and pancreas-specific perioperative complications, recovery and mortality, oncological outcomes, and cost-effectiveness. Again, we have no randomized data to compare the two techniques relying on retrospective comparisons instead. The majority of the comparisons have come from high-volume, dedicated LPD practices and departments, therefore again questioning the generalizability of the results.

It is expected that patients with less advanced disease as well as those with better functional status were selected for LPD. As these characteristics are not commonly described, comparisons in early studies showed few significant differences in baseline patient characteristics such as age, sex, and comorbidity burden. LPD groups did have a lower percentage of patients with malignant diagnosis [70, 73] and lower BMI even when matched for several other factors [74]. Described conversion to open rates were just under 10% in most series with wide variability from 1 to 19% [67, 70, 73, 75]. LPD was associated with decreased intraoperative blood loss to 110–500 ccs in most series [67, 68, 73, 76] that resulted in decreased rates of transfusions [76]. LPD procedures typically lasted between 310 and 540 min that were longer than OPD [67, 68, 73, 74]. Most importantly, LPD was not associated with inferior outcomes when margin status was assessed, although patient selection may have played a role. It was either equivalent to open resection [70] or was associated with improved rates of margin negativity [73, 77]. Similarly lymph node harvest was either equivalent [70, 73] or higher in LPD [68, 77].

Postoperative outcomes assessing safety of the procedure showed mortality rates between 1 and 5% that were similar to open procedures [67, 70, 73, 78, 79]. Mortality rates almost twice as high were observed when less than 10 LPD procedures were performed annually (7.5 vs. 3.4%) [77]. Overall, complications occurred in 25–45% of patients and were similar to open in respective series [67, 70, 76, 79]. One matched comparison by Dokmak et al. [74] did show significantly higher rates of postoperative bleeding (24% vs. 7%), grade C POPF (24% vs. 6%), as well as the need for reoperation (24% vs. 11%) in the laparoscopic group. That inferiority of LPD was not observed in other studies and reviews where overall POPF and clinically relevant POPF rates (Grade B and C) as well as reoperations and readmissions were not statistically different [73, 76]. LPD has been associated with reduced rates of delayed gastric emptying [73], postoperative pain levels [80], and a length of stay that was on average 8–15 days, 1–3 days less than open PDs [67–69, 73, 77, 79]. Also quality of life at 6 months postoperatively was higher in the laparoscopic patients [81].

Oncological outcomes included a shorter time between the surgery and start of adjuvant chemotherapy in the laparoscopic group [69, 81] as well as longer progression-free survival [69] in LPD patients. However, overall survival was not different [69].

Assessment of cost-effectiveness of laparoscopic procedures is another important topic. In general, increased upfront cost is a reason for many surgeons to criticize the technique for unnecessary resource wasting. However, for most procedures, the shorter postoperative length of stay decreases the overall cost. Also, when we take into account also earlier return to work after minor procedures, such as appendectomy or cholecystectomy, the initial increased cost can be justified in the light of the financial burden to the patient and the society. As expected, LPD was associated with increased procedural cost, but the decreased cost of postoperative care resulted in an overall similar overall cost to OPD [82].

With the development of the robotic surgical platform [17], several centers saw the potential of this technology to supply improved visualization and added degrees of freedom compared to laparoscopy. In published studies there has been a gradual improvement in conversion rates, OR time, and patient outcomes with increasing experience [83]. In experienced high-volume centers, robotic pancreaticoduodenectomy (RPD) outcomes have mirrored the results of LPD. RPD was associated with increased OR times, decreased intraoperative blood loss, shorter postoperative length of stay, and similar fistula rates and complications [83–86]. To date, LPD and RPD have never been compared prospectively in a proper clinical trial setting.

Minimally invasive pancreaticoduodenectomy (MIPD) is a procedure with a significant learning curve. As opposed to distal pancreatectomy, where only 20–40 laparoscopic procedures were associated with improved outcomes [26, 27], the number of procedures required for MIPD proficiency is double or roughly 40–80 [25, 29]. Considering the typical annual number of PDs performed by a high-volume HPB surgeon is between 10 and 12, it becomes obvious that the learning curve of 80 MIPDs is difficult to reach. Coupled with the significant difference in mortality between centers performing less than 10 versus 10 or more LPDs per year [77], there is a need for ongoing high annual number of LPD to maintain proficiency. Therefore, incorporation of laparoscopy into practice of PD is more complex. It is important to discourage occasional attempts to try MIPD. In our institution we continue to be relatively selective with inclusion for LPD, and we do not perform RPD. Patients with high BMI and those with extensive disease likely to require multivisceral resection or vascular resection/reconstruction are generally not considered for LPD irrespective of diagnosis. However, it is important to maintain a high volume of LPD per year in order to offer a safe procedure with potentially improved outcomes in terms of length of stay, ability to receive early adjuvant chemotherapy, and improved quality of life.

Other Pancreatic Resections

In addition to MIPD and MIDP that have been the main focus of literature describing minimally invasive pancreatic resections, other procedures are occasionally described although it is rare to see them compared to their open counterparts. These include parenchymal-sparing resections such as central pancreatectomy (CP) and total pancreatectomy (TP).

The rationale to perform a central pancreatectomy is parenchymal preservation in order to minimize the risk of postoperative endocrine or exorine insufficiency in patients with lesions in close proximity to main pancreatic duct that would be otherwise considered for enucleation. Because of two transection lines, this procedure is associated with increased perioperative risk, mainly driven by the fact that there are two sites of potential leak. Also, the typically soft pancreatic gland in nonmalignant indications for CP is associated with further increase in the risk of a leak. Therefore, the potential benefit of functional preservation has to be weighed against the substantial potential for pancreatic fistula.

Despite this downside and the significant technical demand to perform minimally invasive CP, there are several cases and series described in the literature. They consist of well-selected patients, and the procedures were performed in centers dedicated to laparoscopy. Therefore, without the ability to make generalized suggestions for HPB centers, we can conclude that in selected cases, laparoscopic [87–91] and robotic [83, 90, 92, 93] central pancreatectomy can be performed safely with no postoperative mortality, with overall morbidity below 40%, and with CR-POPF rate of 20–35%. No postoperative exocrine or endocrine insufficiency was found during subsequent follow-up of these cases [94].

Total pancreatectomy is an uncommon procedure. It is associated with significant morbidity and 30-day mortality of over 8% [95]. Despite the high risk associated with the open procedure, laparoscopic and robotic TP have been described in the literature.

Choi et al. [96] and Dallemagne et al. [97] described three and two laparoscopic TPs, respectively. Out of the three patients in the first series [96], one experienced a major complication; there was no postoperative complication and length of postoperative stay was 17–22 days. In the second series [97] neither of the two patients experienced a major complication and there was no mortality. Length of stay was 8 days for both studies. Two series describe the experience with robotic TP [83, 98] and describe five cases each. There was no postoperative mortality in either series; major morbidity was 20 and 40%, and patients recovered after 7–18 days in the hospital. One case-matched comparison of 11 laparoscopic robot-assisted TP versus 11 open TP [99] showed association between longer OR time and decreased EBL in the MITP group. Differences in major morbidity (18% in MITP and 27% OTP), mortality (0% both), reoperation rate (9% both), length of stay (12–88 days in MITP and 12–34 on OTP), and rate of R0 resection (100% for both) did not reach statistical significance.

As a result we can conclude that in selected cases, it is possible to perform major complex cases associated with significant intraoperative potential pitfalls and technical demand using minimally invasive techniques. Also, the procedure safety and postoperative recovery can achieve outcomes similar to open surgical technique. These demanding cases performed at properly developed MIS centers also aid in the development of new ways of utilizing existing technologies and discovery of new avenues that may serve our patients in the future.

Surgical Technique

There are multiple ways that minimally invasive pancreatic resections are described and performed. In this section we describe our technique of LDP and LPD in treatment of both benign and malignant diseases of the pancreas. Preoperative assessment and patient selection were described above. As for our practice and our institution, we consider virtually every patient requiring distal pancreatectomy for a laparoscopic procedure. The only exception is the need for vascular resection and reconstruction recognized preoperatively on pancreas protocol CT scan. With pancreaticoduodenectomy we are more likely to consider patients with benign disease or malignant disease that is not bulky and, again, will be unlikely to require formal vascular resection and reconstruction. Although we do consider some patients after neoadjuvant chemotherapy, patients who underwent neoadjuvant radiation are also less likely to be resected using minimally invasive approach due to the presumed vascular involvement.

Each procedure for malignant disease starts with diagnostic laparoscopy and a detailed laparoscopic ultrasound of the liver and pancreas. All suspicious lesions are biopsied and sent for intraoperative pathology examination.

Laparoscopic Distal Pancreatectomy With or Without Splenic Preservation

We place the patient supine with both arms out. For more central tumors, the operating surgeon is standing on the patient's left side, for more distal masses on the right side. Our trocar placement is not completely predefined; exact position of ports changes based on patient habitus and exact organ location on laparoscopy. In general we start with a periumbilical 12-port insertion using a Veress technique. At the final stages of the procedure, this port will be upsized to 15 mm in order to accommodate the stapler for pancreatic transection. Supra- or infraumbilical location is chosen depending on the distance of the umbilicus from the xiphoid process. While majority of patients are well suited for a supraumbilical port, occasionally with a short distance between the xiphoid process and the umbilicus (especially in patients with low BMI), the port would be directly over the pancreas which makes the procedure more challenging, and therefore the port is moved caudally. We use a 10 mm 30° laparoscope in this location. Another 12 mm port is then inserted at the left lateral border of the left rectus muscle for the ultrasound probe. After examination another two 5 mm ports are inserted, one in left subcostal location and one in right paramedian. If necessary,

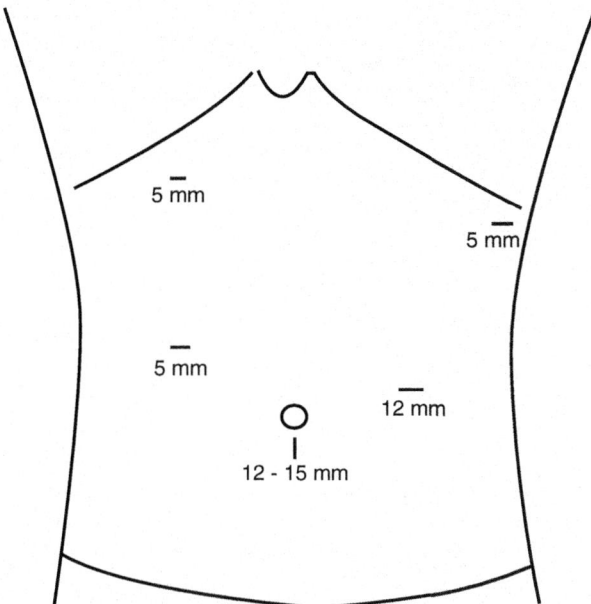

Fig. 11.1 Port placement for distal pancreatectomy

another 5 mm port may be inserted in right paramedian location cranial to the previous one for additional retraction (Fig. 11.1). We use either LigaSure™ Maryland (Covidien) or ENSEAL™ (Ethicon) energy devices for dissection.

Our first move is typically to enter the lesser sac through the gastrocolic ligament just below the gastroepiploic arcade so that the omentum attached to the stomach does not obscure visualization during subsequent steps. This dissection is carried beyond the midline on the right and all the way up through short gastric vessels on the left. We do not typically utilize the Warshaw splenic preservation technique. After separation of the stomach from the pancreas, we place a retractor to help with the visualization – either a Diamond-Flex retractor through the right subcostal 5 mm port or a thin diameter Nathanson retractor through a subxiphoid approach without a port. After repeat ultrasound to confirm location of the tumor, we start a broad dissection along the inferior edge of the pancreas at the area suitable for transection. We aim for a negative margin, not necessarily planning to transect at the neck of the pancreas. With a combination of blunt dissection and energy devices, the pancreas is lifted from the retroperitoneum, and splenic vein and IMV are identified. The splenic vein is then carefully dissected off of the posterior pancreas. The tunnel behind the pancreas is completed, and the artery is dissected free from the pancreas using combination of anterior and posterior dissection. The vein, artery, and pancreas are looped separately.

At that point we confirm that our loop is around the splenic artery. Especially with the surgeon on the left side operating through the left-sided ports, it is possible that the posterior dissection has been carried too far to the right and the common

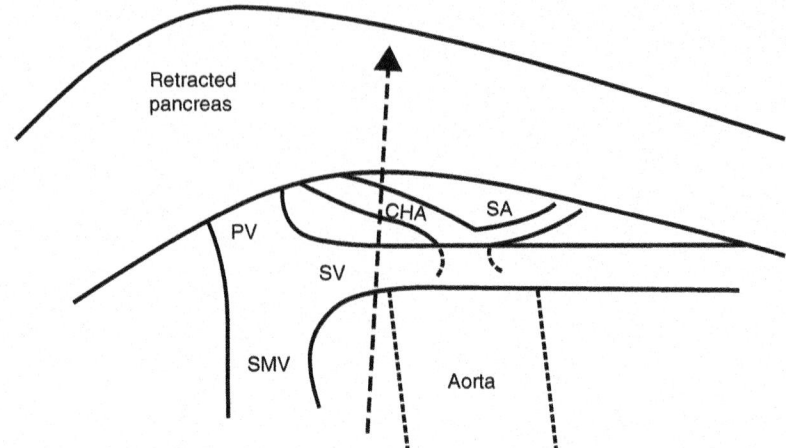

Fig. 11.2 Risk of incorporation of common hepatic artery (CHA) in staple line during pancreatic transection (pancreas retracted anteriorly with a vessel loop, visualization of retropancreatic tunnel). *PV* portal vein, *SMV* superior mesenteric vein, *SV* splenic vein, *SA* splenic artery

hepatic artery has been confused for the splenic artery and is inadvertently looped (Fig. 11.2). In case of splenic preservation, we preserve these vessels; otherwise, after confirmation of anatomy and ultrasonographically safe negative margin on the pancreas, three firings of laparoscopic stapler are used to transect the structures separately. To transect the pancreas, we use a firing of the Endo GIA™ Reinforced Reload 60 mm black Tri-Staple™. The dissection then continues distally. The splenic flexure is mobilized off of the inferior pancreas and spleen, and the retroperitoneal dissection is completed. The specimen is then placed in a retrieval bag oriented so the pancreas is delivered through the somewhat enlarged periumbilical incision first. After pancreas extraction, we transect through the hilum of the spleen, and the spleen is then morcellated and extracted.

A single 15 Fr round hubless Blake Drain is inserted through the right 5 mm port and placed across the lesser sac all the way to the left subphrenic space, making sure it passes along the pancreatic transection margin.

Laparoscopic Pancreaticoduodenectomy

We position the patient supine with both arms out on the arm boards. The procedure starts similarly to distal pancreatectomy with the first two ports and assessment to rule out metastatic disease. After that another 12 mm port is inserted at the right lateral edge of the right rectus muscle and finally two 5 mm ports in the subcostal areas bilaterally (Fig. 11.3).

The procedure then mimics the way we perform open PD. We start by opening the gastrocolic ligament and mobilizing the right colon. Full kocherization of the duodenum (including D3 and D4) and pancreatic head ensues. Dissection of the

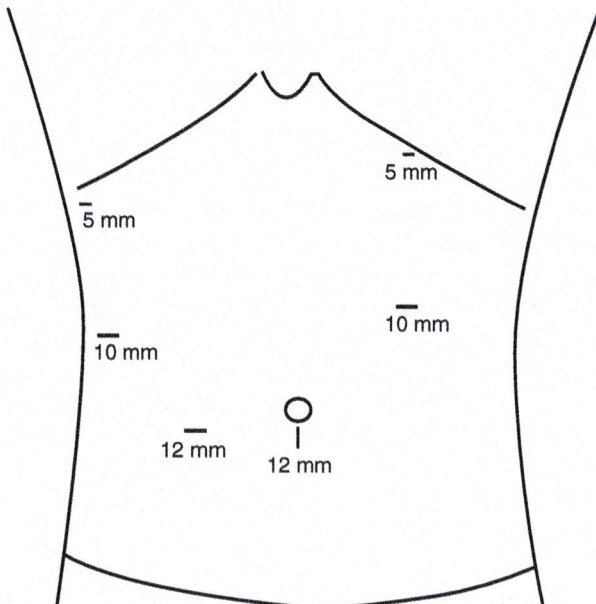

Fig. 11.3 Port placement for pancreaticoduodenectomy

SMV from the pancreatic head starting anterior to D3 and continuing toward the neck of the pancreas with assessment of the SMA using ultrasound confirms resectability. During the assessment we again confirm the presence or lack of replaced arterial anatomy based on preoperative imaging. Subsequently, we move to the hepatoduodenal ligament. The gallbladder is dissected from the liver bed, and the dissection continues down the cystic duct to the CBD. After circumferential dissection it is transected to help with identification of the portal vein. The CBD margin is sent for intraoperative assessment by pathology. The dissection continues medially, and the common hepatic artery lymph node is removed. Hepatic artery and GDA are dissected. Flow before and after occlusion of GDA is assessed with Doppler ultrasound, and the vessel is divided between ties. The tunnel between the pancreas and the SMV/PV is completed.

We perform predominantly a pylorus-preserving PD, but in cases of involvement of D1, a classic PD with antrectomy at the level of incisura is performed. For a PPPD after division of right gastroepiploic vessels and right gastric artery, the soft tissue around D1 is circumferentially dissected, and using an Endo GIA™ stapler, the duodenum is transected approximately 2 cm distal to the pylorus. The pancreas is then looped.

After repositioning the retraction to elevate the transverse colon, the proximal jejunum is identified and transected. The proximal jejunum and the ligament of Treitz are then completely mobilized to the level of D4. The duodenum and proximal jejunum are pulled underneath the superior mesenteric vessels to the right upper quadrant to allow for retraction while dissecting the uncinate process. The pancreas is then transected, and the margin is shaved off and sent for intraoperative frozen section assessment. Then the uncinate process is dissected free from the SMV and SMA that are completely exposed to resect all lymphatic tissue with the specimen from the caudal end going cephalad.

The reconstruction phase starts with pulling the proximal jejunum through an opening in the transverse mesocolon and creation of a pancreaticojejunostomy. We perform the invagination technique with posterior interrupted 3–0 Vicryl sutures, followed by posterior running 5–0 PDS layer. Subsequently a running anterior 5–0 PDS and finally anterior interrupted 3–0 Vicryl sutures are placed. Hepaticojejunostomy is performed using interrupted 5–0 PDS sutures in the usual fashion. Finally a duodenojejunostomy is fashioned using a single layer 3–0 PDS running suture in an antecolic position. Depending on the assessment of risk of leak using a pancreas risk score calculator, no drains are left for patients with negligible risk; in other patients, we typically leave a 15 Fr round hubless drain through a right-sided 5 mm port through the right paracolic gutter posterior to the HJ and posterior to the PJ anastomoses. We do not leave an NG tube in, and we do not place surgical J-tubes in any of our patients.

References

1. McMahon AJ, Baxter J, Anderson J, Ramsay G, O'Dwyer P, Russell I, et al. Laparoscopic versus minilaparotomy cholecystectomy: a randomised trial. Lancet. 1994;343(8890):135–8.
2. Kiviluoto T, Sirén J, Luukkonen P, Kivilaakso E. Randomised trial of laparoscopic versus open cholecystectomy for acute and gangrenous cholecystitis. Lancet. 1998;351(9099):321–5.
3. Attwood SE, Hill AD, Murphy PG, Thornton J, Stephens RB. A prospective randomized trial of laparoscopic versus open appendectomy. Surgery. 1992;112(3):497–501.
4. Frazee RC, Roberts JW, Symmonds RE, Snyder SK, Hendricks JC, Smith RW, et al. A prospective randomized trial comparing open versus laparoscopic appendectomy. Ann Surg. 1994;219(6):725–8. discussion 728–31
5. Puzziferri N, Austrheim-Smith IT, Wolfe BM, Wilson SE, Nguyen NT. Three-year follow-up of a prospective randomized trial comparing laparoscopic versus open gastric bypass. Ann Surg. 2006;243(2):181–8.
6. Huscher CG, Mingoli A, Sgarzini G, Sansonetti A, Di Paola M, Recher A, et al. Laparoscopic versus open subtotal gastrectomy for distal gastric cancer: five-year results of a randomized prospective trial. Ann Surg. 2005;241(2):232–7.
7. Hasegawa H, Kabeshima Y, Watanabe M, Yamamoto S, Kitajima M. Randomized controlled trial of laparoscopic versus open colectomy for advanced colorectal cancer. Surg Endosc Other Int Tech. 2003;17(4):636–40.
8. Lujan J, Valero G, Hernandez Q, Sanchez A, Frutos M, Parrilla P. Randomized clinical trial comparing laparoscopic and open surgery in patients with rectal cancer. Br J Surg. 2009;96(9):982–9.
9. McDermott Jr WV, Bartlett MK. Pancreaticoduodenal cancer. N Engl J Med. 1953;248(22):927–31.
10. Morris PJ, Nardi GL. Pancreaticoduodenal cancer. Experience from 1951 to 1960 with a look ahead and behind. Arch Surg. 1966;92(6):834–7.
11. McDowell BD, Chapman CG, Smith BJ, Button AM, Chrischilles EA, Mezhir JJ. Pancreatectomy predicts improved survival for pancreatic adenocarcinoma: results of an instrumental variable analysis. Ann Surg. 2015;261(4):740–5.

12. Kairaluoma MI, Stahlberg M, Kiviniemi H. Pancreatic resection for carcinoma of the pancreas and the periampullary region. A twenty-year experience. HPB Surgery. 1990. discussion 66–7;2(1):57–66.
13. Cameron JL, Riall TS, Coleman J, Belcher KA. One thousand consecutive pancreaticoduodenectomies. Ann Surg. 2006;244(1):10–5.
14. Birkmeyer JD, Stukel TA, Siewers AE, Goodney PP, Wennberg DE, Lucas FL. Surgeon volume and operative mortality in the United States. N Engl J Med. 2003;349(22):2117–27.
15. Gagner M, Pomp A. Laparoscopic pylorus-preserving pancreatoduodenectomy. Surg Endosc. 1994;8(5):408–10.
16. Gagner M, Pomp A, Herrera MF. Early experience with laparoscopic resections of islet cell tumors. Surgery. 1996;120(6):1051–4.
17. Melvin WS, Needleman B, Krause K, Ellison E. Robotic resection of pancreatic neuroendocrine tumor. J Laparoendosc Adv Surg Tech. 2003;13(1):33–6.
18. Giulianotti PC, Sbrana F, Bianco FM, Elli EF, Shah G, Addeo P, et al. Robot-assisted laparoscopic pancreatic surgery: single-surgeon experience. Surg Endosc. 2010;24(7):1646–57.
19. Okunrintemi V, Gani F, Pawlik TM. National trends in postoperative outcomes and cost comparing minimally invasive versus open liver and pancreatic surgery. J Gastrointest Surg. 2016;20(11):1836–43.
20. Begg CB, Cramer LD, Hoskins WJ, Brennan MF. Impact of hospital volume on operative mortality for major cancer surgery. Surv Anesthesiol. 1999;43(6):368–9.
21. Birkmeyer JD, Finlayson SR, Tosteson AN, Sharp SM, Warshaw AL, Fisher ES. Effect of hospital volume on in-hospital mortality with pancreaticoduodenectomy. Surgery. 1999;125(3):250–6.
22. Kennedy TJ, Cassera MA, Wolf R, Swanstrom LL, Hansen PD. Surgeon volume versus morbidity and cost in patients undergoing pancreaticoduodenectomy in an academic community medical center. J Gastrointest Surg. 2010;14(12):1990–6.
23. Killeen S, O'sullivan M, Coffey J, Kirwan W, Redmond H. Provider volume and outcomes for oncological procedures. Br J Surg. 2005;92(4):389–402.
24. Hardacre JM. Is there a learning curve for pancreaticoduodenectomy after fellowship training? HPB Surg. 2010;2010:230287.
25. Boone BA, Zenati M, Hogg ME, Steve J, Moser AJ, Bartlett DL, et al. Assessment of quality outcomes for robotic pancreaticoduodenectomy: identification of the learning curve. JAMA Surg. 2015;150(5):416–22.
26. Braga M, Ridolfi C, Balzano G, Castoldi R, Pecorelli N, Di Carlo V. Learning curve for laparoscopic distal pancreatectomy in a high-volume hospital. Updat Surg. 2012;64(3):179–83.
27. Ricci C, Casadei R, Buscemi S, Taffurelli G, D'Ambra M, Pacilio CA, et al. Laparoscopic distal pancreatectomy: what factors are related to the learning curve? Surg Today. 2015;45(1):50–6.
28. Shakir M, Boone BA, Polanco PM, Zenati MS, Hogg ME, Tsung A, et al. The learning curve for robotic distal pancreatectomy: an analysis of outcomes of the first 100 consecutive cases at a high-volume pancreatic centre. HPB. 2015;17(7):580–6.
29. Speicher PJ, Nussbaum DP, White RR, Zani S, Mosca PJ, Blazer DG III, et al. Defining the learning curve for team-based laparoscopic pancreaticoduodenectomy. Ann Surg Oncol. 2014;21(12):4014–9.
30. de Rooij T, van Hilst J, Boerma D, Bonsing BA, Daams F, van Dam RM, et al. Impact of a Nationwide training program in minimally invasive distal pancreatectomy (LAELAPS). Ann Surg. 2016;264(5):754–62.
31. Zeng X, Zhong S, Zhu Y, Fei L, Wu W, Cai L. Insulinoma: 31 years of tumor localization and excision. J Surg Oncol. 1988;39(4):274–8.
32. Fernández-Cruz L, Molina V, Vallejos R, Jiménez Chavarria E, López-Boado M, Ferrer J. Outcome after laparoscopic enucleation for non-functional neuroendocrine pancreatic tumours. HPB. 2012;14(3):171–6.
33. Crippa S, Bassi C, Salvia R, Falconi M, Butturini G, Pederzoli P. Enucleation of pancreatic neoplasms. Br J Surg. 2007;94(10):1254–9.

34. Zhang T, Xu J, Wang T, Liao Q, Dai M, Zhao Y. Enucleation of pancreatic lesions: indications, outcomes, and risk factors for clinical pancreatic fistula. J Gastrointest Surg. 2013;17(12):2099–104.
35. Chua TC, Yang TX, Gill AJ, Samra JS. Systematic review and meta-analysis of enucleation versus standardized resection for small pancreatic lesions. Ann Surg Oncol. 2016;23(2):592–9.
36. Briggs CD, Mann CD, Irving GR, Neal CP, Peterson M, Cameron IC, et al. Systematic review of minimally invasive pancreatic resection. J Gastrointest Surg. 2009;13(6):1129–37.
37. Beger H, Siech M, Poch B, Mayer B, Schoenberg M. Limited surgery for benign tumours of the pancreas: a systematic review. World J Surg. 2015;39(6):1557–66.
38. Dedieu A, Rault A, Collet D, Masson B, Cunha AS. Laparoscopic enucleation of pancreatic neoplasm. Surg Endosc. 2011;25(2):572–6.
39. Song KB, Kim SC, Hwang DW, Lee JH, Lee DJ, Lee JW, et al. Enucleation for benign or low-grade malignant lesions of the pancreas: single-center experience with 65 consecutive patients. Surgery. 2015;158(5):1203–10.
40. Weinstein S, Morgan T, Poder L, Shin L, Jeffrey RB, Aslam R, et al. Value of intraoperative sonography in pancreatic surgery. J Ultrasound Med. 2015;34(7):1307–18.
41. Bencini L, Annecchiarico M, Farsi M, Bartolini I, Mirasolo V, Guerra F, et al. Minimally invasive surgical approach to pancreatic malignancies. World J Gastrointest Oncol. 2015;7(12):411–21.
42. Nappo G, Perinel J, El Bechwaty M, Adham M. Minimally invasive pancreatic resection: is it really the future? Dig Surg. 2016;33(4):284–9.
43. Giulianotti PC, Coratti A, Angelini M, Sbrana F, Cecconi S, Balestracci T, et al. Robotics in general surgery: personal experience in a large community hospital. Arch Surg. 2003;138(7):777–84.
44. Cao HST, Lopez N, Chang DC, Lowy AM, Bouvet M, Baumgartner JM, et al. Improved perioperative outcomes with minimally invasive distal pancreatectomy: results from a population-based analysis. JAMA Surg. 2014;149(3):237–43.
45. Ejaz A, Sachs T, He J, Spolverato G, Hirose K, Ahuja N, et al. A comparison of open and minimally invasive surgery for hepatic and pancreatic resections using the Nationwide inpatient sample. Surgery. 2014;156(3):538–47.
46. Eom B, Jang J, Lee S, Han H, Yoon Y, Kim S. Clinical outcomes compared between laparoscopic and open distal pancreatectomy. Surg Endosc. 2008;22(5):1334–8.
47. de Rooij T, Jilesen AP, Boerma D, Bonsing BA, Bosscha K, van Dam RM, et al. A nationwide comparison of laparoscopic and open distal pancreatectomy for benign and malignant disease. J Am Coll Surg. 2015;220(3):263–70. e1
48. DiNorcia J, Schrope BA, Lee MK, Reavey PL, Rosen SJ, Lee JA, et al. Laparoscopic distal pancreatectomy offers shorter hospital stays with fewer complications. J Gastrointest Surg. 2010;14(11):1804–12.
49. Jayaraman S, Gonen M, Brennan MF, D'Angelica MI, DeMatteo RP, Fong Y, et al. Laparoscopic distal pancreatectomy: evolution of a technique at a single institution. J Am Coll Surg. 2010;211(4):503–9.
50. Casadei R, Ricci C, D'Ambra M, Marrano N, Alagna V, Rega D, et al. Laparoscopic versus open distal pancreatectomy in pancreatic tumours: a case–control study. Updat Surg. 2010;62(3–4):171–4.
51. Limongelli P, Belli A, Russo G, Cioffi L, D'Agostino A, Fantini C, et al. Laparoscopic and open surgical treatment of left-sided pancreatic lesions: clinical outcomes and cost-effectiveness analysis. Surg Endosc. 2012;26(7):1830–6.
52. Nakamura M, Wakabayashi G, Miyasaka Y, Tanaka M, Morikawa T, Unno M, et al. Multicenter comparative study of laparoscopic and open distal pancreatectomy using propensity score-matching. J Hepatobiliary Pancreat Sci. 2015;22(10):731–6.
53. Khaled YS, Malde DJ, Packer J, De Liguori Carino N, Deshpande R, O'Reilly DA, et al. A case-matched comparative study of laparoscopic versus open distal pancreatectomy. Surg Laparosc Endosc Percutan Tech. 2015;25(4):363–7.

54. Baker MS, Sherman KL, Stocker S, Hayman AV, Bentrem DJ, Prinz RA, et al. Defining quality for distal pancreatectomy: does the laparoscopic approach protect patients from poor quality outcomes? J Gastrointest Surg. 2013;17(2):273–80.
55. Aly MY, Tsutsumi K, Nakamura M, Sato N, Takahata S, Ueda J, et al. Comparative study of laparoscopic and open distal pancreatectomy. J Laparoendosc Adv Surg Tech. 2010;20(5):435–40.
56. Chung JC, Kim HC, Song OP. Laparoscopic distal pancreatectomy for benign or borderline malignant pancreatic tumors. Turk J Gastroenterol. 2014;25(1):162–6.
57. Riviere D, Gurusamy KS, Kooby DA, Vollmer CM, Besselink MG, Davidson BR, et al. Laparoscopic versus open distal pancreatectomy for pancreatic cancer. Cochrane Libr. 2016:4.
58. Ricci C, Casadei R, Taffurelli G, Toscano F, Pacilio CA, Bogoni S, et al. Laparoscopic versus open distal pancreatectomy for ductal adenocarcinoma: a systematic review and meta-analysis. J Gastrointest Surg. 2015;19(4):770–81.
59. Venkat R, Edil BH, Schulick RD, Lidor AO, Makary MA, Wolfgang CL. Laparoscopic distal pancreatectomy is associated with significantly less overall morbidity compared to the open technique: a systematic review and meta-analysis. Ann Surg. 2012;255(6):1048–59.
60. Hilal MA, Hamdan M, Di Fabio F, Pearce NW, Johnson CD. Laparoscopic versus open distal pancreatectomy: a clinical and cost-effectiveness study. Surg Endosc. 2012;26(6):1670–4.
61. Fox AM, Pitzul K, Bhojani F, Kaplan M, Moulton C, Wei AC, et al. Comparison of outcomes and costs between laparoscopic distal pancreatectomy and open resection at a single center. Surg Endosc. 2012;26(5):1220–30.
62. Daouadi M, Zureikat AH, Zenati MS, Choudry H, Tsung A, Bartlett DL, et al. Robot-assisted minimally invasive distal pancreatectomy is superior to the laparoscopic technique. Ann Surg. 2013;257(1):128–32.
63. Waters JA, Canal DF, Wiebke EA, Dumas RP, Beane JD, Aguilar-Saavedra JR, et al. Robotic distal pancreatectomy: cost effective? Surgery. 2010;148(4):814–23.
64. Kang CM, Kim DH, Lee WJ, Chi HS. Conventional laparoscopic and robot-assisted spleen-preserving pancreatectomy: does da Vinci have clinical advantages? Surg Endosc. 2011;25(6):2004–9.
65. Duran H, Ielpo B, Caruso R, Ferri V, Quijano Y, Diaz E, et al. Does robotic distal pancreatectomy surgery offer similar results as laparoscopic and open approach? A comparative study from a single medical center. Int J Med Rob Comput Assisted Surg. 2014;10(3):280–5.
66. Butturini G, Damoli I, Crepaz L, Malleo G, Marchegiani G, Daskalaki D, et al. A prospective non-randomised single-center study comparing laparoscopic and robotic distal pancreatectomy. Surg Endosc. 2015;29(11):3163–70.
67. Wright GP, Zureikat AH. Development of minimally invasive pancreatic surgery: an evidence-based systematic review of laparoscopic versus robotic approaches. J Gastrointest Surg. 2016;20(9):1658–65.
68. Asbun HJ, Stauffer JA. Laparoscopic vs open pancreaticoduodenectomy: overall outcomes and severity of complications using the accordion severity grading system. J Am Coll Surg. 2012;215(6):810–9.
69. Croome KP, Farnell MB, Que FG, Reid-Lombardo KM, Truty MJ, Nagorney DM, et al. Total laparoscopic pancreaticoduodenectomy for pancreatic ductal adenocarcinoma: oncologic advantages over open approaches? Ann Surg. 2014;260(4):633–8. discussion 638–40
70. Gumbs AA, Croner R, Rodriguez A, Zuker N, Perrakis A, Gayet B. 200 consecutive laparoscopic pancreatic resections performed with a robotically controlled laparoscope holder. Surg Endosc. 2013;27(10):3781–91.
71. Kim SC, Song KB, Jung YS, Kim YH, Park DH, Lee SS, et al. Short-term clinical outcomes for 100 consecutive cases of laparoscopic pylorus-preserving pancreatoduodenectomy: improvement with surgical experience. Surg Endosc. 2013;27(1):95–103.
72. Senthilnathan P, Srivatsan Gurumurthy S, Gul SI, Sabnis S, Natesan AV, Palanisamy NV, et al. Long-term results of laparoscopic pancreaticoduodenectomy for pancreatic and periampullary cancer—experience of 130 cases from a tertiary-care center in South India. J Laparoendosc Adv Surg Tech. 2015;25(4):295–300.

73. de Rooij T, MZ L, Steen MW, Gerhards MF, Dijkgraaf MG, Busch OR, et al. Minimally invasive versus open pancreatoduodenectomy: systematic review and meta-analysis of comparative cohort and registry studies. Ann Surg. 2016;264(2):257–67.
74. Dokmak S, Ftériche FS, Aussilhou B, Bensafta Y, Lévy P, Ruszniewski P, et al. Laparoscopic pancreaticoduodenectomy should not be routine for resection of periampullary tumors. J Am Coll Surg. 2015;220(5):831–8.
75. Boggi U, Amorese G, Vistoli F, Caniglia F, De Lio N, Perrone V, et al. Laparoscopic pancreaticoduodenectomy: a systematic literature review. Surg Endosc. 2015;29(1):9–23.
76. Kuroki T, Adachi T, Okamoto T, Kanematsu TA. Non-randomized comparative study of laparoscopy-assisted pancreaticoduodenectomy and open pancreaticoduodenectomy. Hepato-Gastroenterology. 2012;59(114):570–3.
77. Sharpe SM, Talamonti MS, Wang CE, Prinz RA, Roggin KK, Bentrem DJ, et al. Early national experience with laparoscopic pancreaticoduodenectomy for ductal adenocarcinoma: a comparison of laparoscopic pancreaticoduodenectomy and open pancreaticoduodenectomy from the National Cancer Data Base. J Am Coll Surg. 2015;221(1):175–84.
78. Adam MA, Choudhury K, Dinan MA, Reed SD, Scheri RP, Blazer DG III, et al. Minimally invasive versus open pancreaticoduodenectomy for cancer: practice patterns and short-term outcomes among 7061 patients. Ann Surg. 2015;262(2):372–7.
79. Tran TB, Dua MM, Worhunsky DJ, Poultsides GA, Norton JA, Visser BC. The first decade of laparoscopic pancreaticoduodenectomy in the United States: costs and outcomes using the nationwide inpatient sample. Surg Endosc. 2016;30(5):1778–83.
80. Song KB, Kim SC, Hwang DW, Lee JH, Lee DJ, Lee JW, et al. Matched case-control analysis comparing laparoscopic and open pylorus-preserving Pancreaticoduodenectomy in patients with Periampullary tumors. Ann Surg. 2015;262(1):146–55.
81. Langan RC, Graham JA, Chin AB, Rubinstein AJ, Oza K, Nusbaum JA, et al. Laparoscopic-assisted versus open pancreaticoduodenectomy: early favorable physical quality-of-life measures. Surgery. 2014;156(2):379–84.
82. Mesleh MG, Stauffer JA, Bowers SP, Asbun HJ. Cost analysis of open and laparoscopic pancreaticoduodenectomy: a single institution comparison. Surg Endosc. 2013;27(12):4518–23.
83. Zureikat AH, Moser AJ, Boone BA, Bartlett DL, Zenati M, Zeh HJ 3rd. 250 robotic pancreatic resections: safety and feasibility. Ann Surg. 2013;258(4):554–9. discussion 559–62
84. Buchs NC, Addeo P, Bianco FM, Ayloo S, Benedetti E, Giulianotti PC. Robotic versus open pancreaticoduodenectomy: a comparative study at a single institution. World J Surg. 2011;35(12):2739–46.
85. Chalikonda S, Aguilar-Saavedra J, Walsh RM. Laparoscopic robotic-assisted pancreaticoduodenectomy: a case-matched comparison with open resection. Surg Endosc. 2012;26(9):2397–402.
86. Lai EC, Yang GP, Tang CN. Robot-assisted laparoscopic pancreaticoduodenectomy versus open pancreaticoduodenectomy–a comparative study. Int J Surg. 2012;10(9):475–9.
87. Cunha AS, Rault A, Beau C, Collet D, Masson B. Laparoscopic central pancreatectomy: single institution experience of 6 patients. Surgery. 2007;142(3):405–9.
88. Rotellar F, Pardo F, Montiel C, Benito A, Regueira FM, Poveda I, et al. Totally laparoscopic Roux-en-Y duct-to-mucosa pancreaticojejunostomy after middle pancreatectomy: a consecutive nine-case series at a single institution. Ann Surg. 2008;247(6):938–44.
89. Chen X, Zhang Y, Sun D. Laparoscopic central pancreatectomy for solid pseudopapillary tumors of the pancreas: our experience with ten cases. World J Surg Oncol. 2014;12(1):1.
90. Machado MA, Surjan RC, Epstein MG, Makdissi FF. Laparoscopic central pancreatectomy: a review of 51 cases. Surg Laparosc Endosc Percutan Tech. 2013;23(6):486–90.
91. Senthilnathan P, Gul SI, Gurumurthy SS, Palanivelu PR, Parthasarathi R, Palanisamy NV, et al. Laparoscopic central pancreatectomy: our technique and long-term results in 14 patients. J Minim Access Surg. 2015;11(3):167.
92. Abood GJ, Can MF, Daouadi M, Huss HT, Steve JY, Ramalingam L, et al. Robotic-assisted minimally invasive central pancreatectomy: technique and outcomes. J Gastrointest Surg. 2013;17(5):1002–8.

93. Kang CM, Kim DH, Lee WJ, Chi HS. Initial experiences using robot-assisted central pancreatectomy with pancreaticogastrostomy: a potential way to advanced laparoscopic pancreatectomy. Surg Endosc. 2011;25(4):1101–6.
94. Kuroki T, Eguchi S. Laparoscopic parenchyma-sparing pancreatectomy. J Hepatobiliary Pancreat Sci. 2014;21(5):323–7.
95. Murphy MM, Knaus I, William J, Ng SC, Hill JS, McPhee JT, et al. Total pancreatectomy: a national study. HPB. 2009;11(6):476–82.
96. Choi SH, Hwang HK, Kang CM, Yoon CI, Lee WJ. Pylorus- and spleen-preserving total pancreatoduodenectomy with resection of both whole splenic vessels: feasibility and laparoscopic application to intraductal papillary mucin-producing tumors of the pancreas. Surg Endosc. 2012;26(7):2072–7.
97. Dallemagne B, Oliveira A, Lacerda CF, D'Agostino J, Mercoli H, Marescaux J. Full laparoscopic total pancreatectomy with and without spleen and pylorus preservation: a feasibility report. J Hepatobiliary Pancreat Sci. 2013;20(6):647–53.
98. Giulianotti PC, Addeo P, Buchs NC, Bianco FM, Ayloo SM. Early experience with robotic total pancreatectomy. Pancreas. 2011;40(2):311–3.
99. Boggi U, Palladino S, Massimetti G, Vistoli F, Caniglia F, De Lio N, et al. Laparoscopic robot-assisted versus open total pancreatectomy: a case-matched study. Surg Endosc. 2015;29(6):1425–32.

Jordan M. Cloyd and Matthew H.G. Katz

Introduction

The superior mesenteric artery (SMA) courses just to the left of the uncinate process, along its path from the aorta into the root of the small bowel mesentery. Tumors of the proximal pancreas therefore closely approach the SMA, and cancer cells from the primary tumor may infiltrate the surrounding perineural and lymphatic tissues of the retroperitoneum. Thorough clearance of the soft tissues located to the right of the SMA is required to enhance the likelihood of a margin-negative (R0) resection [1]. However, access to the SMA is impeded by the overlying superior mesenteric vein-portal vein (SMV-PV) confluence, its major branches, and the pancreatic parenchyma [2]. For these reasons, a meticulous uncinate dissection is simultaneously the most oncologically critical and technically challenging part of a pancreatoduodenectomy (PD).

Because the tissue between the uncinate process and the SMA is the most likely location of macroscopic (R2) or microscopic (R1) residual disease after PD, meticulous attention to this area and routine clearance of all of its fibrofatty tissue maximize the likelihood of an R0 resection in correctly staged patients. This may be accomplished by skeletonizing the right lateral aspect of the SMA using sharp, ultrasonic, or thermal dissection. In this chapter, we describe and illustrate technical approaches to retroperitoneal dissection during PD for patients with pancreatic ductal adenocarcinoma (PDAC) and discuss important considerations regarding the resection of tumors with vascular involvement.

J.M. Cloyd, MD (✉)
Department of Surgery, The Ohio State University Medical Center, Columbus, OH, USA
e-mail: jordan.cloyd@osumc.edu

M.H.G. Katz, MD (✉)
Department of Surgical Oncology, The University of Texas MD Anderson Cancer Center, Houston, TX, USA
e-mail: mhgkatz@mdanderson.org

© Springer International Publishing AG 2018
F.G. Rocha, P. Shen (eds.), *Optimizing Outcomes for Liver and Pancreas Surgery*, DOI 10.1007/978-3-319-62624-6_12

Important Considerations

Radiographic Staging

All patients with PDAC should be evaluated with high-quality, pancreatic protocol computed tomography (CT), not only to rule out distant metastatic disease but also to evaluate locoregional extension and to characterize local vascular anatomy. The ability to safely perform complex resections of tumors that involve the major mesenteric vasculature has led to radiographic categorizations based on the anatomic relationship of the tumor to its nearby vascular structures [3]. Broadly termed potentially resectable (PR), borderline resectable (BR), and locally advanced (LA), these categories predict a surgeon's ability to successfully complete a margin-negative resection, as well as the need for vascular resection. Furthermore, they may be used to guide decisions regarding the delivery of preoperative therapy. For example, patients with borderline resectable disease are typically offered preoperative chemotherapy and/or chemoradiation therapy because these patients have been shown to be at high risk for margin-positive resection and the development of early metastatic disease when surgery is conducted de novo [3].

Important aspects of the preoperative CT to consider include the location, size, and extent of the primary tumor. A systematic review of the liver, peritoneal surfaces, and regional lymph nodes should be conducted for signs of metastatic disease. Abutment or encasement of venous and arterial structures should be noted, and the exact circumferential interface between the primary tumor and each major vessel (e.g., ≤ or >180°) should be measured. In addition, the regional arterial and venous anatomy should be thoroughly examined. This review should include an inspection of the pattern and distribution of the branches of the SMV, identification of the insertion of the inferior mesenteric vein (IMV), and evaluation of hepatic artery variants that will influence the operative strategy [2].

Histopathologic Evaluation

Margin status at the time of pancreatectomy is an important prognostic factor in patients with PDAC. Published R1 resection rates from large institutional series range from 20 to 40% [4]; however, recent studies using meticulous histopathologic protocols have shown evidence of cancer cells in at least one surgical margin in close to 90% of resected specimens from patients who had undergone PD [5]. This finding may account for the observation that up to 80% of patients who die as a result of PDAC after undergoing PD have evidence of locoregional recurrence at the time of autopsy [6]. Clearly, the margin status may be influenced as much by the histopathologic analysis than by the surgery itself. Thus, in addition to routine analysis of the primary tumor and regional lymph nodes, a meticulous histopathologic evaluation of the surgical margins should be performed. Although the pancreatic neck and bile duct margins are inked en face and considered positive if tumor cells are identified at the inked margin, special consideration must be given to the SMA margin, given its oncologic importance and high likelihood of positivity. The entire inked SMA margin should be submitted perpendicularly for microscopic evaluation after fixation overnight. Previous studies have demonstrated similar outcomes among patients with microscopically positive SMA margins and those with tumor cells within 1 mm of the SMA; therefore, a positive SMA margin is generally defined as one with tumor cells at or within 1 mm of the ink [7].

It is important to understand the implications of the dissection technique in terms of the consequences of a positive margin. First, only the surgeon can make the distinction between an R2 and R1 resection because pathologists' interpretations will be similar in either case; therefore, information regarding residual disease should be clearly documented by the surgeon in the operative report. Second, in contrast to positive pancreatic neck and bile duct margins, for which re-excision to achieve negative margins may or may not be possible, an R1 SMA margin cannot be further excised because all the tissue to the right of the SMA will have already been exhausted.

It is critical that surgeons and pathologists work together to ensure correct specimen orientation. A PD specimen is extraordinarily complex ex vivo. With multiple transection sites and a lack of normal retroperitoneal structures that serve as landmarks in vivo, correct orientation of the specimen ex vivo is challenging, especially for less-experienced pathologists. Guidelines from the American Joint Committee on Cancer, the College of American Pathologists, and the American College of Surgeons/Alliance for Clinical Trials in Clinical Oncology recommend immediate inking of the bile duct, the SMV-PV groove, the uncinate/SMA margins, the neck, and the anterior and posterior/retropancreatic surface of the pancreas at the time of resection [8]. This procedure is best performed collaboratively by the surgeon and pathologist at the time of specimen removal.

Preoperative Therapy

Increasingly, patients with PDAC are being treated with preoperative chemotherapy and/or chemoradiation therapy. In fact, national guidelines now recommend the use of neoadjuvant therapy in patients with borderline resectable or locally advanced disease and acknowledge that the administration of preoperative therapy is an acceptable alternative treatment strategy for patients with technically resectable tumors [9, 10]. The potential advantages of preoperative therapy include the opportunity to identify patients who are most likely to benefit from major surgery, guarantee the delivery of multimodality therapy to all patients, provide early treatment of micrometastatic disease, and facilitate a successful margin-negative resection [11].

Several important considerations should be noted in patients who have received preoperative therapies. First, previous studies have found that radiographic evidence of downstaging is unlikely to occur [12]. In fact, several authors have demonstrated that posttreatment scans overestimate the degree of residual carcinoma [13]. Accordingly, surgeons should focus on the absence of local or distant progression, as well as on the optimization of nutritional and physiologic parameters, to make decisions regarding surgery after preoperative therapy. Second, surgical, medical, and radiation oncologists should communicate frequently to ensure that patients receive the appropriate duration of therapy, because extended regiments of cytotoxic chemotherapy may lead to significant treatment-related toxicities. Third, although anecdotally surgeons have reported a more difficult dissection following radiation, evidence suggests that preoperative therapy does not adversely influence postoperative morbidity and mortality [14]. In fact, preoperative radiation has the surreptitious advantage of being associated with reduced rates of postoperative pancreatic fistula [14, 15]. Finally, pathologists should evaluate and document the percentage of residual carcinoma—i.e., the response to preoperative therapy—in the primary tumor because this information has important prognostic implications.

Technical Details

The retroperitoneal dissection is classically the final step before removal of the PD specimen and subsequent reconstruction. PD begins in the standard fashion; once the stomach or duodenum, jejunum, bile duct, and neck of the pancreas have been divided, attention is turned to the uncinate dissection. This critical field of dissection extends from the caudal border of the uncinate process to the level of the takeoff of the SMA from the aorta. Because the proximal SMA lies directly posterior to the SMV-PV, complete mobilization of the SMV-PV is required. When the primary tumor does not adhere to the vein, the SMV-PV may be retracted to the left with vessel loops or vein retractors. With the freed SMV-PV retracted toward the left and the surgical specimen retracted toward the right, the proximal SMA is maximally exposed (Fig. 12.1). Next, all fat, fibrous, perineural, and lymphatic tissues are swept to the right by dissecting along the periadventitial plane of the SMA (Fig. 12.2a, b). The dissection should be carried cephalad from the level of the first jejunal branch of the SMV to the takeoff of the artery from the aorta. Inferior pancreaticoduodenal arteries should be individually ligated with clips and ties or divided with ultrasonic or thermal devices. Importantly, circumferential dissection of the SMA should be avoided to prevent disruption of the sympathetic nerve plexuses, which can lead to chronic diarrhea [16]. Finally, the relatively avascular retroperitoneal connections can be divided, and the specimen may be removed. Meticulous dissection of the SMA ensures that cancer cells that infiltrate from the primary tumor through the retroperitoneum and into the perineural tissues surrounding the artery are cleared, but even when a thorough dissection is conducted, a margin-positive resection may occur (Fig. 12.3) [17].

SMV-PV Involvement

In cases in which the tumor and the SMV-PV are inseparable, exposure of the SMA by leftward retraction of the SMV-PV is not possible. In such cases, the proper plane of dissection along the SMA can be established by dissecting between the

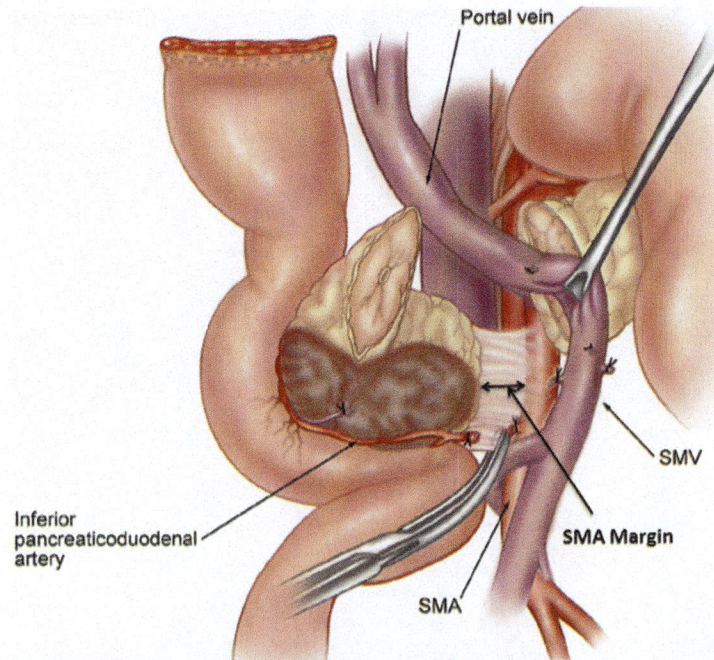

Fig. 12.1 During standard pancreatoduodenectomy, the SMV-PV should be completely mobilized, freed from the tumor, and reflected to the left, exposing the optimal plane of dissection along the periadventitial plane of the SMA (From Katz et al. [17])

SMV and SMA (Fig. 12.2a, b). Several veins, including one or more anterior jejunal branches, the IMV, and various combinatory trunks, cross superficial to this plane; they course from the mesentery and drain into the SMV below the SMV-PV confluence, and each represents an obstacle to dissection. Often, simple ligation of these vessels represents the easiest approach to the retroperitoneum, but the potential repercussions of ligating each branch should be considered. Ideally, the pattern of portal venous drainage from the small bowel should already be known from a thorough evaluation and interpretation of the preoperative CT, and whether each vessel should be left intact or could be a candidate for ligation should be determined prior to surgery. For example, if preoperative imaging shows that most venous drainage from the small bowel occurs through proximal jejunal branches, every attempt should be made to leave these branches intact. If, however, several distal venous branches exist, then ligation of the proximal branches can likely be performed without significant clinical sequelae. Ligation of these vessels permits progressive rightward retraction of the SMV with the specimen and, therefore, greater exposure of the SMA. The surgeon can then begin caudal-to-cephalad dissection along the SMA to the level of the splenic vein (Fig. 12.4), as described above.

Because the splenic vein also courses anterior to the SMA, the splenic vein likewise may inhibit access to the plane of dissection. Often, the splenic vein can be

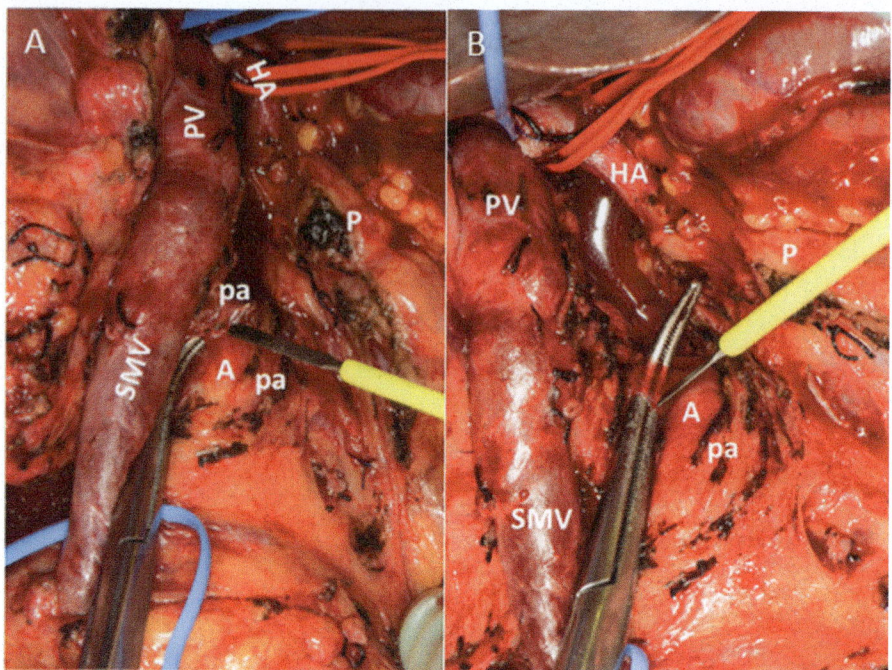

Fig. 12.2 Intraoperative photographs of the optimal dissection plane along the right periadventitial plane of the superior mesenteric artery (SMA). (**a**) The plane is accessed sharply, and all periarterial nerves and fibrofatty tissues (pa) are elevated away from the SMA. (**b**) The right lateral aspect of the SMA is progressively skeletonized, leaving periarterial tissues along the *left* lateral aspect of the artery. *A* SMA, *HA* hepatic artery, *P* pancreas, *PV* portal vein, *SMV* superior mesenteric vein

retracted cephalad and caudad to expose the caudal and cephalad aspects, respectively, of the dissection. Sometimes, however, ligation of the splenic vein offers the safest approach to an oncologically complete operation. This is most commonly the case when a tumor engulfs the portosplenic confluence and extends into the pancreatic neck. In this circumstance, the pancreatic body can be meticulously divided superficial to the splenic vein, and then the vein can be ligated at the confluence. This step allows the retroperitoneum to open up "like a book," facilitating dissection along the SMA to its takeoff (Fig. 12.4).

Splenorenal Shunt

When splenic vein ligation is performed, maintenance of gastrosplenic outflow must be considered. In most cases, outflow is either maintained through the coronary vein or retrograded through the IMV if it drains into the splenic vein. However, although the IMV typically inserts into the splenic vein, it inserts into the SMV caudal to the confluence in up to one-third of patients. In such cases,

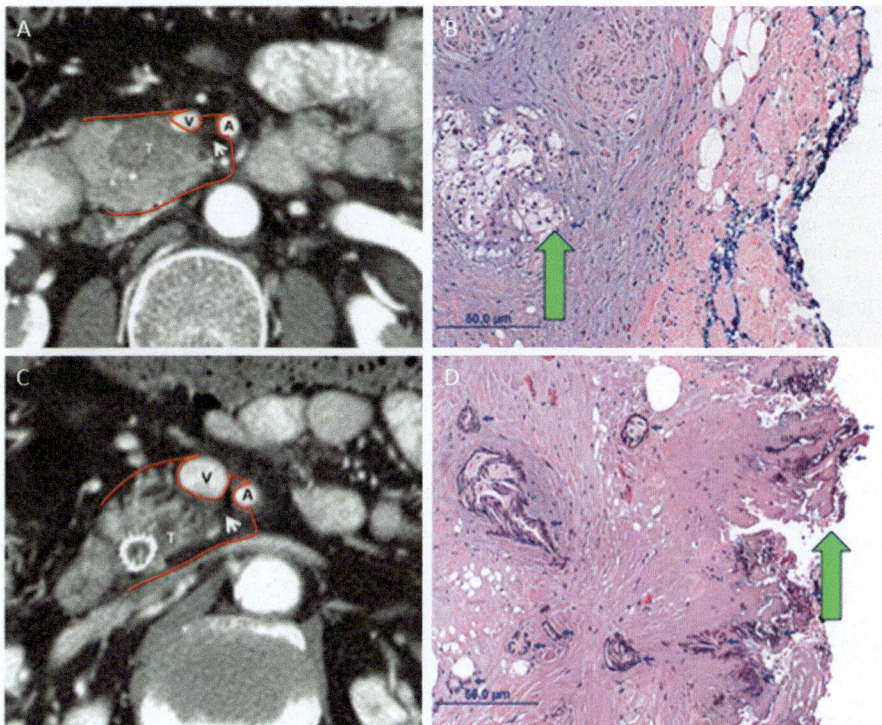

Fig. 12.3 Superior mesenteric artery margin distance estimated radiographically and measured histopathologically in two patients. Preoperative imaging typically overestimates the margin. (**a, b**) A patient who underwent pancreatoduodenectomy with tangential vein resection and who had tumor cells within 1 mm of the inked retroperitoneal margin. (**c, d**) A patient who underwent pancreatoduodenectomy with a positive retroperitoneal margin. *A* SMA, *T tumor*, *V* SMV. *Red line* depicts path of surgical resection. *Small arrow* highlights tissue between SMA and tumor; *large arrow* demonstrates cancer cells proximity to inked margin (From Katz et al. [17])

splenic vein division may cause inadequate gastrosplenic outflow, particularly if the coronary vein has also been divided. In this scenario, we typically construct a distal splenorenal shunt (Fig. 12.5). The need for splenorenal shunting should be anticipated prior to splenic vein ligation because dissection of a length of splenic vein sufficient to create a splenorenal shunt is easiest prior to splenic vein division. Again, a comprehensive analysis of the preoperative CT study should have alerted the surgeon to the possibility of needing a shunt. To construct the shunt, the surgeon should expose the left renal vein to the left of the SMA. The left gonadal and/or adrenal vein may be divided if necessary to facilitate the placement of vascular clamps.

After the SMA dissection is completed and the deep retroperitoneal tissues have been divided, the surgical specimen should be left suspended in the abdomen only at the site of venous adherence. Venous resection and subsequent reconstruction are then conducted as the last step of the resection.

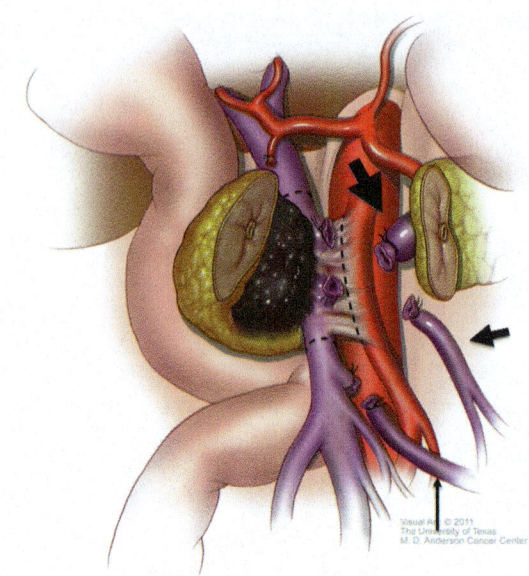

Fig. 12.4 When a tumor involves the superior mesenteric vein-portal vein, the superior mesenteric artery dissection may be facilitated by dividing the splenic vein (*large wide arrow*), the inferior mesenteric vein (*small wide arrow*), or the first jejunal branch (*long arrow*), reflecting the specimen to the *right* (From Katz et al. [1])

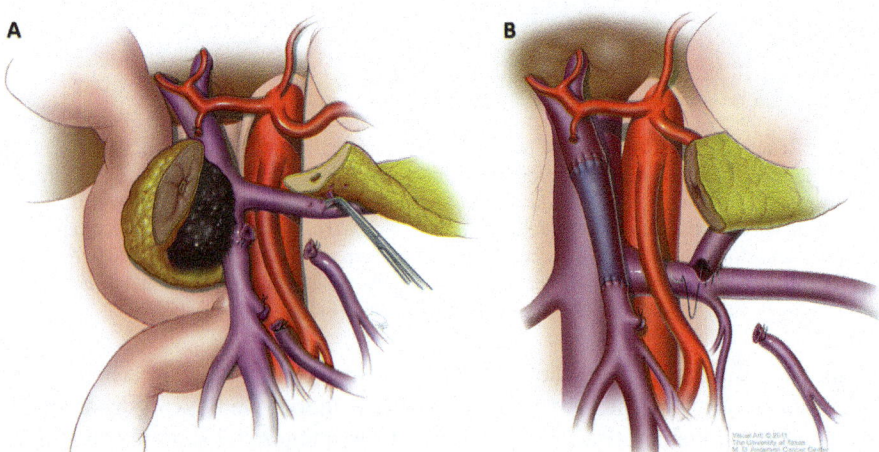

Fig. 12.5 When division of the splenic vein is required during pancreatoduodenectomy and the inferior mesenteric vein enters the superior mesenteric vein, left-sided portal hypertension may occur owing to inadequate gastrosplenic outflow. Creation of a splenorenal shunt is recommended and performed by (**a**) mobilizing the splenic vein from the pancreas and (**b**) creating an anastomosis between the splenic vein and the left renal vein (From Katz et al. [1])

SMA Abutment

Since meticulous dissection along the SMA is required for an oncologic resection, tumors that abut the SMA represent a unique challenge. Tumor extension into this area typically involves encasement of the inferior pancreaticoduodenal arteries, because they enter the uncinate process directly from the SMA. In this situation, dissection along the plane just to the right of the SMA could lead to uncontrollable hemorrhage. Therefore, safe dissection typically requires total vascular control of the SMA. Because tumors that abut the SMA typically have concomitant SMV-PV involvement, the initial approach should be made as described above. After division of the pancreatic neck and splenic vein with rightward retraction of the tumor to provide maximal SMA exposure, vascular clamps are placed directly on the SMA to obtain proximal and distal control (Fig. 12.6). Dissection along the periadventitial plane of the SMA ensues while individually dividing the inferior pancreaticoduodenal arteries. Heparin is administered systemically prior to clamp placement, and reversal is not typically required. Again, circumferential dissection of the SMA is avoided. Venous resection and reconstruction are then performed as the final step before reconstruction.

Posterior Approach

In many cases, dissection along the periadventitial plane of the SMA may be facilitated by a posterior approach. In this method, the kocherization is extended until the left renal vein is evident as it passes anterior to the abdominal aorta. The surgeon retracts the duodenum and pancreatic head to the left until the SMA is exposed on the undersurface of the specimen. The perivascular connective tissue along the lateral plane of the SMA is then divided from cephalad to caudad. The attachments to the uncinate are released, and the inferior pancreaticoduodenal arteries and other feeding branches may be ligated individually. The lateral border of the SMV is then released, and venous resection and reconstruction follow. Often the posterior approach is most effectively used in tandem with the traditional SMA dissection (as described above).

A distinct advantage of the posterior approach is the ability to assess whether the SMA is involved prior to pancreatic neck transection, i.e., before taking any irreversible steps. As venous involvement no longer represents an absolute contraindication to PD, the criterion for unresectability has shifted (leftward) to the SMA. Therefore, methods of early evaluation of SMA involvement are needed because radiographic findings after neoadjuvant therapy do not reliably predict SMA resectability. The posterior approach is one of several "artery-first" approaches that have recently been developed and allow an early SMA assessment.

Hepatic Artery Involvement

Tumors of the head of the pancreas may extend along the gastroduodenal artery to abut or encase the common hepatic artery (CHA). Vascular control, resection, and reconstruction are typically performed early in the operation, prior to pancreatic neck division and retroperitoneal dissection (Fig. 12.7). Proximal and distal control of the CHA should be obtained; in some cases, the area of involvement may extend distally to the proper hepatic artery, as well. Next, heparin is administered systemically and vascular clamps are applied. For tumors that involve the proximal

Fig. 12.6 When a tumor involving the superior mesenteric vein-portal vein closely abuts the superior mesenteric artery, proximal and distal control of the artery facilitates safe dissection along the periadventitial plane (From Katz et al. [1])

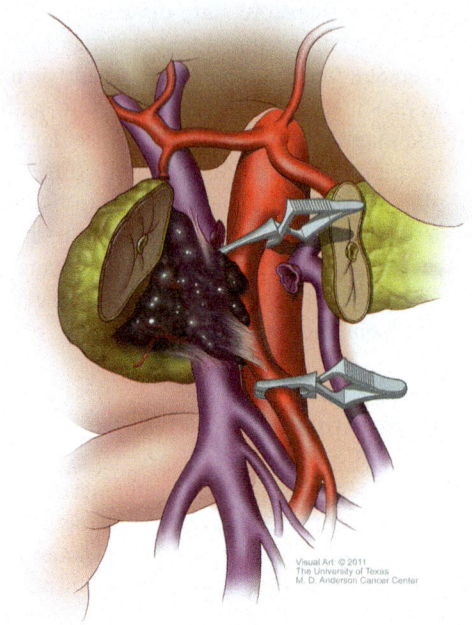

Visual Art: © 2011
The University of Texas
M. D. Anderson Cancer Center

gastroduodenal artery, this artery may be divided at its origin on the CHA and the subsequent defect repaired primarily. When a segment of the CHA must be resected en bloc with the tumor, the artery should be reconstructed with an interposition graft. A reversed saphenous vein graft, internal jugular vein graft, or allograft may be used. In rare instances, when total pancreatectomy is required, the splenic artery can be transposed to the right for CHA reconstruction. Reconstruction of smaller, more distal branches of the proper hepatic artery may require microsurgical techniques.

Arterial Aberrancy

Not infrequently, a replaced or accessory common (RCHA) or replaced right hepatic artery (RRHA) may arise from the SMA and course posterior to the head of the pancreas before entering the porta hepatis. Therefore, it is not uncommon for tumors of the pancreatic head or uncinate process to involve the aberrant artery. Although accessory arteries can often be ligated, replaced vessels typically need to be reconstructed if the tumor cannot be separated from the vessel (Fig. 12.8). The origin of a RRHA or RCHA is best approached during the retroperitoneal dissection. Vascular control is obtained proximally at its origin on the SMA and distally in the porta hepatis. A routine SMA dissection is then performed, and the encased replaced hepatic artery is resected en bloc with the tumor. Reconstruction with a venous interposition graft is then performed in a standard fashion. Bifurcated grafts to the

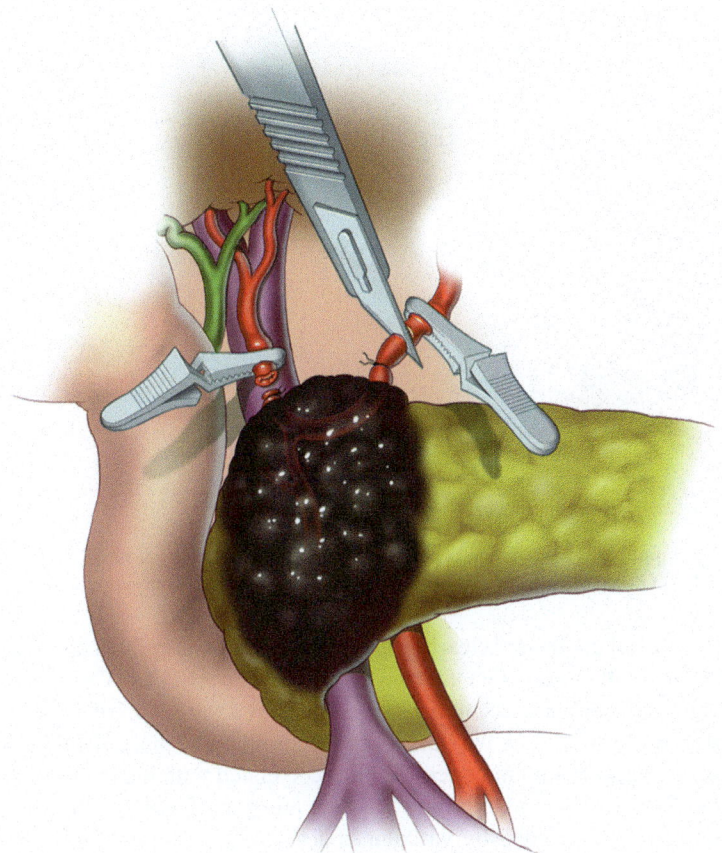

Fig. 12.7 En bloc resection of a common hepatic artery involved by tumor early in the operation. Reconstruction will entail interposition grafting (From Katz et al. [1])

left and right hepatic arteries may be appropriate in the case of RCHA, in order to minimize the consequences of vascular thrombosis, should it occur. Preoperative embolization of a RRHA is an alternative strategy that may lead to sufficient collateralization that reconstruction is not necessary at the time of PD.

Lymphadenectomy

Extent of Lymphadenectomy

PDAC has a strong propensity for both locoregional infiltration and lymph node involvement. In fact, lymph node involvement and lymphovascular invasion are two of the most important prognostic factors for PDAC. Therefore, performing a standardized lymphadenectomy during PD is critically important for proper staging and

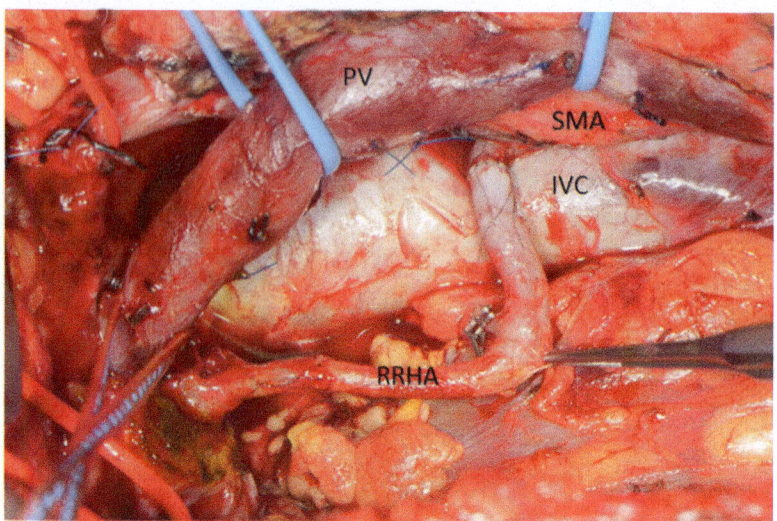

Fig. 12.8 Intraoperative photograph demonstrating the reconstruction of a replaced right hepatic artery (RRHA). *IVC* inferior vena cava, *PV* portal vein, *SMA* superior mesenteric artery

may improve local control by clearing the extrapancreatic lymphatic pathways in the retroperitoneal soft tissues that frequently harbor cancer cells. Current American Joint Committee on Cancer recommendations are for a minimum of 12 lymph nodes to be analyzed following PD, but others have recommended that at least 15 be examined because higher lymph node retrieval has correlated with better survival [18].

Because most peripancreatic lymph nodes are not visible intraoperatively, the lymphadenectomy is guided by vascular and visceral anatomic landmarks, rather than by visualized lymphatics. A standard lymphadenectomy should include the regional lymph node basins: CHA (8), common bile duct (12b), gallbladder (12c), PV (12p), posterior (13) and anterior (17) pancreaticoduodenal arcades, SMV (14v), and right lateral wall of the SMA (14a) (Fig. 12.9) [8]. Several randomized controlled trials have failed to demonstrate a survival advantage with a more extensive lymphadenectomy than that described here [19–21].

Technical Aspects

The retropancreatic and retroduodenal tissues anterior to the inferior vena cava are first mobilized during the Kocher maneuver. This mobilization should extend medially until the left renal vein is exposed. The aortocaval lymph nodes (16) are not necessarily included in a standard lymphadenectomy, but they may be sampled if specific concern exists as involvement of these lymph nodes portends an extremely poor outcome [22]. During the portal dissection, lymph nodes can be either resected en bloc with the final specimen or taken separately. In the latter case, the lymph nodes should be labeled and submitted on the basis of their anatomic lymph node basin. After the removal of the gallbladder and division of the common hepatic duct, the pericholedochal tissues are

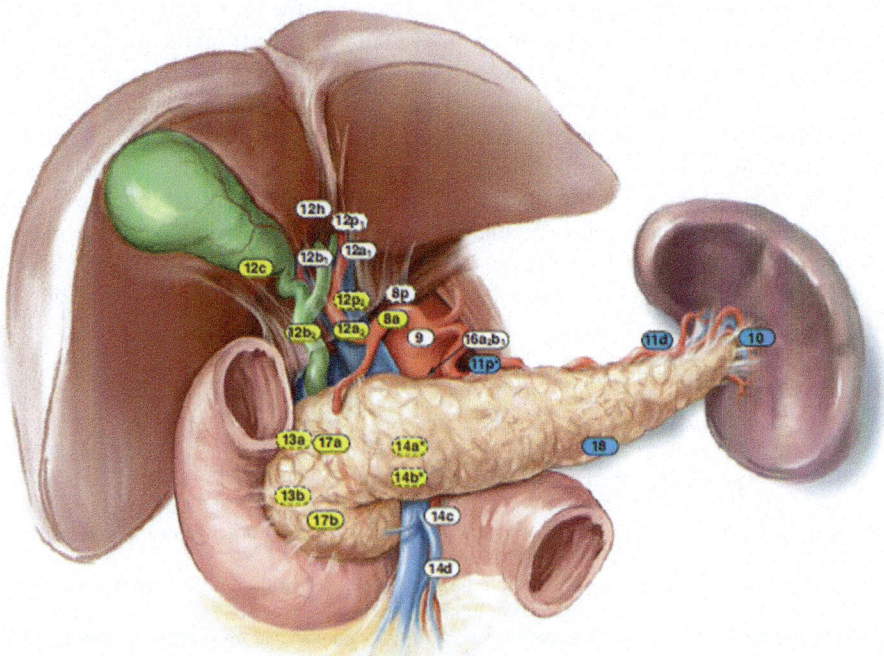

Fig. 12.9 Lymph node basins that should be resected as part of a standard pancreatoduodenectomy (*yellow*) (From Hunt [8])

swept inferiorly, and all soft tissues adjacent to the proper hepatic artery, as well as those anterior and lateral to the PV, are dissected. A prominent CHA lymph node is often encountered and should be resected. Dissection of lymph nodes proximal to this (7, 9) is not specifically required, but we routinely skeletonize the hepatic artery and retrieve both stations 8a and 8p nodes en bloc with the specimen, passing them posterior to the hepatoduodenal ligament structures for removal. Next, dissection of the perigastric and paraduodenal tissues is performed up to the level of the proximal transection, depending on whether pylorus preservation is planned. Finally, after division of the pancreatic neck, the uncinate dissection is performed as described above in detail. This includes all lymphatic tissues adjacent to the SMV and right lateral wall of the SMA, and this completes the standard lymphadenectomy. Note that lymph nodes in the root of the mesentery beyond the first jejunal branch and middle colic lymph nodes are not routinely resected.

Conclusions

Given its propensity for early metastasis, multimodality therapy is thought to be essential for nearly all patients with PDAC. Therefore, a surgeon's most important contribution to the multidisciplinary care of these patients is the performance of a margin-negative resection and a standardized regional lymph node dissection.

Because of the infiltrative nature of PDAC, as well as the proximity of the SMA to the head and uncinate process of the pancreas, cancer cells from the primary tumor frequently infiltrate into the surrounding perineural and lymphatic tissues of the retroperitoneum toward the SMA. Thorough clearance of these soft tissues, which may be accomplished by skeletonizing along the right lateral aspect of the SMA, is therefore required to enhance the likelihood of a margin-negative resection. As is evident in the scenarios depicted in this chapter, a meticulous uncinate dissection is essential even for tumors with complex vascular involvement. When combined with contemporary multimodality therapy, the use of advanced surgical techniques may contribute to optimized locoregional control and hopefully improve long-term survival.

References

1. Katz MHG, et al. Retroperitoneal dissection in patients with borderline resectable pancreatic cancer: operative principles and techniques. J Am Coll Surg. 2012;215:e11–8.
2. Katz MHG, Fleming JB, Pisters PWT, Lee JE, Evans DB. Anatomy of the superior mesenteric vein with special reference to the surgical management of first-order branch involvement at pancreaticoduodenectomy. Ann Surg. 2008;248:1098–102.
3. Katz MHG, et al. Borderline resectable pancreatic cancer: the importance of this emerging stage of disease. J Am Coll Surg. 2008;206:833–46. discussion 846–848.
4. Neoptolemos JP, et al. Influence of resection margins on survival for patients with pancreatic cancer treated by adjuvant chemoradiation and/or chemotherapy in the ESPAC-1 randomized controlled trial. Ann Surg. 2001;234:758–68.
5. Verbeke CS, Gladhaug IP. Resection margin involvement and tumour origin in pancreatic head cancer. Br J Surg. 2012;99:1036–49.
6. Iacobuzio-Donahue CA, et al. DPC4 gene status of the primary carcinoma correlates with patterns of failure in patients with pancreatic cancer. J Clin Oncol Off J Am Soc Clin Oncol. 2009;27:1806–13.
7. Liu L, et al. Superior mesenteric artery margin of posttherapy pancreaticoduodenectomy and prognosis in patients with pancreatic ductal adenocarcinoma. Am J Surg Pathol. 2015;39:1395–403.
8. Hunt K. Operative standards for cancer surgery, Breast, lung, pancreas, colon, vol. 1. Philadelphia: Wolters Kluwer; 2015.
9. National Comprehensive Cancer Network. NCCN practice guidelines for pancreatic cancer. Available at: http://www.nccn.org/professionals/physician_gls/pdf/pancreatic.pdf. Accessed 1 Mar 2016.
10. Khorana AA, et al. Potentially curable pancreatic cancer: American Society of Clinical Oncology clinical practice guideline. J Clin Oncol Off J Am Soc Clin Oncol. 2016;34:2541–56.
11. Cloyd JM, et al. Preoperative therapy and pancreatoduodenectomy for pancreatic ductal adenocarcinoma: a 25-year single-institution experience. J Gastrointest Surg Off J Soc Surg Aliment Tract. 2017;21:164–74.
12. Katz MHG, et al. Response of borderline resectable pancreatic cancer to neoadjuvant therapy is not reflected by radiographic indicators. Cancer. 2012;118:5749–56.
13. Ferrone CR, et al. Radiological and surgical implications of neoadjuvant treatment with FOLFIRINOX for locally advanced and borderline resectable pancreatic cancer. Ann Surg. 2015;261:12–7.
14. Denbo J, et al. Preoperative chemoradiation for pancreatic adenocarcinoma does not increase 90-day postoperative morbidity or mortality. J Gastrointest Surg. 2016;20(12):1975–85.
15. Takahashi H, et al. Preoperative chemoradiation reduces the risk of pancreatic fistula after distal pancreatectomy for pancreatic adenocarcinoma. Surgery. 2011;150:547–56.

16. Kurosaki I, Minagawa M, Takano K, Takizawa K, Hatakeyama K. Left posterior approach to the superior mesenteric vascular pedicle in pancreaticoduodenectomy for cancer of the pancreatic head. JOP. 2011;12:220–9.
17. Katz MHG, et al. Effect of neoadjuvant chemoradiation and surgical technique on recurrence of localized pancreatic cancer. J Gastrointest Surg Off J Soc Surg Aliment Tract. 2012;16:68–78. discussion 78–79.
18. Tomlinson JS, et al. Accuracy of staging node-negative pancreas cancer: a potential quality measure. Arch Surg Chic Ill 1960. 2007;142:767–23. discussion 773–774
19. Farnell MB, et al. A prospective randomized trial comparing standard pancreatoduodenectomy with pancreatoduodenectomy with extended lymphadenectomy in resectable pancreatic head adenocarcinoma. Surgery. 2005;138:618–628.; discussion 628–630.
20. Yeo CJ, et al. Pancreaticoduodenectomy with or without distal gastrectomy and extended retroperitoneal lymphadenectomy for periampullary adenocarcinoma, part 2: randomized controlled trial evaluating survival, morbidity, and mortality. Ann Surg. 2002;236:355–366.; discussion 366–368.
21. Jang J-Y, et al. A prospective randomized controlled study comparing outcomes of standard resection and extended resection, including dissection of the nerve plexus and various lymph nodes, in patients with pancreatic head cancer. Ann Surg. 2014;259:656–64.
22. Shimada K, Sakamoto Y, Sano T, Kosuge T. The role of paraaortic lymph node involvement on early recurrence and survival after macroscopic curative resection with extended lymphadenectomy for pancreatic carcinoma. J Am Coll Surg. 2006;203:345–52.

Early Recovery After Surgery Pathways for Pancreatectomy

13

Daniel J. Kagedan and Alice C. Wei

Introduction

ERaS Background

Initially described in the colorectal literature, enhanced recovery after surgery (ERaS) is a concept that emphasizes minimization of the physiologic disturbances produced by surgery – and focuses on interventions that minimize surgical stress – and promotes rapid recovery to presurgical levels of function. The introduction of ERaS protocols also provides a prime opportunity to additionally improve perioperative quality of care by systemizing the processes of care for patients according to the best available evidence. These protocols lay out an uncomplicated patient's

The authors have no conflicts of interest or disclosures.

D.J. Kagedan
Division of General Surgery, Department of Surgery, University of Toronto, Toronto, ON, Canada

Institute of Health Policy, Management, and Evaluation, University of Toronto, Toronto, ON, Canada
e-mail: dkagedan@gmail.com

A.C. Wei (✉)
Department of Surgery, Princess Margaret Cancer Centre, University Health Network, Toronto, ON, Canada

Department of Surgery, Toronto General Hospital, University Health Network, Toronto, ON, Canada

Division of General Surgery, Department of Surgery, University of Toronto, Toronto, ON, Canada

Institute of Health Policy, Management, and Evaluation, University of Toronto, Toronto, ON, Canada
e-mail: Alice.Wei@uhn.ca

© Springer International Publishing AG 2018
F.G. Rocha, P. Shen (eds.), *Optimizing Outcomes for Liver and Pancreas Surgery*, DOI 10.1007/978-3-319-62624-6_13

expected course in the hospital and recommend when certain process of care events is to occur (e.g., catheter removal, dietary advancement). Independent of individual ERaS elements, standardization of care has been shown to improve the quality of care and increase the efficiency of care, generating economic cost savings in addition as well as the same or superior patient outcomes compared to conventional care. In the current healthcare landscape with emphasis on maximizing the value obtained for each dollar expended, standardized postoperative recovery protocols such as ERaS have generated considerable interest.

Standardized postoperative recovery protocols, such as ERaS, are a type of surgical process improvement tool (SPIT) [1]. Other examples of SPITs include checklists and patient safety initiatives. SPITs are based on the theory of improving quality of care by minimizing variability through direct interventions in the processes of care implemented at the point of care. The most widely utilized SPITs are surgical checklists, which have been shown to reduce perioperative mortality and are now mandatory in all Canadian hospitals [2, 3]. We believe that standardized postoperative recovery protocols such as ERaS protocols, postoperative clinical pathways (CPWs), fast-track algorithms, and critical pathways can make a comparable contribution to improving patient care. Encouraging results from ERaS implementation in other areas, in particular following colorectal surgery, have prompted the application of ERaS protocols to myriad operations from cardiovascular to complex cancer procedures such as pancreatectomy [4].

Several recent studies examining the effects of ERaS protocols following pancreatic surgery have demonstrated that they are safe and effective at decreasing postoperative length of stay (LoS) without compromising morbidity, mortality, or readmission rates [5–8]. Enhanced recovery protocols are hypothesized to attenuate the postoperative stress and inflammatory response following surgery, minimizing physiologic disruption in homeostasis and enabling an earlier return to baseline function [9, 10]. Examples of specific interventions promoting earlier return to normal function following pancreatic surgery include minimizing drain use, mobilizing patients early in the postoperative period, multimodality opioid-sparing pain control, and resuming normal enteral alimentation as soon as possible following surgery. Patient engagement is also a key component of postoperative recovery protocols. Education regarding interventions and anticipated milestones begins in the preoperative period, ensuring that patients are aware of the expected pace of postoperative recovery, are motivated to actively participate in activities designed to facilitate recovery, and are able to make necessary arrangements and mentally prepare for discharge.

ERaS protocols are inherently multidisciplinary and benefit from the involvement of surgeons, anesthesiologists, nurses, physiotherapists, dietitians, and on occasion others such as intensivists, occupational therapists, homecare nurses, pharmacists, and discharge planners. To optimize engagement and participation in the protocol, we recommend involving representatives from these disciplines early in ERaS protocol development and implementation processes and continually soliciting feedback from each on opportunities for improvement. The success of an ERaS protocol requires that each healthcare team member understands not only their own role but how their role fits within the overall postoperative care plan; accordingly, the importance of educating each healthcare provider on the specifics of the protocol prior to implementation cannot be overemphasized.

While ERaS initially gained traction in the colorectal surgery literature, the first attempts to apply the principles of fast-track recovery to pancreatic surgery occurred in the mid-1990s [11]. A post-pancreaticoduodenectomy pathway was found to decrease postoperative LoS as well as hospital and physician costs, without increasing mortality or readmission rates [11, 12]. While prospective randomized trials of ERaS protocols in pancreatic surgery are lacking, similarly encouraging findings have been reported by several other retrospective and prospective cohort studies, as well as systematic reviews and meta-analyses [7, 13–15]. The ERaS Society has published evidence-based guidelines to serve as a foundation for post-pancreatectomy-enhanced recovery protocols (http://erassociety.org/specialties/pancreas/) [16].

At our own institution, a post-pancreaticoduodenectomy ERaS protocol has been in use since 2013. The ERaS protocol guidelines have been summarized in Table 13.1. This protocol was developed following a systematic needs assessment, with input from a working group of HPB surgeons from hospitals across Ontario. We have had great success with the protocol, and it is currently the standard of care at our institution. Also, it is currently being used at other high-volume HPB centers across Ontario with appropriate modifications based on local resources and practice patterns.

ERaS represents a standardized approach to postoperative care, and many of the benefits conferred by its utilization relate to the decrease in variability of care provided. The use of a standardized protocol and attendant clinical tools such as electronic order sets can reduce errors of omission and force a healthcare provider to think carefully before placing an order that deviates from the protocol. Evolving postoperative complications may initially manifest as a patient's inability to meet the goals of the protocol, which can trigger investigations to diagnose a complication, and facilitate early interventions to treat it, rescuing the patient from more severe sequelae. Thus, the protocol can act as a tool for alerting clinicians to patients who may be developing postoperative morbidity.

In summary, ERaS protocols and related surgical process improvement tools have the potential to reduce length of hospital stay and hospital costs with no deleterious impact on readmission rates, morbidity, and mortality; therefore, ERaS should be utilized to improve the quality of care for patients undergoing pancreatic surgery.

Preoperative Care

Preoperative Education and Evaluation

As the primary participant in the postoperative recovery process, patients should receive education and counseling regarding the anticipated sequence of events, target milestones and when each milestone is expected to be achieved, and ways in which the patient can actively participate in the ERaS protocol. This provides an opportunity to clarify patient expectations and also to ensure they are aware of

Table 13.1 Summary of enhanced recovery after surgery (ERaS) guidelines for the treatment of patients undergoing pancreatic surgery

Preoperative	
Evaluation and education	
Discharge planning	Discharge planning should commence during the preoperative evaluation, including informing the patient of the anticipated date of discharge and assessing the potential need for discharge to an assisted-living or rehabilitation environment, particularly for elderly patients or those with multiple comorbidities
Smoking cessation	Cigarette smoking is an accepted risk factor for postoperative complications following pancreatic resection, and efforts should be made to encourage smoking cessation prior to surgery
Nutritional considerations	
Carbohydrate loading	Particular attention should be paid to patient nutritional status, and strong consideration should be given to preoperative carbohydrate loading
Nutritional supplementation	Consideration should be given to a short course (5 days) of preoperative nutritional supplementation (enteral route preferred over parenteral) for patients with pancreatic exocrine insufficiency
Iron supplementation	As both preoperative anemia and perioperative transfusion of allogeneic red blood cells have been associated with increased morbidity, mortality, and LoS, strategies to address anemia should be undertaken prior to surgery
Perioperative care	
Surgical site infections	Preoperative administration of antimicrobial agents within 1 h of making an incision is accepted as standard practice, with re-dosing of antibiotics every 3–4 h during prolonged procedures
Venous thromboembolism events	Perioperative venous thromboembolism prophylaxis is recommended for patients undergoing pancreatic surgery, using either unfractionated or fractionated low-molecular-weight heparin (LMWH), initiated 2–12 h before surgery
Fluid management	Intraoperative fluid management should be goal directed based on the metrics commonly monitored (heart rate, blood pressure, urine output) and, if more invasive assessment is employed, stroke volume and cardiac output
Blood transfusion	Allogeneic blood transfusions are associated with inferior short- and long-term postoperative outcomes. Consistent application of accepted transfusion triggers (hemoglobin <70, estimated blood loss >1 L, hemodynamic instability) may decrease perioperative transfusion rates
Multimodal pain control	
Opioid-sparing techniques	Opioid analgesia, the foundation of postoperative pain control, is associated with postoperative nausea, vomiting, and gastrointestinal ileus; therefore, strategies to minimize opiate utilization are essential
Epidural analgesia	Currently, patients undergoing pancreatic resections are recommended to have epidurals placed at the mid-thoracic level (T5–T8) at the discretion of the treating anesthesiologist and surgeon

(continued)

Table 13.1 (continued)

Transversus abdominis plane blocks	Currently have not been evaluated in pancreatic surgery, although data from patients undergoing other abdominal procedures suggests that they may be effective in improving pain control and reducing opiate consumption
Patient-controlled analgesia	Patients who do not receive an epidural should be initially managed postoperatively with intravenous infusion of opioids using a patient-controlled analgesia (PCA) approach
Intraoperative placement of abdominal drains, enteric tubes, and urinary catheters	
Intra-abdominal drains	Use of surgical drains remains controversial, selective drainage is recommended at the discretion of the treating physician, and early removal is advocated when drains are present
Enteric tubes	Routine nasogastric decompression is not indicated in the postoperative period, and their usage may in fact increase the likelihood of delayed gastric emptying and prolong LoS following pancreatic resection
Urinary catheters	Urinary catheters placed at the time of surgery should be removed early in the postoperative period to prevent urinary tract infections and encourage patient mobilization
Postoperative care	
Nutritional considerations	
Early oral feeding	Patients are likely to benefit from early oral feeding during the postoperative recovery period following pancreatic surgery
Nasogastric (NG) tube avoidance	Routine use of NG tubes should be avoided following pancreatic surgery If present, NG tubes should be removed on POD#1 when PO intake is commenced
Gastrointestinal motility	
Gum chewing	Gum chewing activates the cephalic phase of digestion and has been demonstrated to speed the recovery of gastrointestinal function and to decrease the time to first bowel movement following gastrointestinal surgery
Prokinetic agents	There is insufficient evidence to recommend routine use of prokinetic agents
Somatostatin analogues	The use of routine use of somatostatin analogues for the prevention of postoperative pancreatic fistulae is recommended; however, the evidence supporting this recommendation remains controversial Some authors have recommended selective somatostatin use in patients at high risk of fistula development based on the pancreatic fistula score or other assessment
Activity	
Early mobilization	Data suggests early mobilization after surgery is safe and may provide benefits such as decreased ileus
Patient education	
Discharge planning	Early discharge planning by the entire team is important for each patient Discharge planning should begin prior to surgery, so that patients with barriers to discharge can be identified and arrangements can be initiated well in advance of discharge

specific tasks that they are expected to perform (i.e., mobilization on the day of surgery). Preoperative counseling should occur in person during outpatient appointments and be reinforced with educational brochures and/or audiovisual multimedia applications describing the procedure in question and the anticipated postoperative recovery protocol presented in a language and format accessible to the average reader. Preoperative education and counseling have been postulated to be one of the single most important components of ERaS-type initiatives and furthermore may alleviate patient anxiety and uncertainty regarding the operation and subsequent hospitalization [16–18]. These counseling appointments can also be used as an opportunity to evaluate the patient preoperatively for specific conditions which may be optimized prior to surgery, identify the need for further preoperative investigations, assess patient appropriateness for management according to an ERaS protocol, and identify anticipated challenges to protocol completion [18].

Discharge planning should commence during the preoperative evaluation, including informing the patient of the anticipated date of discharge and assessing the potential need for discharge to an assisted-living or rehabilitation environment, particularly for elderly patients or those with multiple comorbidities [19]. Early identification of patients who may require increased levels of care following discharge from hospital (i.e., patients >75 years old, those lacking supports in the community, frail patients) enables the preemptive involvement of social workers in determining appropriate placements and helps manage patient expectations of their transitions from hospital to convalescent facility to home [20–22]. Some institutions employ dedicated healthcare professionals, discharge planners, and patient navigators who assist with this aspect of perioperative care.

Nutritional Considerations

Particular attention should be paid to patient nutritional status, and strong consideration should be given to preoperative carbohydrate loading [23, 24]. Assessment of preoperative nutritional status includes measurement of serum albumin and identification of patients with >10% weight loss in the preceding 6 months [25]. Preoperative nutritional supplementation should be administered in select cases to those requiring it, with the enteral route preferred over parenteral administration [16, 26]. Preoperative sarcopenia, a novel metric of frailty, has been associated with postoperative pancreatic fistula formation and may be amenable to correction with preoperative rehabilitation and nutrition optimization [27].

Oral carbohydrate intake shortly prior to surgery is recommended based on data from several studies of patients undergoing elective abdominal surgery, and a Cochrane review of preoperative carbohydrate loading suggests that it may reduce postoperative LoS [16, 23]. Carbohydrate loading may not be appropriate for patients with impaired glucose metabolism. Also, patients should not be required to fast from midnight onward on the day of surgery; clear fluids may be consumed up to 2 h prior to surgery and provide an additional opportunity for preoperative carbohydrate intake [28].

General Preoperative Patient Optimization

Cigarette smoking is an accepted risk factor for postoperative complications following surgery, and efforts should be made to encourage smoking cessation prior to pancreatectomy [29, 30]. Ideally, smoking cessation interventions should begin 4–8 weeks before surgery. Nevertheless, each day of smoking avoidance can reduce perioperative complications so even when the perioperative period is short, smoking cessation is important. Most successful smoking cessation programs combine scheduled behavioral counseling sessions as well as pharmacologic nicotine replacement therapy [30].

Preoperative anemia has similarly been identified as a risk factor for morbidity following pancreatic surgery [31]. As both preoperative anemia and perioperative transfusion of allogeneic red blood cells have been associated with increased morbidity, mortality, and LoS, strategies to address anemia should be undertaken prior to surgery [32, 33]. Despite a lack of high-quality evidence supporting their use, perioperative iron supplementation (oral or intravenous) and erythropoiesis-stimulating agent administration have been recommended by some for the treatment of preoperative anemia [33–35]. Consideration may also be given to routine supplementation with folic acid and vitamin B12, to prevent anemia secondary to their deficiency [33]. As strategies to minimize perioperative blood transfusions are pondered, discontinuation of anticoagulant and antiplatelet medications and the need for bridging with short-acting anticoagulants should be considered. Lastly, patients should be assessed for usage of complementary and alternative medicines, as some of these may produce unexpected reactions intraoperatively and postoperatively [36, 37].

Preoperative Considerations Specific to Pancreatic Surgery

Patients undergoing pancreatic surgery may present with syndromes secondary to their underlying disease process, including obstructive jaundice, new-onset diabetes mellitus, and pancreatic exocrine insufficiency [38, 39]. Traditionally, preoperative biliary decompression was recommended for jaundiced patients with hyperbilirubinemia secondary to periampullary obstruction, based partly on the theory that hyperbilirubinemia increased the risks associated with surgery and was detrimental to postoperative healing [40, 41]. However, high-quality randomized controlled trial evidence has cast doubt on this assumption. In fact preoperative biliary decompression increased rates of infectious complications and other serious postoperative morbidity [42, 43]. Currently, routine preoperative biliary drainage is not recommended for patients presenting with obstructive jaundice secondary to a periampullary neoplasm, except in cases of concomitant sepsis [42]. Among patients who do undergo preoperative stenting, metallic stents are associated with fewer stent-related and postoperative complications than plastic stents [44, 45].

Diabetes mellitus commonly coexists with pancreatic cancer, as it can be both a risk factor for and a consequence of pancreatic cancer development [38]. Though somewhat controversial, pancreatic cancer patients with diabetes likely have increased risk of postoperative complications, as well as inferior long-term survival [38]. In addition to screening newly diagnosed pancreatic cancer patients for impaired glucose tolerance, emphasis should be placed on optimizing glycemic control preceding, during, and following surgery while taking care to avoid hypoglycemia. Among patients with new-onset diabetes secondary to their pancreatic tumor, between 20 and 40% experience resolution of their diabetes following surgical resection and must be carefully monitored for postoperative hypoglycemia [46–48].

Pancreatic exocrine insufficiency is most often seen in patients with chronic pancreatitis, although it may also occur in cystic fibrosis, pancreatic cancer, acute pancreatitis, and critical illness. These patients are much more likely to be malnourished, and in select cases consideration may be given to a short course (5 days) of preoperative nutritional supplementation although data supporting this practice are controversial [49, 50]. Patients should also be counseled preoperatively regarding the possibility of worsening exocrine function following surgery and the potential need for pancreatic enzyme replacement therapy.

Neoadjuvant Treatment

As interest in neoadjuvant treatment of pancreatic cancer grows, potential consequences for the perioperative period must be anticipated. While preliminary reports suggest that administration of neoadjuvant therapy is not associated with increased rates of postoperative complications, data from the colorectal literature has reported that neoadjuvant therapy is associated with increased rates of hospital readmission after discharge according to an ERaS-type protocol [51, 52]. The period of neoadjuvant treatment may also afford a longer duration of time for preoperative optimization.

Perioperative Care

Perioperative Antimicrobial and Venous Thromboembolism Prophylaxis

Preoperative administration of antimicrobial agents within 1 h of skin incision is accepted as standard practice, with redosing of antibiotics every 3–4 h during prolonged procedures [16]. Commonly administered antibiotics include cefazolin plus metronidazole, cefoxitin, ampicillin-sulbactam, and clindamycin, although some groups have reported decreased rates of post-pancreaticoduodenectomy surgical site infections with the use of prophylactic piperacillin-tazobactam [53, 54]. Patients who have undergone preoperative biliary drainage should receive perioperative antibiotics with activity against biliary microorganisms, based on antimicrobial sensitivities from cultures obtained at the time of biliary instrumentation [55, 56]. Also, antibiotics may be tailored based on local antimicrobial sensitivity and resistance patterns.

Major abdominal surgery including pancreatectomy is associated with an increased risk for venous thromboembolic (VTE) events. The presence of malignancy is an independent risk for thromboembolic disease [57–59]. Perioperative VTE prophylaxis is recommended for patients undergoing pancreatic surgery, using either unfractionated or fractionated low-molecular-weight heparin (LMWH), initiated 2–12 h before surgery [16, 60–62]. Thromboprophylaxis should be continued during the postoperative hospitalization. Recent evidence suggests that extending pharmacologic prophylaxis for 4 weeks postoperatively may be beneficial without increasing the risk of major postoperative hemorrhage [63–65].

Fluid Management

Intraoperative fluid management should be goal-directed based on standard measures such as heart rate, blood pressure, and urine output. If more invasive monitoring is available, stroke volume and cardiac output may be used to guide therapy [66–68]. Caution should be exercised in interpreting hypotension in the context of epidural analgesia, as hypotension may reflect vasodilation rather than genuine hypovolemia. Perioperative heart rate and blood pressure should be considered relative to each individual patient's baseline values, and changes of <20% are most often acceptable [69].

When hypovolemia is suspected, small-volume fluid challenges of 250 mL of crystalloid or colloid should be administered; improvement in the patient's hemodynamic parameters (heart rate, blood pressure, pulse pressure variability, stroke volume) should prompt additional fluid administration, until no further improvements are observed. According to the ERaS guidelines for pancreaticoduodenectomy, the goal should be a near-zero fluid balance [16].

Acute blood loss during surgery may be replaced with crystalloid or colloid solutions [70]. Colloids have the added advantage of facilitating intravascular fluid compartment expansion with comparatively less fluid volume than crystalloids [71, 72].

Much of the evidence favoring restrictive fluid administration is derived from the colorectal literature; studies conducted on patients undergoing pancreatic procedures suggest that fluid restriction is not detrimental to outcomes and may improve them [68, 73–76]. Notably, the volume of intraoperative fluids recommended for fluid restriction (1–2 mL/kg/hr) is based on colorectal procedures, whereas the studies examining fluid restriction in pancreatic surgery utilized maintenance fluid rates of 5–10 mL/kg/hr [73, 74, 76, 77]. Isotonic crystalloid solutions are the recommended intravenous fluids, with balanced salt solutions (Ringer's lactate, Plasmalyte) preferred over normal saline, so as not to cause hyperchloremic acidosis [16, 78]. In instances of hyponatremia or hypochloremia, normal saline may be utilized.

Perioperative Blood Transfusion

Allogeneic blood transfusions are associated with inferior short- and long-term postoperative outcomes [79–82]. Historically, pancreatic surgery was associated with rates of transfusion ranging from 40 to 60%; however, rates as low as 6% have been reported in the modern era [83, 84]. Consistent application of accepted transfusion triggers (hemoglobin <70, estimated blood loss >1 L, hemodynamic instability) may decrease perioperative transfusion rates [79]. Preoperative detection and correction of anemia are also indicated, as discussed above. Acute normovolemic hemodilution failed to reduce blood transfusions following pancreaticoduodenectomy in a randomized trial and was associated with increased anastomotic complications, possibly related to the increased fluid volumes delivered [85]. While other groups have reported success with normovolemic hemodilution, it is not considered to be the standard of care at this time [86].

Multimodality Pain Control

Effective control of postoperative pain is a crucial component of enhanced recovery after surgery, enabling early mobilization, deep breathing, and oral alimentation [10]. Opioid analgesia, the foundation of postoperative pain control, is associated with postoperative nausea, vomiting, and gastrointestinal ileus; therefore, strategies to minimize opiate utilization are essential [87]. Multi-institutional population-based analyses have demonstrated improved outcomes (decreased LoS, improved mortality) among patients undergoing pancreatectomy associated with epidural analgesia [88, 89]. In spite of this, epidural analgesia was employed in only a minority of pancreatic resections in the United States between 2000 and 2012, according to a study querying the Nationwide Inpatient Sample database (9.4% of pancreaticoduodenectomies and 7.1% of distal pancreatectomies) [89]. This poor uptake may be related to reports from single institutions demonstrating inferior or equivalent outcomes of epidural analgesia compared to standard narcotic regimens [90–92]. A randomized trial is currently underway to determine the superiority of epidural vs patient-controlled intravenous analgesia on postoperative complications following pancreaticoduodenectomy [93]. Currently, patients undergoing pancreatic resections are recommended to have epidurals placed at the mid-thoracic level (T5–T8) at the discretion of the treating anesthesiologist and surgeon [16, 94].

Patients who do not receive an epidural should be initially managed postoperatively with intravenous infusion of opioids using a patient-controlled analgesia (PCA) approach [95, 96]. Evidence suggests that PCA is superior to non-patient-controlled opioid analgesia in terms of providing effective pain relief and is also preferred by patients due to the increased autonomy afforded [97].

Other strategies reported in perioperative pancreatic surgery pain management include pre-incisional infusion of medications such as sufentanil, clonidine, and ketamine via epidural catheters, intrathecal morphine administered intraoperatively, and continuous local infusion of anesthetics; however, due to limited evidence, none of these are recommended at this time [98–100]. Transversus abdominis plane (TAP) blocks, which anesthetize the anterior abdominal wall via infusion of local anesthetics through a catheter placed intraoperatively, have not been evaluated in pancreatic surgery, although data from patients undergoing other abdominal procedures suggests that they may be effective in improving pain control and reducing opiate consumption [101].

Intraoperative Placement of Abdominal Drains, Enteric Tubes, and Urinary Catheters

A fundamental tenet underlying enhanced recovery is the principle of minimizing physiologic disruptions accompanying operative intervention and returning the postoperative patient to their preoperative homeostatic state as rapidly as is safely feasible [10]. Accordingly, routine placement of foreign devices is generally discouraged, and when necessary, early removal is advocated [16].

Abdominal Drains

Substantial controversy persists regarding the routine intraoperative placement of prophylactic abdominal drains among patients undergoing pancreatic resection. Several systematic reviews have analyzed the effect of prophylactic abdominal drainage on patient outcomes following pancreatic surgery [102–105]. Each evaluated variations of the same nine primary studies, which included two randomized controlled trials [106, 107] and seven retrospective studies [108–114]. Dou et al. concluded that prophylactic abdominal drainage did not affect the risk of postoperative abdominal abscess but that omitting drain placement might result in higher mortality after pancreatectomy and pancreaticoduodenectomy [102]. Conversely, Nitsche et al. reported decreased overall morbidity following any type of pancreatic resection managed without drains, but found no significant difference in mortality rates [103]. When restricted to patients undergoing pancreaticoduodenectomy, increased rates of intra-abdominal abscesses and mortality were observed when intraperitoneal drains were not routinely placed [103]. Rondelli et al. reported that intra-abdominal drainage may increase pancreatic fistulae rates, overall postoperative complications, and readmission rates, but did not identify an association with overall mortality [104]. Wang et al. suggested that patients managed without prophylactic drainage after pancreaticoduodenectomy might have higher mortality, but fewer major complications (Clavien grades III-IV) and readmissions [105, 115].

A total of three randomized controlled trials have been reported, routine intraperitoneal drain vs no-drain placement for pancreatectomy. The oldest is a single-center randomized controlled trial [106], and two more recent studies are multicenter randomized controlled trial [107, 116]. Similar to the observational data, the randomized controlled trial data have reported conflicting results of routine drainage. Van Buren et al. conducted a multicenter North American trial that compared routine intraperitoneal drain vs no drain for pancreaticoduodenectomies which was notable because it was terminated early as a result of increased mortality (3% vs

12%) in the no-drain study arm [107]. In addition, the number and severity of the complications were significantly higher in the no drainage arm. As a result of these data, the authors concluded that drain omission may be harmful. The results of this study impact the recommendations made in the systematic reviews to date.

A more recent randomized controlled trial reported in 2016 found different results and is not included in the aforementioned systematic reviews [116]. In a large multicenter randomized controlled trial European study, Witzigmann et al. compared 395 patients undergoing pancreatic surgery with pancreaticojejunal anastomosis. Patients were randomized to receive either no drain or intra-abdominal drainage. There was no significant difference between surgical, medical, and overall morbidity. Grade B/C pancreatic fistula was significantly lower in the no-drain group. Fistula-associated complications were significantly increased in the drain group. The reintervention rate was lower in the no-drain group. However, postoperative ascites was significantly higher in the no-drain group. The authors concluded the abandonment of drains did not increase reintervention rates, mortality, and overall morbidity. The results of this study suggest routine prophylactic drainage should not be recommended for patients undergoing pancreatic resection with pancreatico-jejunal anastomosis.

In conclusion, there is mixed evidence with respect to prophylactic intra-abdominal drainage of patients undergoing pancreatic resection. Placement of surgical drains in select patients following pancreatic surgery may reduce postoperative complications. Therefore, routine omission of intra-abdominal surgical drains cannot be advocated, and selective drainage at the discretion of the treating physician is recommended [107] (Table 13.2).

Early removal (within 72 h) of prophylactic abdominal drains is recommended based on prospective trials demonstrating a reduction in postoperative complications overall and pancreatic fistulae specifically, with no significant difference in mortality [117, 118]. If fluid is present in the drain, the amylase level should be checked prior to drain removal [16].

Enteric Tubes

Routine nasogastric decompression is not indicated in the postoperative period, and their usage may in fact increase the likelihood of delayed gastric emptying and prolong LoS following pancreatic resection [119, 120]. While nasogastric tubes may be placed intraoperatively to decompress the stomach and facilitate the operation, these should be removed upon reversal of anesthesia, or with the initiation of oral intake on the first postoperative day [16]. Early enteral feeding via a nasojejunal tube is not recommended based on the results of a recent randomized controlled trial [121]. Routine placement of feeding jejunostomy tubes is not recommended and may infrequently cause bowel strangulation [122]. Even patients with preoperative symptoms of gastric outlet obstruction may be fed orally after pancreaticoduodenectomy [123]. Oral feeding is considered the preferred route for alimentation following pancreatic surgery [124].

Table 13.2 Summary of data reporting mixed evidence with respect to prophylactic intra-abdominal drainage of patients undergoing pancreatic resection

Publication type	Number of studies or patients	Outcomes		Conclusions
Witzigmann et al. (2016) No need for routine drainage after pancreatic head resection: The dual-center, randomized, controlled PANDRA trial [116]				
Randomized controlled trial	395 patients Drain vs no drain: 202 vs 193	*No drain* ≈Overall complications		Results do not support routine prophylactic drainage after pancreatic resection with pancreaticojejunal anastomosis. Abandoning intraperitoneal drains did not increase reintervention rates, morbidity, or mortality
		↓Reintervention rates	$p = 0.0004$	
		↓Grade B/C pancreatic fistulas	$p = 0.03$	
		↓ Fistula-associated complications	$p = 0.0008$	
		≈Length of stay ≈In-hospital mortality		
Dou et al. (2015) Systematic review and meta-analysis of prophylactic abdominal drainage after pancreatic resection [102]				
Systematic review and meta-analysis	9 studies 7 OCS [108–114] 2 RCT [106, 107] 2794 patients Drain vs no drain: 1373 vs 1421 patients	*No drain* ↓Length of stay	$p = 0.02$	Prophylactic abdominal drainage after pancreatic resection is still necessary, but more evidence is needed
		↓Morbidity	$p = 0.01$	
		≈Reoperation rates ≈Mortality		
Wang et al. (2015) Prophylactic intraperitoneal drain placement following pancreaticoduodenectomy: A systematic review and meta-analysis [105]				
Systematic review and meta-analysis	5 studies 4 OCS [109–111, 114] 1 RCT [107] 1728 patients Drain vs no drain: 783 vs 945 patients	*No drain* ↓Overall complications	$p < 0.01$	Indiscriminate abandonment of intra-abdominal drainage following pancreatic surgery is associated with greater mortality, but lower complication rates
		↓Major complications	$p = 0.01$	
		≈Pancreatic fistula ≈Delayed gastric emptying		
		↑Mortality	$p = 0.02$	
		↓Readmission	$p = 0.04$	
Nitsche et al. (2014) The evidence-based dilemma of intraperitoneal drainage for pancreatic resection: a systematic review and meta-analysis [103]				

(continued)

Table 13.2 (continued)

Publication type	Number of studies or patients	Outcomes		Conclusions
Systematic review and meta-analysis	8 studies 6 OCS [108–113] 2 RCT [106, 107] 2773 patients Drain vs no drain: 1359 vs 1414 patients	*No drain* ≈Minor complications ≈Major complications ≈Pancreatic fistula ≈Mortality ≈Length of stay		Routine omission of drains cannot be advocated, especially after pancreatic surgery
Rondelli et al. (2014) Intra-abdominal drainage after pancreatic resection: Is it really necessary? A meta-analysis of short-term outcomes [104]				
Systematic review and meta-analysis	7 studies 5 OCS [108–111, 113] 2 RCT [106, 107] 2704 patients Drain vs no drain: 1320 vs 1384 patients	*No drain* ↓Total complications ≈Wound infection ≈Mortality ↓Pancreatic fistula	$p < 0.00001$ $p < 0.0001$	The presence of an intra-abdominal drainage does not improve the postoperative outcome after pancreatic resection

≈ no significant change ($p > 0.05$) ↓ significantly decreased ($p \le 0.05$) ↑ significantly increased ($p \le 0.05$) *RCT* randomized controlled trial, *OCS* observational comparative study

Urinary Catheters

Urinary catheters placed at the time of surgery should be removed early in the postoperative period to prevent urinary tract infections and encourage patient mobilization [16, 125]. A recent study using the National Surgical Quality Improvement Program database observed increased rates of urinary tract infections among patients whose urinary catheters were maintained for >2 days postoperatively [126]. Among patients with a thoracic epidural in situ, early removal of the urinary catheter is still recommended [127].

Postoperative Care

Early Oral Intake

Following pancreatectomy, patients were traditionally kept nil per os (NPO) pending return of bowel function, as demonstrated by flatus or bowel movements. Until recently, jejunal feeding tubes were routinely placed intraoperatively. As enhanced recovery principles have permeated postoperative management, early oral feeding has gained broad acceptance following pancreatic resection, including pancreaticoduodenectomy. At our center, patients are routinely given clear fluids on the first postoperative day.

The data supporting early feeding following upper gastrointestinal surgery includes patients who have undergone myriad procedures, primarily esophageal or gastric operations with the creation of esophagojejunal or gastrojejunal anastomoses [128–135]. Randomized controlled trials have reported that patients fed early had decreased time to passing flatus, more rapid dietary advancement, and decreased LoS [135, 136]. There is a paucity of data examining pancreatic resections alone. However, published studies on ERaS after pancreatectomy advocate early oral intake [7]. As no signal of harm due to early oral intake is apparent (i.e., major complications; anastomotic leaks do not appear elevated among patients receiving early oral intake following pancreatectomy), it is our interpretation of the available data that early oral intake is safe following gastrojejunal anastomoses. Therefore, patients are likely to benefit from early oral feeding during the postoperative recovery period following pancreatic surgery.

Role of Prokinetic Agents

Many institutions use prokinetic agents to minimize delayed gastric emptying. However, at this time there is no evidence to support the routine administration of prokinetic agents for gastrointestinal motility recovery following major abdominal surgery [137]. As a result, we do not recommend their inclusion in ERaS protocols at this time given their potential for side effects and lack of demonstrated efficacy [137–140].

Gum Chewing

Gum chewing activates the cephalic phase of digestion and has been demonstrated to speed the recovery of gastrointestinal function and to decrease the time to first bowel movement following gastrointestinal surgery (primarily colorectal operations) [141]. Following pancreatic surgery, a small randomized controlled trial demonstrated a trend toward more rapid return of gastrointestinal function, although no significant differences in LoS or other measures of gastrointestinal function were identified [142]. Despite poor-quality evidence specifically for pancreatectomy, gum chewing has been demonstrated to be effective following other gastrointestinal and abdominal procedures. As it is a low risk, we recommend gum chewing be included after pancreatectomy as part of the intervention bundle for ileus reduction.

Early Mobilization

Early return to mobility is a standard recommendation for enhanced recovery protocols in many areas of surgery. This is in keeping with the underlying rationale of ERaS, to return patients back to their physiologic baseline as rapidly as possible. Few studies in mobilization have included patients undergoing pancreatectomy. Studies in other major abdominal procedures report that early mobilization appears safe and well tolerated. In the context of a multimodal enhanced postoperative rehabilitation approach, early mobilization was associated with shorter duration of narcotic analgesia utilization and decreased time to overall recovery, with no increase in pain scores, quality of life metrics, complications, or readmissions [143]. Another prospective study reported that early patient mobilization decreased the rate of postoperative paralytic ileus following colorectal and urologic operations [144]. In summary, data suggests early mobilization after surgery is safe and may provide benefits such as decreased ileus, particularly when used as a bundle with other ERaS interventions.

Somatostatin Analogues

The routine use of somatostatin analogues for the prevention of postoperative pancreatic fistulae remains controversial. There is substantial heterogeneity in the published literature with respect to patient population examined, pancreas procedures included, and the specific somatostatin analogue administered (Table 13.3). A systematic review of 21 randomized trials concluded that while somatostatin analogues decreased the overall rate of postoperative pancreatic fistulae, no correlation was seen between somatostatin analogue administration and the development of clinically significant pancreatic fistulae, or perioperative mortality [145]. Nevertheless, the authors concluded that routine use of prophylactic somatostatin analogues was indicated following pancreatic surgery [145].

Recently, Allen et al. conducted a randomized controlled trial comparing the somatostatin analogue pasireotide vs placebo for patients undergoing pancreatic

Table 13.3 Summary of data regarding the routine use of somatostatin analogues for the prevention of postoperative pancreatic fistulae following pancreatic surgery

Publication type	Number of studies or patients	Outcomes		Conclusions
Allen et al. (2014) Pasireotide for postoperative pancreatic fistula [146]				
Randomized controlled trial	300 patients Pasireotide vs placebo: 152 vs 148 patients	*Somatostatin* ≈Length of stay		Perioperative treatment with pasireotide decreased the rate of clinically significant postoperative pancreatic fistula, leak, or abscess
		↓≥ grade 3 pancreatic fistulas, leak, or abscess	$p = 0.01$	
		↓ Readmission	$p = 0.02$	
Gurusamy et al. (2013) Somatostatin analogues for pancreatic surgery [145]				
Systematic review and meta-analysis	21 studies 21 RCT 2348 patients	*Somatostatin* ≈Length of stay ≈Perioperative mortality ≈Reoperation rates		Somatostatin analogues reduced overall complication rates and decreased incidents of pancreatic fistulas without impacting length of stay, mortality, or reoperation rates
		↓Overall postoperative complications	$p < 0.0001$	
		≈Treatment withdrawal		
		↑Treatment adverse effects	$p = 0.003$	
		≈Anastomotic leak		
		↓Pancreatic fistula	$p < 0.00001$	
		≈Pancreatitis		
		↓Sepsis	$p = 0.002$	
		≈Renal failure ≈Delayed gastric emptying ≈Pulmonary complications ≈Infected abdominal collections		

≈ no significant change ($p > 0.05$) ↓ significantly decreased ($p \leq 0.05$) ↑ significantly increased ($p \leq 0.05$) *RCT* randomized controlled trial

resection and reported decreased rates of pancreatic fistulae and readmission to hospital among patients treated with pasireotide [146]. Additionally, routine administration of pasireotide appears to be cost-effective [147].

Based on our interpretation of the evidence, at our institution, we routinely utilize somatostatin analogues. Other authors have recommended selective somatostatin use in patients at high risk of fistula development based on the pancreatic fistula score or other assessment [148]. At this time, evidence does not clearly support either approach. As a result, we recommend local review of the best available evidence and adoption of a prospective standardized approach when managing these patients according to an ERaS protocol.

Early Discharge Planning

Active discharge planning will facilitate ERaS success and should commence at the time that surgery is offered with identification of patients as risk of delayed recovery. We have found that poor or absent discharge planning on the part of the medical team often contributes to prolonged LoS in otherwise well patients. A proactive discharge planning process provides more time to make necessary arrangements which may include mobilizing social supports, obtaining specialized equipment, or arranging rehabilitation services for patients when they are ready to leave the acute care setting.

Implementation and Outcomes

Introducing an ERaS protocol into clinical practice requires a planned, active implementation process in order to achieve optimal results [149]. The use of formal knowledge translation strategies and quality improvement concepts to launch an ERaS program for pancreatectomy will help promote quick acceptance and use of ERaS protocols, improve compliance among clinical team members responsible for implementing ERaS elements, and facilitate optimal outcomes related to the bundle of changes that ERaS may bring to the current clinical care of post-pancreatectomy patients.

We successfully introduced an ERaS protocol for pancreatectomy patients at ten high-volume HPB sites in Ontario, Canada, using a formal implementation process. The knowledge-to-action cycle described by Graham et al. [150] was used as the framework for developing an ERaS-based clinical pathway. The knowledge-to-action cycle is used to develop and implement evidence-based knowledge tools for implementation into clinical practice. Key steps include identifying a knowledge gap; adapting knowledge use for the local context; assessing barriers/enablers to successful implementation; tailoring a knowledge intervention – i.e., an ERaS protocol; and monitoring use and evaluating outcomes.

We first sought and obtained buy-in for an ERaS protocol prior to introducing the tool. All HPB sites were made aware and agreed strongly on the need for an ERaS approach. Next we established best evidence recommendations for each intervention mapped by the CPW. High-quality knowledge synthesis products (meta-analysis/systematic reviews) were sought when available, or through expert review of primary data if high-quality evidence was lacking or inconclusive. CPW materials developed included multidisciplinary CPW tool, preprinted/electronic order templates, and evidentiary support for the best practice recommendations.

ERaS protocols were reviewed by the clinicians prior to its introduction into clinical care, and approval to initiate ERaS-based care in all eligible patients was obtained. In-service education of clinicians, allied healthcare professionals, and trainees was undertaken. The protocol was introduced with a 3-month roll-out period before becoming part of standard care.

Once the ERaS protocol was established in clinical use, we undertook an audit and feedback process that included clinical outcomes as well as a staff satisfaction survey. There were 42 respondents, all of whom had used the EraS protocol. The majority of staff liked the protocol (88%) and believed the patients could achieve its goals (79%). In terms of clinical outcomes, introduction of the ERaS protocol was associated with a significantly decreased LoS to 8 days, whereas readmission rates, complication rates including reoperation and mortality, remained unchanged. These outcomes were presented to the clinical team responsible for pancreatectomy patients in order to promote compliance with ERaS use.

In our experience the keys to successful introduction of an ERaS protocol are clinical engagement and audit feedback of clinical outcomes. Since the introduction of ERaS at most institutions performing pancreatectomy will require changes in the management of most patients undergoing pancreatectomy, a considered approach to change management should be employed. Clinical engagement both prior to and during ERaS protocol development facilitated the change management necessary for ERaS introduction. Some of the ERaS recommendations differed from established clinical practices. In particular, early feeding and minimization of drain use were new for several clinicians. Clinical involvement and approval prior to making ERaS mandatory were very useful at promoting adherence to the standardized ERaS approach. We believe the use and availability of high-quality evidence to support ERaS recommendations in an easily digestible format were particularly helpful in encouraging clinicians to change their long-established practices.

Also, the presentation of ERaS results and staff satisfaction with ERaS protocols was highly effective in emphasizing the safety and positive clinical outcomes achievable with a standardized ERaS approach. Thus, we strongly recommend that if one is considering the introduction of ERaS, these implementation principles should be used.

Conclusions

An enhanced recovery after surgery approach is an advance in the science of surgical recovery. Each element of an enhanced recovery protocol aims to minimize the physiologic disturbances that result from surgical stress and/or promotes a return to normal physiology. The use of surgical bundles of care, as opposed to individual ERaS elements in isolation, is more effective, particularly when introduced in a standardized manner. A standardized approach to perioperative patient care minimizes errors of omission and/or errors of commission, which allows a higher number of patients to receive more elements of ERaS care, than if ERaS concepts are applied ad hoc. Furthermore, a standardized ERaS approach can be responsive to future developments in perioperative pancreatectomy care. As new evidence becomes available, changes can be transmitted to all care providers simultaneously through the ERaS protocol materials.

Thus, an ERaS approach to pancreatectomy can help achieve important clinical and quality goals for patients post-pancreatectomy. They can safely reduce length of stay and resource utilization and, most importantly, support patient recovery.

References

1. Wei AC, Urbach DR, Devitt KS, Wiebe M, Bathe OF, McLeod RS, et al. Improving quality through process change: a scoping review of process improvement tools in cancer surgery. BMC Surg. 2014;14:45. Epub 2014/07/21
2. Children's Hospital of Eastern Ontario. Surgical safety checklist – biannual report. Ottawa 2012, 1 Feb 2013. Available from: http://www.cheo.on.ca/en/surgicalsafetychecklist.
3. Haynes AB, Weiser TG, Berry WR, Lipsitz SR, Breizat AH, Dellinger EP, et al. A surgical safety checklist to reduce morbidity and mortality in a global population. N Engl J Med. 2009;360(5):491–9. Epub 2009/01/16
4. Kehlet H, Wilmore DW. Multimodal strategies to improve surgical outcome. Am J Surg. 2002;183(6):630–41.
5. Kobayashi S, Ooshima R, Koizumi S, Katayama M, Sakurai J, Watanabe T, et al. Perioperative care with fast-track management in Patients undergoing pancreaticoduodenectomy. World J Surg. 2014;38:2430–7.
6. Williamsson C, Karlsson N, Sturesson C, Lindell G, Andersson R, Tingstedt B. Impact of a fast-track surgery programme for pancreaticoduodenectomy. Br J Surg. 2015;102:1133–41.
7. Kagedan DJ, Ahmed M, Devitt KS, Wei AC. Enhanced recovery after pancreatic surgery: a systematic review of the evidence. HPB (Oxford). 2015;17(1):11–6. Epub 2014/04/23
8. Coolsen MM, van Dam RM, van der Wilt AA, Slim K, Lassen K, Dejong CH. Systematic review and meta-analysis of enhanced recovery after pancreatic surgery with particular emphasis on pancreaticoduodenectomies. World J Surg. 2013;37(8):1909–18.
9. Wilmore DW, Kehlet H. Management of patients in fast track surgery. BMJ. 2001;322(7284):473–6.
10. Kehlet H. Multimodal approach to control postoperative pathophysiology and rehabilitation. Br J Anaesth. 1997;78(5):606–17.
11. Porter GA, Pisters PWT, Mansyur C, Bisanz A, Reyna K, Stanford P, et al. Cost and utilization impact of a clinical pathway for patients undergoing pancreaticoduodenectomy. Ann Surg Oncol. 2000;7(7):484–9.
12. Basse L, Hjort Jakobsen D, Billesbolle P, Werner M, Kehlet H. A clinical pathway to accelerate recovery after colonic resection. Ann Surg. 2000;232(1):51–7.
13. Bond-Smith G, Belgaumkar AP, Davidson BR, Gurusamy KS. Enhanced recovery protocols for major upper gastrointestinal, liver and pancreatic surgery. Cochrane Database Syst Rev. 2016;2:CD011382.
14. Pecorelli N, Nobile S, Partelli S, Cardinali L, Crippa S, Balzano G, et al. Enhanced recovery pathways in pancreatic surgery: state of the art. World J Gastroenterol. 2016;22(28):6456–68.
15. Xiong J, Szatmary P, Huang W, de la Iglesia-Garcia D, Nunes QM, Xia Q, et al. Enhanced recovery after surgery program in patients undergoing pancreaticoduodenectomy: a PRISMA-compliant systematic review and meta-analysis. Medicine (Baltimore). 2016;95(18):e3497.
16. Lassen K, Coolsen MM, Slim K, Carli F, de Aguilar-Nascimento JE, Schafer M, et al. Guidelines for perioperative care for pancreaticoduodenectomy: enhanced recovery after surgery (ERAS(R)) society recommendations. Clin Nutr. 2012;31(6):817–30.
17. Forsmo HM, Pfeffer F, Rasdal A, Ostgaard G, Mohn AC, Korner H, et al. Compliance with enhanced recovery after surgery criteria and preoperative and postoperative counselling reduces length of hospital stay in colorectal surgery: results of a randomized controlled trial. Color Dis. 2016;18(6):603–11.
18. Halaszynski TM, Juda R, Silverman DG. Optimizing postoperative outcomes with efficient preoperative assessment and management. Crit Care Med. 2004;32(4 Suppl):S76–86.

19. Ehlenbach CC, Tevis SE, Kennedy GD, Oltmann SC. Preoperative impairment is associated with a higher postdischarge level of care. J Surg Res. 2015;193(1):1–6.
20. Lithner M, Klefsgard R, Johansson J, Andersson E. The significance of information after discharge for colorectal cancer surgery-a qualitative study. BMC Nurs. 2015;14:36.
21. Carroll A, Dowling M. Discharge planning: communication, education and patient participation. Br J Nurs. 2007;16(14):882–6.
22. Li LT, Barden GM, Balentine CJ, Orcutt ST, Naik AD, Artinyan A, et al. Postoperative transitional care needs in the elderly: an outcome of recovery associated with worse long-term survival. Ann Surg. 2015;261(4):695–701.
23. Smith MD, McCall J, Plank L, Herbison GP, Soop M, Nygren J. Preoperative carbohydrate treatment for enhancing recovery after elective surgery. Cochrane Database Syst Rev. 2014(8):CD009161.
24. Lohsiriwat V. The influence of preoperative nutritional status on the outcomes of an enhanced recovery after surgery (ERAS) programme for colorectal cancer surgery. Tech Coloproctol. 2014;18(11):1075–80.
25. van Stijn MF, Korkic-Halilovic I, Bakker MS, van der Ploeg T, van Leeuwen PA, Houdijk AP. Preoperative nutrition status and postoperative outcome in elderly general surgery patients: a systematic review. JPEN J Parenter Enteral Nutr. 2013;37(1):37–43.
26. Goonetilleke KS, Siriwardena AK. Systematic review of peri-operative nutritional supplementation in patients undergoing pancreaticoduodenectomy. JOP. 2006;7(1):5–13.
27. Nishida Y, Kato Y, Kudo M, Aizawa H, Okubo S, Takahashi D, et al. Preoperative sarcopenia strongly influences the risk of postoperative pancreatic fistula formation after Pancreaticoduodenectomy. J Gastrointest Surg. 2016;20(9):1586–94.
28. Practice guidelines for preoperative fasting and the use of pharmacologic agents to reduce the risk of pulmonary aspiration: application to healthy patients undergoing elective procedures: an updated report by the American Society of Anesthesiologists Task Force on preoperative fasting and the use of pharmacologic agents to reduce the risk of pulmonary aspiration. Anesthesiology. 2017.
29. Okano K, Hirao T, Unno M, Fujii T, Yoshitomi H, Suzuki S, et al. Postoperative infectious complications after pancreatic resection. Br J Surg. 2015;102(12):1551–60.
30. Thomsen T, Villebro N, Moller AM. Interventions for preoperative smoking cessation. Cochrane Database Syst Rev. 2014(3):CD002294.
31. Hughes C, Hurtuk MG, Rychlik K, Shoup M, Aranha GV. Preoperative liver function tests and hemoglobin will predict complications following pancreaticoduodenectomy. J Gastrointest Surg. 2008;12(11):1822–7. discussion 7–9
32. Hallet J, Mahar AL, Tsang ME, Lin Y, Callum J, Coburn NG, et al. The impact of perioperative blood transfusions on post-pancreatectomy short-term outcomes: an analysis from the American College of Surgeons National Surgical Quality Improvement Program. HPB (Oxford). 2015;17(11):975–82.
33. Munoz M, Gomez-Ramirez S, Campos A, Ruiz J, Liumbruno GM. Pre-operative anaemia: prevalence, consequences and approaches to management. Blood Transfus. 2015;13(3):370–9.
34. Ng O, Keeler BD, Mishra A, Simpson A, Neal K, Brookes MJ, et al. Iron therapy for preoperative anaemia. Cochrane Database Syst Rev. 2015;12:CD011588.
35. Lin DM, Lin ES, Tran MH. Efficacy and safety of erythropoietin and intravenous iron in perioperative blood management: a systematic review. Transfus Med Rev. 2013;27(4):221–34.
36. Ang-Lee MK, Moss J, Yuan CS. Herbal medicines and perioperative care. JAMA. 2001;286(2):208–16.
37. Lu WI, Lu DP. Impact of chinese herbal medicine on american society and health care system: perspective and concern. Evid Based Complement Alternat Med. 2014;2014:251891.
38. Raghavan SR, Ballehaninna UK, Chamberlain RS. The impact of perioperative blood glucose levels on pancreatic cancer prognosis and surgical outcomes: an evidence-based review. Pancreas. 2013;42(8):1210–7.
39. Olson SH, Xu Y, Herzog K, Saldia A, DeFilippis EM, Li P, et al. Weight loss, diabetes, fatigue, and depression preceding pancreatic cancer. Pancreas. 2016;45(7):986–91.

40. Iacono C, Ruzzenente A, Campagnaro T, Bortolasi L, Valdegamberi A, Guglielmi A. Role of preoperative biliary drainage in jaundiced patients who are candidates for pancreatoduodenectomy or hepatic resection: highlights and drawbacks. Ann Surg. 2013;257(2):191–204.
41. Kloek JJ, Heger M, van der Gaag NA, Beuers U, van Gulik TM, Gouma DJ, et al. Effect of preoperative biliary drainage on coagulation and fibrinolysis in severe obstructive cholestasis. J Clin Gastroenterol. 2010;44(9):646–52.
42. Fang Y, Gurusamy KS, Wang Q, Davidson BR, Lin H, Xie X, et al. Pre-operative biliary drainage for obstructive jaundice. Cochrane Database Syst Rev. 2012;9:CD005444.
43. van der Gaag NA, Rauws EA, van Eijck CH, Bruno MJ, van der Harst E, Kubben FJ, et al. Preoperative biliary drainage for cancer of the head of the pancreas. N Engl J Med. 2010;362(2):129–37.
44. Crippa S, Cirocchi R, Partelli S, Petrone MC, Muffatti F, Renzi C, et al. Systematic review and meta-analysis of metal versus plastic stents for preoperative biliary drainage in resectable periampullary or pancreatic head tumors. Eur J Surg Oncol. 2016;42(9):1278–85.
45. Tol JA, van Hooft JE, Timmer R, Kubben FJ, van der Harst E, de Hingh IH, et al. Metal or plastic stents for preoperative biliary drainage in resectable pancreatic cancer. Gut. 2016;65(12):1981–7.
46. Kang MJ, Jung HS, Jang JY, Jung W, Chang J, Shin YC, et al. Metabolic effect of pancreatoduodenectomy: resolution of diabetes mellitus after surgery. Pancreatology. 2016;16(2):272–7.
47. JM W, Ho TW, Kuo TC, Yang CY, Lai HS, Chiang PY, et al. Glycemic change after pancreaticoduodenectomy: a population-based study. Medicine (Baltimore). 2015;94(27):e1109.
48. JM W, Kuo TC, Yang CY, Chiang PY, Jeng YM, Huang PH, et al. Resolution of diabetes after pancreaticoduodenectomy in patients with and without pancreatic ductal cell adenocarcinoma. Ann Surg Oncol. 2013;20(1):242–9.
49. Ockenga J. Importance of nutritional management in diseases with exocrine pancreatic insufficiency. HPB (Oxford). 2009;11(Suppl 3):11–5.
50. Burden S, Todd C, Hill J, Lal S. Pre-operative nutrition support in patients undergoing gastrointestinal surgery. Cochrane Database Syst Rev. 2012;11:CD008879.
51. Francis NK, Mason J, Salib E, Allanby L, Messenger D, Allison AS, et al. Factors predicting 30-day readmission after laparoscopic colorectal cancer surgery within an enhanced recovery programme. Color Dis. 2015;17(7):O148–54.
52. Tzeng CW, Tran Cao HS, Lee JE, Pisters PW, Varadhachary GR, Wolff RA, et al. Treatment sequencing for resectable pancreatic cancer: influence of early metastases and surgical complications on multimodality therapy completion and survival. J Gastrointest Surg. 2014;18(1):16–24. discussion -5
53. Ueno T, Yamamoto K, Kawaoka T, Takashima M, Oka M. Current antibiotic prophylaxis in pancreatoduodenectomy in Japan. J Hepato-Biliary-Pancreat Surg. 2005;12(4):304–9.
54. Donald GW, Sunjaya D, Lu X, Chen F, Clerkin B, Eibl G, et al. Perioperative antibiotics for surgical site infection in pancreaticoduodenectomy: does the SCIP-approved regimen provide adequate coverage? Surgery. 2013;154(2):190–6.
55. Sudo T, Murakami Y, Uemura K, Hashimoto Y, Kondo N, Nakagawa N, et al. Perioperative antibiotics covering bile contamination prevent abdominal infectious complications after pancreatoduodenectomy in patients with preoperative biliary drainage. World J Surg. 2014;38(11):2952–9.
56. Fong ZV, McMillan MT, Marchegiani G, Sahora K, Malleo G, De Pastena M, et al. Discordance between perioperative antibiotic prophylaxis and wound infection cultures in patients undergoing pancreaticoduodenectomy. JAMA Surg. 2016;151(5):432–9.
57. Ansari D, Ansari D, Andersson R, Andren-Sandberg A. Pancreatic cancer and thromboembolic disease, 150 years after trousseau. Hepatobiliary Surg Nutr. 2015;4(5):325–35.
58. Osborne NH, Wakefield TW, Henke PK. Venous thromboembolism in cancer patients undergoing major surgery. Ann Surg Oncol. 2008;15(12):3567–78.
59. Spyropoulos AC, Brotman DJ, Amin AN, Deitelzweig SB, Jaffer AK, McKean SC. Prevention of venous thromboembolism in the cancer surgery patient. Cleve Clin J Med. 2008;75(Suppl 3):S17–26.

60. Reinke CE, Drebin JA, Kreider S, Kean C, Resnick A, Raper S, et al. Timing of preoperative pharmacoprophylaxis for pancreatic surgery patients: a venous thromboembolism reduction initiative. Ann Surg Oncol. 2012;19(1):19–25.
61. Lyman GH, Khorana AA, Falanga A, Clarke-Pearson D, Flowers C, Jahanzeb M, et al. American Society of Clinical Oncology guideline: recommendations for venous thromboembolism prophylaxis and treatment in patients with cancer. J Clin Oncol. 2007;25(34):5490–505.
62. Akl EA, Kahale L, Sperati F, Neumann I, Labedi N, Terrenato I, et al. Low molecular weight heparin versus unfractionated heparin for perioperative thromboprophylaxis in patients with cancer. Cochrane Database Syst Rev. 2014;6:CD009447.
63. Fagarasanu A, Alotaibi GS, Hrimiuc R, Lee AY, Wu C. Role of extended thromboprophylaxis after abdominal and pelvic surgery in cancer patients: a systematic review and meta-analysis. Ann Surg Oncol. 2016;23(5):1422–30.
64. Farge D, Debourdeau P, Beckers M, Baglin C, Bauersachs RM, Brenner B, et al. International clinical practice guidelines for the treatment and prophylaxis of venous thromboembolism in patients with cancer. J Thromb Haemost. 2013;11(1):56–70.
65. Rasmussen MS, Jorgensen LN, Wille-Jorgensen P. Prolonged thromboprophylaxis with low molecular weight heparin for abdominal or pelvic surgery. Cochrane Database Syst Rev. 2009;1:CD004318.
66. Rollins KE, Lobo DN. Intraoperative goal-directed fluid therapy in elective major abdominal surgery: a meta-analysis of randomized controlled trials. Ann Surg. 2016;263(3):465–76.
67. Weinberg L, Wong D, Karalapillai D, Pearce B, Tan CO, Tay S, et al. The impact of fluid intervention on complications and length of hospital stay after pancreaticoduodenectomy (Whipple's procedure). BMC Anesthesiol. 2014;14:35.
68. Healy MA, McCahill LE, Chung M, Berri R, Ito H, Obi SH, et al. Intraoperative fluid resuscitation strategies in Pancreatectomy: results from 38 hospitals in Michigan. Ann Surg Oncol. 2016;23(9):3047–55.
69. Bundgaard-Nielsen M, Secher N, Kehlet H. 'liberal' vs. 'restrictive' perioperative fluid therapy--a critical assessment of the evidence. Acta Anaesthesiol Scand. 2009;57(7):843–51.
70. Kozek-Langenecker SA, Afshari A, Albaladejo P, Santullano CA, De Robertis E, Filipescu DC, et al. Management of severe perioperative bleeding: guidelines from the European Society of Anaesthesiology. Eur J Anaesthesiol. 2013;30(6):270–382.
71. Rasmussen KC, Secher NH, Pedersen T. Effect of perioperative crystalloid or colloid fluid therapy on hemorrhage, coagulation competence, and outcome: a systematic review and stratified meta-analysis. Medicine (Baltimore). 2016;95(31):e4498.
72. Rasmussen KC, Johansson PI, Hojskov M, Kridina I, Kistorp T, Thind P, et al. Hydroxyethyl starch reduces coagulation competence and increases blood loss during major surgery: results from a randomized controlled trial. Ann Surg. 2014;259(2):249–54.
73. Grant F, Brennan MF, Allen PJ, DeMatteo RP, Kingham TP, D'Angelica M, et al. Prospective randomized controlled trial of liberal vs restricted perioperative fluid management in patients undergoing pancreatectomy. Ann Surg. 2016;264(4):591–8.
74. van Samkar G, Eshuis WJ, Bennink RJ, van Gulik TM, Dijkgraaf MG, Preckel B, et al. Intraoperative fluid restriction in pancreatic surgery: a double blinded randomised controlled trial. PLoS One. 2015;10(10):e0140294.
75. Grant FM, Protic M, Gonen M, Allen P, Brennan MF. Intraoperative fluid management and complications following pancreatectomy. J Surg Oncol. 2013;107(5):529–35.
76. Eng OS, Melstrom LG, Carpizo DR. The relationship of perioperative fluid administration to outcomes in colorectal and pancreatic surgery: a review of the literature. J Surg Oncol. 2015;111(4):472–7.
77. Lavu H, Sell NM, Carter TI, Winter JM, Maguire DP, Gratch DM, et al. The HYSLAR trial: a prospective randomized controlled trial of the use of a restrictive fluid regimen with 3% hypertonic saline versus lactated ringers in patients undergoing pancreaticoduodenectomy. Ann Surg. 2014;260(3):445–53. discussion 53–5
78. Rizoli S. PlasmaLyte. J Trauma. 2011;70(5 Suppl):S17–8.

79. Ross A, Mohammed S, Vanburen G, Silberfein EJ, Artinyan A, Hodges SE, et al. An assessment of the necessity of transfusion during pancreatoduodenectomy. Surgery. 2013;154(3):504–11.
80. Benson D, Barnett CC Jr. Perioperative blood transfusions promote pancreas cancer progression. J Surg Res. 2011;166(2):275–9.
81. Sutton JM, Kooby DA, Wilson GC, Squires MH 3rd, Hanseman DJ, Maithel SK, et al. Perioperative blood transfusion is associated with decreased survival in patients undergoing pancreaticoduodenectomy for pancreatic adenocarcinoma: a multi-institutional study. J Gastrointest Surg. 2014;18(9):1575–87.
82. Mavros MN, Xu L, Maqsood H, Gani F, Ejaz A, Spolverato G, et al. Perioperative blood transfusion and the prognosis of pancreatic cancer surgery: systematic review and meta-analysis. Ann Surg Oncol. 2015;22(13):4382–91.
83. Singer MB, Sheckley M, Menon VG, Sundaram V, Donchev V, Voidonikolas G, et al. Can transfusions be eliminated in major abdominal surgery? Analysis of a five-year experience of blood conservation in patients undergoing pancreaticoduodenectomy. Am Surg. 2015;81(10):983–7.
84. Sun RC, Button AM, Smith BJ, Leblond RF, Howe JR, Mezhir JJ. A comprehensive assessment of transfusion in elective pancreatectomy: risk factors and complications. J Gastrointest Surg. 2013;17(4):627–35.
85. Fischer M, Matsuo K, Gonen M, Grant F, Dematteo RP, D'Angelica MI, et al. Relationship between intraoperative fluid administration and perioperative outcome after pancreaticoduodenectomy: results of a prospective randomized trial of acute normovolemic hemodilution compared with standard intraoperative management. Ann Surg. 2010;252(6):952–8.
86. Jeon YB, Yun S, Ok SY, Kim HJ, Choi D. Impact of a transfusion-free program on patients undergoing pancreaticoduodenectomy. Am Surg. 2016;82(2):140–5.
87. Senagore AJ. Pathogenesis and clinical and economic consequences of postoperative ileus. Clin Exp Gastroenterol. 2010;3:87–9.
88. Sanford DE, Hawkins WG, Fields RC. Improved peri-operative outcomes with epidural analgesia in patients undergoing a pancreatectomy: a nationwide analysis. HPB (Oxford). 2015;17(6):551–8.
89. Amini N, Kim Y, Hyder O, Spolverato G, CL W, Page AJ, et al. A nationwide analysis of the use and outcomes of perioperative epidural analgesia in patients undergoing hepatic and pancreatic surgery. Am J Surg. 2015;210(3):483–91.
90. Shah DR, Brown E, Russo JE, Li CS, Martinez SR, Coates JM, et al. Negligible effect of perioperative epidural analgesia among patients undergoing elective gastric and pancreatic resections. J Gastrointest Surg. 2013;17(4):660–7.
91. Pratt WB, Steinbrook RA, Maithel SK, Vanounou T, Callery MP, Vollmer CM Jr. Epidural analgesia for pancreatoduodenectomy: a critical appraisal. J Gastrointest Surg. 2008;12(7):1207–20.
92. Choi DX, Schoeniger LO. For patients undergoing pancreatoduodenectomy, epidural anesthesia and analgesia improves pain but increases rates of intensive care unit admissions and alterations in analgesics. Pancreas. 2010;39(4):492–7.
93. Klotz R, Hofer S, Schellhaass A, Dorr-Harim C, Tenckhoff S, Bruckner T, et al. Intravenous versus epidural analgesia to reduce the incidence of gastrointestinal complications after elective pancreatoduodenectomy (the PAKMAN trial, DRKS 00007784): study protocol for a randomized controlled trial. Trials. 2016;17:194.
94. Guay J, Nishimori M, Kopp S. Epidural local anaesthetics versus opioid-based analgesic regimens for postoperative gastrointestinal paralysis, vomiting and pain after abdominal surgery. Cochrane Database Syst Rev. 2016;7:CD001893.
95. De Pietri L, Montalti R, Begliomini B. Anaesthetic perioperative management of patients with pancreatic cancer. World J Gastroenterol. 2014;20(9):2304–20.
96. Hughes MJ, Ventham NT, McNally S, Harrison E, Wigmore S. Analgesia after open abdominal surgery in the setting of enhanced recovery surgery: a systematic review and meta-analysis. JAMA Surg. 2014;149(12):1224–30.

97. McNicol ED, Ferguson MC, Hudcova J. Patient controlled opioid analgesia versus non-patient controlled opioid analgesia for postoperative pain. Cochrane Database Syst Rev. 2015;(6):CD003348.
98. Gottschalk A, Freitag M, Steinacker E, Kreissl S, Rempf C, Staude HJ, et al. Pre-incisional epidural ropivacaine, sufentanil, clonidine, and (S)+−ketamine does not provide pre-emptive analgesia in patients undergoing major pancreatic surgery. Br J Anaesth. 2008;100(1):36–41.
99. Dichtwald S, Ben-Haim M, Papismedov L, Hazan S, Cattan A, Matot I. Intrathecal morphine versus intravenous opioid administration to impact postoperative analgesia in hepato-pancreatic surgery: a randomized controlled trial. J Anesth. 2017;31(2):237–45.
100. Thompson TK, Hutchison RW, Wegmann DJ, Shires GT 3rd, Beecherl E. Pancreatic resection pain management: is combining PCA therapy and a continuous local infusion of 0.5% ropivacaine beneficial? Pancreas. 2008;37(1):103–4.
101. Charlton S, Cyna AM, Middleton P, Griffiths JD. Perioperative transversus abdominis plane (TAP) blocks for analgesia after abdominal surgery. Cochrane Database Syst Rev. 2010;(12):CD007705.
102. Dou C, Liu Z, Jia Y, Zheng X, Tu K, Yao Y, et al. Systematic review and meta-analysis of prophylactic abdominal drainage after pancreatic resection. Worl J Gastroenterol. 2015;21(18):5719–34.
103. Nitsche U, Müller T, Späth C, Cresswell L, Wilhelm D, Friess H, et al. The evidence based dilemma of intraperitoneal drainage for pancreatic resection – a systematic review and meta-analysis. BMC Surg. 2014;14:76.
104. Rondelli F, Desio M, Vedovati M, Balzarotti Canger R, Sanguinetti A, Avenia N, et al. Intra-abdominal drainage after pancreatic resection: is it really necessary? A meta-analysis of short-term outcomes. Int J Surg. 2014;12(Suppl 1):S40–7.
105. Wang YC, Szatmary P, Zhu JQ, Xiong JJ, Huang W, Gomatos I, Nunes QM, Sutton R, Liu XB. Prophylactic intra-peritoneal drain placement following pancreaticoduodenectomy: a systematic review and meta-analysis. World J Gastroenterol. 2015;21(8):2150–21.
106. Conlon KC, Labow D, Leung D, Smith A, Jarnagin W, Coit DG, et al. Prospective randomized clinical trial of the value of intraperitoneal drainage after pancreatic resection. Ann Surg. 2001;234(4):487–93.
107. Van Buren G 2nd, Bloomston M, Hughes SJ, Winter J, Behrman SW, Zyromski NJ, et al. A randomized prospective multicenter trial of pancreaticoduodenectomy with and without routine intraperitoneal drainage. Ann Surg. 2014;259(4):605–12. Epub 2014/01/01
108. Fisher W, Hodges S, Silberfein E, Artinyan A, Ahern C, Jo E, et al. Pancreatic resection without routine intraperitoneal drainage. HPB. 2011;13(7):503–10.
109. Mehta VV, Fisher SB, Maithel SK, Sarmiento JM, Staley CA, Kooby DA. Is it time to abandon routine operative drain use? A single institution assessment of 709 consecutive pancreaticoduodenectomies. J Am Coll Surg. 2013;216(4):635–42.
110. Heslin MJ, Harrison LE, Brooks AD, Hochwald SN, Coit DG, Brennan MFI. Intra-abdominal drainage necessary after pancreaticoduodenectomy? J Gastrointest Surg. 1998;2:373–8.
111. Correa-Gallego C, Brennan M, D'angelica M, Fong Y, Dematteo R, Kingham T, et al. Operative drainage following pancreatic resection: analysis of 1122 patients resected over 5 years at a single institution. Ann Surg. 2013;258(6):1051–8.
112. Paulus E, Zarzaur B, Behrman S. Routine peritoneal drainage of the surgical bed after elective distal pancreatectomy: is it necessary? Am J Surg. 2012;204(4):422–7.
113. Adham M, Chopin-Laly X, Lepilliez V, Gincul R, Valette P, Ponchon T. Pancreatic resection: drain or no drain? Surgery. 2013;154(5):1069–77.
114. Lim C, Dokmak S, Cauchy F, Aussilhou B, Belghiti J, Sauvanet A. Selective policy of no drain after pancreaticoduodenectomy is a valid option in patients at low risk of pancreatic fistula: a case-control analysis. World J Surg. 2013;37(5):1021–7.
115. Dindo D, Demartines N, Clavien PA. Classification of surgical complications: a new proposal with evaluation in a cohort of 6336 patients and results of a survey. Ann Surg. 2004;240(2):205–13.

116. Witzigmann H, Diener M, Kienkötter S, Rossion I, Bruckner T, Bärbel W, et al. No need for routine drainage after pancreatic head resection: the dual-center, randomized, controlled PANDRA trial (ISRCTN04937707). Ann Surg. 2016;264(3):528–37.
117. Bassi C, Molinari E, Malleo G, Grippa S, Butturini G, Salvia R, et al. Early versus late drain removal after standard pancreatic resections – results of a prospective randomized trial. Ann Surg. 2010;252:207–14.
118. Kawai M, Tani M, Terasawa H, Ina S, Hirono S, Nishioka R, et al. Early removal of prophylactic drains reduces the risk of intra-abdominal infections in patients with pancreatic head resection: prospective study for 104 consecutive patients. An Surg. 2006;244:1–7.
119. Kunstman JW, Klemen ND, Fonseca AL, Araya DL, Salem RR. Nasogastric drainage may be unnecessary after pancreaticoduodenectomy: a comparison of routine vs selective decompression. J Am Coll Surg. 2013;217(3):481–8.
120. Roland CL, Mansour JC, Schwarz RE. Routine nasogastric decompression is unnecessary after pancreatic resections. Arch Surg. 2012;147(3):287–9.
121. Perinel J, Mariette C, Dousset B, Sielezneff I, Gainant A, Mabrut JY, et al. Early enteral versus total parenteral nutrition in patients undergoing pancreaticoduodenectomy: a randomized multicenter controlled trial (Nutri-DPC). Ann Surg. 2016;264(5):731–7.
122. Gerritsen A, Besselink MG, Cieslak KP, Vriens MR, Steenhagen E, van Hillegersberg R, et al. Efficacy and complications of nasojejunal, jejunostomy and parenteral feeding after pancreaticoduodenectomy. J Gastrointest Surg. 2012;16(6):1144–51.
123. Gerritsen A, Wennink RA, Busch OR, Borel Rinkes IH, Kazemier G, Gouma DJ, et al. Feeding patients with preoperative symptoms of gastric outlet obstruction after pancreatoduodenectomy: early oral or routine nasojejunal tube feeding? Pancreatology. 2015;15(5):548–53.
124. Gerritsen A, Besselink MG, Gouma DJ, Steenhagen E, Borel Rinkes IH, Molenaar IQ. Systematic review of five feeding routes after pancreatoduodenectomy. Br J Surg. 2013;100(5):589–98. discussion 99
125. Zmora O, Madbouly K, Tulchinsky H, Hussein A, Khaikin M. Urinary bladder catheter drainage following pelvic surgery--is it necessary for that long? Dis Colon Rectum. 2010;53(3):321–6.
126. Trickey AW, Crosby ME, Vasaly F, Donovan J, Moynihan J, Reines HD. Using NSQIP to investigate SCIP deficiencies in surgical patients with a high risk of developing hospital-associated urinary tract infections. Am J Med Qual. 2014;29(5):381–7.
127. Zaouter C, Kaneva P, Carli F. Less urinary tract infection by earlier removal of bladder catheter in surgical patients receiving thoracic epidural analgesia. Reg Anesth Pain Med. 2009;34(6):542–8.
128. Liu X, Wang D, Zheng L, Mou T, Liu H, Li G. Is early oral feeding after gastric cancer surgery feasible? A systematic review and meta-analysis of randomized controlled trials. PLoS One. 2014;9(11):e112062.
129. Feng F, Ji G, Li J, Li X, Shi H, et al. Fast-track surgery could improve postoperative recovery in radical total gastrectomy patients. World J Gastroenterol. 2013;19:3642–8.
130. Chen H, Xin Jiang L, Cai L, Tao Zheng H, Yuan H, et al. Preliminary experience of fast-track surgery combined with laparoscopy-assisted radical distal gastrectomy for gastric cancer. J Gastrointest Surg. 2012;16:1830–9.
131. Hur H, Kim S, Shim J, Song K, Kim W, et al. Effect of early oral feeding after gastric cancer surgery: a result of randomized clinical trial. Surgery. 2011;149:561–8.
132. Kim J, Kim W, Cheong J, Hyung W, Choi S, et al. Safety and efficacy of fast-track surgery in laparoscopic distal gastrectomy for gastric cancer: a randomized clinical trial. World J Surg. 2012;36:2879–87.
133. Liu X, Jiang Z, Wang Z, Li J. Multimodal optimization of surgical care shows beneficial outcome in gastrectomy surgery. JPEN J Parenter Enteral Nutr. 2010;34:313–21.
134. Wang D, Kong Y, Zhong B, Zhou X, Zhou Y. Fast-track surgery improves postoperative recovery in patients with gastric cancer: a randomized comparison with conventional postoperative care. J Gastrointest Surg. 2010;14:620–7.

135. Mahmoodzadeh H, Shoar S, Sirati F, Khorgami Z. Early initiation of oral feeding following upper gastrointestinal tumor surgery: a randomized controlled trial. Surg Today. 2015;45(2):203–8.
136. Hosseini S, Mousavinasab S, Rahmanpour H, Sotodeh S. Comparing early oral feeding with traditional oral feeding in upper gastrointestinal surgery. Turk J Gastroenterol. 2010;21(2):119–24.
137. Traut U, Brugger L, Kunz R, Pauli-Magnus C, Haug K, Bucher HC, et al. Systemic prokinetic pharmacologic treatment for postoperative adynamic ileus following abdominal surgery in adults. Cochrane Database Syst Rev. 2008;1:CD004930.
138. Narita K, Tsunoda A, Takenaka K, Watanabe M, Nakao K, Kusano M. Effect of mosapride on recovery of intestinal motility after hand-assisted laparoscopic colectomy for carcinoma. Dis Colon Rectum. 2008;51(11):1692–5.
139. Shaw M, Pediconi C, McVey D, Mondou E, Quinn J, Chamblin B, et al. Safety and efficacy of ulimorelin administered postoperatively to accelerate recovery of gastrointestinal motility following partial bowel resection: results of two randomized, placebo-controlled phase 3 trials. Dis Colon Rectum. 2013;56(7):888–97.
140. Mochiki E, Ohno T, Yanai M, Toyomasu Y, Andoh H, Kuwano H. Effects of glutamine on gastrointestinal motor activity in patients following gastric surgery. World J Surg. 2011;35(4):805–10.
141. Short V, Herbert G, Perry R, Atkinson C, Ness A, Penfold C, et al. Chewing gum for postoperative recovery of gastrointestinal function. Cochrane Database Syst Rev. 2015;2:CD006506.
142. Andersson T, Bjersa K, Falk K, Olsen M. Effects of chewing gum against postoperative ileus after pancreaticoduodenectomy—a randomized controlled trial. BMC Res Notes. 2015;10(8):37.
143. Lee T, Kang S, Kim D, Hong S, Heo S, Park K. Comparison of early mobilization and diet rehabilitation program with conventional care after laparoscopic colon surgery: a prospective randomized controlled trial. Dis Colon Rectum. 2011;54(1):21–8.
144. Kibler K, Hayes R, Johnson D, Anderson L, Just S, Wells N. Early postoperative ambulation: back to basics a quality improvement project increases postoperative ambulation and decreases patient complications. Cultivating Quality. 2012;112(4):63–9.
145. Gurusamy K, Koti R, Fusai G, Davidson B. Somatostatin analogues for pancreatic surgery. Cochrane Database Syst Rev. 2013;4:CD008370.
146. Allen P, Gonen M, Brennan M, Bucknor A, Robinson L, Pappas M, et al. Pasireotide for postoperative pancreatic fistula. N Engl J Med. 2014;370(21):2014–22.
147. Goyert N, Eeson G, Kagedan DJ, Behman R, Lemke M, Hallet J, et al. Pasireotide for the prevention of pancreatic fistula following pancreaticoduodenectomy: a cost-effectiveness analysis. Ann Surg. 2017;265(1):2–10.
148. Callery MP, Pratt WB, Kent TS, Chaikof EL, Vollmer CM Jr. A prospectively validated clinical risk score accurately predicts pancreatic fistula after pancreatoduodenectomy. J Am Coll Surg. 2013;216(1):1–14.
149. Maessen J, Dejong CH, Hausel J, Nygren J, Lassen K, Andersen J, et al. A protocol is not enough to implement an enhanced recovery programme for colorectal resection. Br J Surg. 2007;94(2):224–31. Epub 2007/01/06
150. Straus S, Tetroe J, Graham I. Knowledge translation in health care: moving from evidence to practice. West Sussex: Wiley-Blackwell; 2009.

Index

© Springer International Publishing AG 2018
F.G. Rocha, P. Shen (eds.), *Optimizing Outcomes for Liver and Pancreas*
Surgery, DOI 10.1007/978-3-319-62624-6

The manufacturer's authorised representative in the EU is Springer
Nature Customer Service Centre GmbH, Europaplatz 3, 69115 Heidelberg,
Germany. If you have any concerns regarding our products, please
contact ProductSafety@springernature.com

Printed and bound by CPI Group (UK) Ltd, Croydon, CR0 4YY
27/04/2026
02097580-0004